Parkinson's Disease
A Multidisciplinary Guide to Management

Parkinson's Disease
A Multidisciplinary Guide to Management

Fiona Lindop, MCSP, PGDip
Specialist Physiotherapist
Parkinson's Foundation Centre of Excellence,
Florence Nightingale Community Hospital
University Hospitals of Derby and Burton NHS Foundation Trust
Derby
United Kingdom

Rob Skelly, MBBS, MMedSci, DTM + H, FRCP
Consultant Geriatrician
Parkinson's Foundation Centre of Excellence,
Royal Derby Hospital
University Hospitals of Derby and Burton NHS Foundation Trust
and Honorary Clinical Assistant Professor
Division of Medical Sciences and Graduate Entry Medicine,
University of Nottingham
Derby
United Kingdom

ELSEVIER

Foreword

Why Multidisciplinary Care Is Essential for People With Parkinson's

Prof. Bastiaan R. Bloem, MD, PhD, FRCPE

Radboud University Medical Centre; Donders Institute for Brain, Cognition and Behaviour; Department of Neurology; Centre of Expertise for Parkinson & Movement Disorders; Nijmegen, Netherlands

Various sources of evidence suggest that Parkinson's is among the fastest-growing neurological diseases in the world.[1,2] Parkinson's is also one of the most debilitating neurological conditions known, which is presumably related to its very complex and changeable clinical presentation: persons living with Parkinson's can experience a wide range of motor symptoms (including the well-known bradykinesia, rigidity, tremor, gait problems, and postural instability) as well as many different non-motor symptoms (including cognitive decline, depression, anxiety, various sorts of pain, constipation, urinary incontinence, orthostatic hypotension, sleep disorders, loss of smell … and the list goes on). Fortunately, Parkinson's is also a treatable condition. For a long time, oral pharmacotherapy in the form of levodopa has been the cornerstone of the treatment approach, but we are increasingly realising that drugs alone are insufficient to support people with Parkinson's and their families. Certainly, levodopa and other dopaminergic drugs can help to suppress motor symptoms and also some of the non-motor symptoms; they can help to reduce disability and improve quality of life. Recent large studies have emphasised that there is no need to fear pharmacotherapy and that persons with Parkinson's deserve to receive symptomatic pharmacotherapy as soon as the symptoms and signs of the disease begin to interfere with daily activities.[3,4] However, not all symptoms respond in a gratifying way to pharmacotherapy; this is particularly true for many of the non-motor symptoms but also for important motor symptoms such as postural instability or dysphagia. Moreover, the drug treatment is increasingly complicated by adverse effects, in particular fluctuations in response but also other adverse effects such as hallucinations and orthostatic hypotension. In a recent and very comprehensive review in *The Lancet*,[5] we have underscored that the optimal management of Parkinson's involves much more than just drugs and should indeed be seen as a table resting on four essential legs: (1) pharmacotherapy, (2) device-aided therapies (such as deep brain stimulation and other neurosurgical techniques), (3) multidisciplinary care and (4) the involvement of a well-informed and engaged person with Parkinson's (plus family and other near ones). Given the extremely complex and multifaceted manifestations of Parkinson's, it should perhaps come as no surprise that the multidisciplinary team approach involves a wide range of professional disciplines—more than 20 different disciplines can potentially offer support to people living with Parkinson's. In the same recent paper in *The Lancet*,[5] we have visualised the multidisciplinary team approach as a universe where the person living with Parkinson's is positioned right at the centre, as the "sun" toward whom all of our supportive efforts should be focused. All the professional disciplines orbit as planets around this sun. Importantly, none of the medical professionals should be regarded a star; no single professional discipline is more important than another. Instead, all should work together as equals within a well-organised team to support the person with Parkinson's to the best of our abilities. Some professional disciplines are nearly always involved as part of the multidisciplinary team; this includes the medical specialist (a neurologist or geriatrician, depending on how care is organised), a Parkinson's nurse, and a general practitioner supported by a community nurse. The second "ring" frequently involves other disciplines that are frequently involved such as the physiotherapist, occupational therapist, or speech-language therapist. The third and outer ring involves a range of professionals that can occasionally be engaged if the situation calls for their support. This includes not only well-recognised professionals such as the psychiatrist but also less usual suspects that are not always intuitively relevant for Parkinson's care, such as a dentist, gastroenterologist or pulmonologist. Crucially, not all professionals will be involved for each individual person with Parkinson's, nor should they be involved continuously. The challenge is to develop a personalised approach, looking very carefully at the needs and wishes of each individual person with Parkinson's, and to build the contours of the multidisciplinary team accordingly. In that regard, personalised medicine should extend well beyond matching the pharmacotherapy to a person's DNA; it should also move toward personalised rehabilitation.[6] Given the enormous complexity of Parkinson's, it is important that the involved professionals are well trained according to the latest guidelines and have accumulated deep experience in supporting people with Parkinson's.[7] These professionals should work efficiently together as a team regardless of their specific workplaces.[8]

In that regard, I very much welcome this new book. It offers extremely helpful guidance for anyone interested in building an optimal multidisciplinary team approach tailored to the unique situation of each individual living with Parkinson's. The authors are well respected for their deep experience in this field and have succeeded extremely well in conveying their knowledge to the readers of this book. I hope that you will enjoy reading this new book as much as I did and that you will keep it closely around as an extremely useful reference and practical guide to support you in your decisions as you strive to offer multidisciplinary support to persons with Parkinson's.

Bastiaan R. Bloem

References

1. Dorsey, E. R., & Bloem, B. R. (2018). The Parkinson pandemic—a call to action. *JAMA Neurology*, *75*(1), 9–10.
2. Dorsey, E. R., Sherer, T., Okun, M. S., & Bloem, B. R. (2018). The emerging evidence of the Parkinson pandemic. *Journal of Parkinson's Disease*, *8*(s1), S3–S8.
3. Armstrong, M. J., & Okun, M. S. (2020). Diagnosis and treatment of Parkinson disease: a review. *JAMA*, *323*(6), 548–560.
4. Lang, A. E., de Bie, R. M. A., Clarke, C. E., Espay, A. J., & Fox, S. H. (2020). Initiating pharmacotherapy in early Parkinson's disease. *Lancet Neurology*, *19*(8), 643–644.
5. Bloem, B. R., Okun, M. S., & Klein, C. (2021). Parkinson's disease. *Lancet*.
6. Nonnekes, J., & Nieuwboer, A. (2018). Towards personalised rehabilitation for gait impairments in Parkinson's disease. *Journal of Parkinson's Disease*, *8*(s1), S101–S106.
7. Bloem, B. R., Rompen, L., Vries, N. M., Klink, A., Munneke, M., Jeurissen, P., & Parkinson-Net: (2017). A low-cost health care innovation with a systems approach from The Netherlands. *Health affairs (Project Hope)*, *36*(11), 1987–1996.
8. Bloem, B. R., Henderson, E. J., Dorsey, E. R., et al. (2020). Integrated and patient-centred management of Parkinson's disease: a network model for reshaping chronic neurological care. *Lancet Neurology*, *19*(7), 623–634.

Acknowledgments

Many people have helped to make this book possible, and we would like to express our sincere thanks to our colleagues, fellow authors and contributors. We would also like to thank the many people with Parkinson's who have helped us to grow in our knowledge and understanding of this condition. We also owe a debt of gratitude to members of our families and the many friends who have offered their support and encouragement.

We would especially like to thank our colleagues in the Multidisciplinary Parkinson's Team at University Hospitals of Derby & Burton NHS Foundation Trust for their dedication and commitment to providing integrated, holistic care for people with Parkinson's. It has been a great pleasure to work with such a fantastic team. We are grateful to the many members of the team who have contributed as named authors to one or more chapters, and to Lakmali Jarman and Alison Hartley for their contributions. We also thank the unsung heroes who ensure the service is welcoming and friendly and runs smoothly.

Thank you to our fellow authors who value and champion multidisciplinary working in Parkinson's. Without their expertise and enthusiasm this book would not have been possible. Thanks for getting chapters in on time (or nearly on time!)

Thank you to Diana Jones, Jane Youde, Chris Taylor, Purba Choudhury and Bushra Khizar who read draft chapters and gave us helpful, constructive feedback. Jonny Acheson has done an amazing job in designing the artwork for the cover and we are so grateful for his inspiration, creativity and ability to deliver much faster than the deadlines we gave him.

We would also like to extend our thanks, along with fellow author Sally Jones, to the QI team at the Heart of England NHS Foundation Trust, as well as Maggie Johnson, Caroline Maries-Tillott, Karen Barber, Ali Bahron and Shahzad Razaq.

The publishing team at Elsevier have kept us on the straight and narrow and provided support along the way. We would especially like to thank Helen Leng, Andrae Akeh, Haritha Dharmarajan and Poppy Garraway for everything they have done to help us and for bringing this book to publication.

And finally, we owe a huge thank you to our families who have put up with us spending much of whatever spare time we had during the pandemic and lockdown of 2020 writing, editing and doing endless Zoom calls. They willingly gave us support and advice, read draft chapters and offered ideas, supplying us with food and refreshments which included endless mugs of tea and coffee and occasionally a glass of something stronger! Thank you, Richard Lindop, Jenny, Pat and Chris Skelly.

Contents

Parkinson's Disease

A Multidisciplinary Guide to Management

Chapter 1

Introduction

Fiona Lindop and Rob Skelly

Provision of best clinical care

Life can be difficult for people with Parkinson's. They can have a wide range of symptoms that change as the condition progresses. Motor problems alone can make everyday tasks a struggle, while cognitive changes, apathy and mood disturbance impair a person's ability to overcome challenges. For caregivers, the burden of looking after a person with Parkinson's can be heavy and may lead to mental health problems. The urgency of the need to find a cure (or cures) for Parkinson's cannot be overstated. Important work on disease mechanisms continues, and new trials of potentially neuroprotective drugs are underway. Meanwhile, people with Parkinson's need good clinical care. This book is intended as a practical guide for doctors, nurses, therapists, dietitians, psychologists and other health professionals who care for people with Parkinson's. Students too should find the text accessible.

A handbook

The guidance we offer in this book is consistent with evidence-based reviews from the International Parkinson's and Movement Disorder Society and guidelines from the United Kingdom's National Institute of Health and Care Excellence. Where relevant evidence exists, it has been referenced. Where evidence is lacking, the authors offer expert opinion and advice. We intend this book to be more of a handbook than an academic tome and have ended each chapter with the authors' "top tips."

dementia and exercise. We also include chapters on the care of hospitalised persons and atypical Parkinsonian syndromes. The final chapter covers the use of technology for the remote assessment of Parkinson's, a field that continues to grow in the wake of the COVID-19 pandemic.

As we were preparing this book, we learned a lot from our fellow authors. We hope you will too.

References

MacMahon, D. G., & Thomas, S. (1998). Practical approach to quality of life in Parkinson's disease: The nurse's role. *Journal of Neurology, 245*(Suppl 1), S19–S22.

WHO International Classification of Functioning, Disability, and Health. Retrieved December 27, 2020, from https://www.who.int/standards/classifications/international-classification-of-functioning-disability-and-health.

Worth, P. F. (2019). Taking the "disease" out of "Parkinson's": Has the disease had its day? *Practical Neurology, 19*, 2–4.

Chapter 2

Parkinson's: Setting the Scene

Rob Skelly

Chapter outline

Introduction

The focus of this book is the multidisciplinary management of people with Parkinson's. Non-etheless, an appreciation of the incidence and prevalence of Parkinson's and of the age, gender, and ethnic profiles of sufferers (epidemiology) will help both in the development of appropriate services and the identification of possible risk factors. A shared understanding of what is abnormal in the brain and elsewhere (pathology) and what has caused it (etiology) will aid in the development and implementation of rational treatment strategies. With development of precision medicine and increasing public uptake of commercially available genetic screening, an understanding of the genetics of Parkinson's is increasingly important. Also, some knowledge of environmental factors linked to the development or progression of Parkinson's could lead to evidence-based lifestyle advice. On the most basic level, the aim of this chapter is to equip the reader to better answer two common questions from patients: "What is Parkinson's?" and "Why me?"

What is Parkinson's?

Parkinson's is the second most common neurodegenerative disease, with an estimated 144,500 cases in the United Kingdom in 2018 (Parkinson's UK, 2017). It is characterised clinically by bradykinesia, rigidity, and tremor at rest. The term *bradykinesia* means slowness of movement and includes both slowness in reaction time and slowness in carrying out the movement. Abnormalities of speech, gait and posture may occur.

Non-motor symptoms are common and include:

- Autonomic problems (constipation, urinary frequency, sexual dysfunction, thermoregulatory dysfunction)
- Sensory disturbance (pain, paresthesia)
- Sleep disturbance (rapid-eye-movement sleep behaviour disorder, insomnia, excessive daytime sleepiness)
- Mental health problems (anxiety, depression, apathy, psychosis, hallucinations, dementia)

Some non-motor problems may appear before the motor problems, including constipation, sleep problems, loss of sense of smell and depression. These may constitute prodromal Parkinson's.

In the brain, Parkinson's is characterised by depigmentation of the substantia nigra due to the loss of dopaminergic neurons and microscopically by intracytoplasmic Lewy bodies. The condition is slowly progressive and, though there is currently no cure, dopaminergic treatments are effective for many of the motor symptoms. A range of medical and therapy treatments can help to ameliorate the wide range of motor and non-motor symptoms; we believe that this care is best delivered by a coordinated multidisciplinary team (MDT).

Epidemiology

Incidence is the number of new cases in a defined population in a year (or other specified time period). It is not affected by duration of the condition or migration from other geographic areas. Estimates of incidence vary, but a useful estimate is 16 to 18 new cases per 100,000 population. This is helpful in estimating the number of new Parkinson's diagnoses a service might expect to make in a year. The lifetime risk for developing Parkinson's is about 2% for men and a little lower for women. Because Parkinson's is a chronic condition lasting a number of years, the prevalence of Parkinson's is higher: about 160 to 180 cases per 100,000 population.

Age

Parkinson's is an age-related condition. Most people with Parkinson's are elderly, above working age, with a recent UK community-based cohort measuring a mean age of onset at 72 years (Caslake et al., 2013). Figure 2.1 shows how

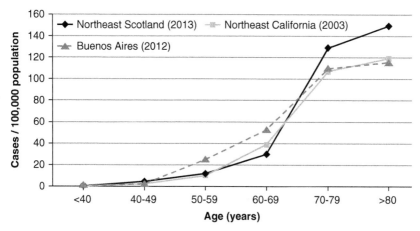

FIGURE 2.1 Age-specific incidence of Parkinson's.

the incidence of Parkinson's increases with age in different populations (Bauso et al., 2012, Caslake et al., 2013, Van Den Eeden et al., 2003).

Although services must serve people of all ages, it is especially important to meet the needs of the elderly. Issues facing older versus younger people with Parkinson's include a greater risk for dementia and comorbidity, relative poverty and difficulty traveling. Comorbidity in Parkinson's is similar to that in age-matched controls and associated with increased mortality. In the general population, by the age of 80 years, 50% of people have at least two chronic conditions. Management may have to be modified to take account of age-related physiologic changes and comorbidities.

On the other hand, 1 in 25 people with Parkinson's are under the age of 50 at the time of diagnosis. Those diagnosed before 65 years of age are more likely to live longer with Parkinson's and have less dementia but more motor fluctuations and dyskinesia than older people with Parkinson's. These younger individuals have special needs in relation to their work. Helping working-age patients stay in employment may be important for society, as such people continue to contribute to the economy; more importantly, ongoing employment may be important for the individual's self-esteem and sense of purpose. Occupational therapists have a crucial role in advising these working-age people, but occupational health doctors and nurses also have a part to play.

It is not uncommon for Parkinson's research studies to have an age profile that does not match the true age profile of Parkinson's in the community (Macleod et al., 2018). Caution should be exercised in applying the outcomes of such research to routine practice.

Gender

Studies consistently find that Parkinson's is 1.5 to 2 times more common in men than in women. The reason for this is not known for certain. Possible explanations include a protective effect of female hormones, greater risk in men of exposure to known environmental risks such as head injury and pesticides, and increased genetic risk mediated via the sex chromosomes. In support of the hormonal hypothesis, there is a positive correlation between age of onset and both age of menopause and length of fertile lifespan. Also, women with greater parity (more children) have a lower incidence of Parkinson's.

The clinical characteristics of Parkinson's (phenotype) may be different in women. Age at onset is later, presentation with tremor is more common, and rigidity is less severe. Women also have earlier dyskinesia, more wearing off, postural issues, anxiety, and depression, and they report a lower quality of life. In comparison, men have more drooling, speech disturbance, taste and olfactory problems, REM-sleep behavioral disturbance, orthostatic hypotension, sexual dysfunction and cognitive impairment (Picillo et al., 2017, Szewczyk-Krolikowski et al., 2014).

Progression of Parkinson's is not slower in women, and trials of estrogen-based hormone replacement therapy showed no benefit. There are also differences in service utilisation. Women experience greater delay between first symptoms and specialist assessment, and they access deep brain stimulation less often.

Ethnicity

Parkinson's may have a greater incidence in Caucasian populations, but this is far from certain (Van Den Eeden et al., 2003). Differences in incidence by country might be due to environmental or genetic factors, but they could also reflect ascertainment bias. For example, the low incidence of Parkinson's in developing countries may be due to the failure to recognise cases because of the patchy provision of medical services. In the United Kingdom, there is evidence that Black and minority ethnic groups are underrepresented among those attending movement disorder clinics. Services should consider why that might be. Reaching out to underserved populations could include contact with community leaders and listening to their perspectives.

Life expectancy/mortality

Before levodopa (L-dopa) therapy became available in the 1960s, mortality among Parkinson's patients was threefold higher than that among populations matched for age, gender, and comorbidity. Since then, there has been some improvement. Longitudinal studies comparing people with Parkinson's to age-matched controls show an average mortality ratio of 1.5. Factors linked to increased mortality are shown in Table 2.1.

In one study, coffee drinking was associated with lower mortality, slower progression of the disease and a lower incidence of dementia (Paul et al., 2019).

TABLE 2.1 Risk factors for early mortality in Parkinson's
Age at diagnosis
Male gender
Postural instability with gait disorder subtype
Symmetry of motor signs
Poor response to L-dopa
Hallucinations
Cognitive impairment
Smoking

Time from key disease milestones (i.e., visual hallucinations, cognitive disability, residential home placement, recurrent falls) to death is shown in relation to age of onset in Fig. 2.2. Sadly, each of these milestones is a harbinger of demise (Kempster et al., 2010).

Other UK studies also inform mortality predictions. In the community-based Parkinsonism Incidence in North-East Scotland (PINE) study, the median time from diagnosis to death was 7.8 years, and 46% of people diagnosed with Parkinson's had died or were dependent 3 years from diagnosis (Fielding et al., 2016). In the Cambridgeshire Parkinson's Incidence from GP to Neurologist (CamPaIGN) study, also community based, the median time to death was 10.3 years. The commonest cause of death was pneumonia (33%), and predictors of death at baseline were age and smoking (Williams-Gray et al., 2013).

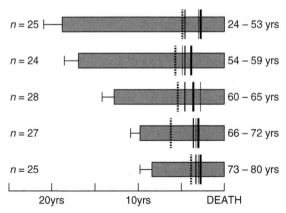

FIGURE 2.2   Disease course and disability milestones for five age-at-onset groups. Disease courses aligned for time of death. Regular falls = fine lines; residential care = heavy lines; cognitive disability = fine dots; visual hallucinations = heavy dots. Error bars show the standard error of the mean disease duration. Figure from Kempster el al., 2010.

Environmental risk factors

Although it is true that you cannot choose your parents, other risk factors for Parkinson's may be modifiable. Some knowledge of environmental risk factors may allow clinicians to give rational advice to those at high risk for developing Parkinson's (Tables 2.2 and 2.3).

First, protective associations are listed in Table 2.2.

TABLE 2.2 Factors associated with a reduced risk for developing Parkinson's
Exercise
Smoking
Coffee drinking (intake of caffeine)
The Mediterranean diet
Vagotomy
Appendicectomy
High level of serum urate
High level of serum cholesterol
Use of calcium antagonists
Use of statins

TABLE 2.3 Factors associated with an increased risk for Parkinson's
Pesticide exposure (paraquat, rotenone)
Rural living
Drinking well water
Solvents (trichloroethylene [TCE])
Head injury
Diabetes
Melanoma
Stress
Vitamin D deficiency
Beta blockers
Methamphetamine

There is good evidence that physical activity protects against Parkinson's and has other health benefits; it can therefore be recommended (see Chapter 11). Smoking has consistently been associated with a lower risk for developing Parkinson's. Smokers may have a lower chance of reaching old age, but correcting for that, the association remains. A dose-response effect has been observed, supporting a possible causal link. The mechanism is speculative; nicotine may play a part. Alternatively, prodromal reductions in brain dopamine may reduce rewards from cigarette smoking, leading to smoking cessation. It has also been suggested that personality types at risk for Parkinson's may include those less likely to smoke, but passive smoking is also associated with reduced risk. Clearly, smoking cannot be recommended because it causes—among others—cancer, stroke, and ischemic heart disease. A study investigating the disease-modifying potential of transdermal NICotine in early Parkinson's Disease (NIC-PD) found no benefit (Oertel et al., 2018). A trial of nicotine patches in those at risk for developing Parkinson's has not yet been undertaken.

Coffee drinking has been linked to slower progression and lower standardised mortality rates (Paul et al., 2019). Coffee drinking and smoking go hand in hand in some cultures, but an inverse association between caffeine consumption and Parkinson's persists after correcting for smoking.

The Mediterranean diet has been linked to a reduced probability of prodromal Parkinson's, but there were potential confounders (Maraki et al., 2019). Non-etheless, other health benefits of such a diet are likely, and it can be cautiously recommended. Diets should be rich in vitamin D, as deficiency is associated with Parkinson's and worse motor outcomes.

Some physiologic variables are linked to Parkinson's risk. There is an inverse association between the serum urate level and Parkinson's. Urate acts as an antioxidant. Those with the highest urate levels have lower rates of progression; therefore the safety in Parkinson's of inosine (a compound that is taken orally, penetrates the central nervous system, and is already taken widely as a nutritional supplement) has been investigated. Inosine effectively raised urate levels, but a phase 3 randomised controlled trial of inosine was terminated early owing to lack of efficacy in slowing disease progression (The Parkinson's Study Group SURE-PD investigators).

Higher cholesterol levels are linked with a lower risk for Parkinson's, but statins (especially simvastatin) have also been linked with lower risk. The beneficial effect of the statin must be independent of its cholesterol-lowering effect, and animal models suggest an anti-inflammatory mechanism. Non-steroidal anti-inflammatory drugs (NSAIDs), however, have not been consistently linked with a reduced risk for Parkinson's. Dihydropyridine calcium channel blockers have also been associated with a lower risk for Parkinson's and with neuroprotective effects in animal models. Beta blockers, on the other hand, are associated with an increased risk of Parkinson's and with lower urinary tract symptoms.

Factors associated with an increased risk for Parkinson's are listed in Table 2.3.

The accidental production and consumption of 1-methyl-4-phenyl-1,2,3,6-tetrahydropyridine (MPTP) by four drug addicts in Santa Clara County, California, in 1983 was a disaster for those who took the drug, as they rapidly developed a severe and irreversible parkinsonism. However, MPTP proved to be a useful model for Parkinson's in the laboratory and was a reminder, if one were needed, that environmental toxins can cause parkinsonism.

Pesticide exposure has consistently been associated with Parkinson's. Drinking well water and rural living may be linked to Parkinson's through pesticide exposure. Rotenone and paraquat have both been associated with an increased risk for Parkinson's. Rotenone is a plant-based pesticide; it has been used for many decades and causes nigrostriatal damage in animal models. Paraquat was developed in the 1960s. It has structural similarities to MPTP and has been banned in many jurisdictions. Where its use is still allowed, local Parkinson's groups should be encouraged to lobby for legislation to ban it. Use of gloves and protective clothing may reduce the risk.

Trichloroethylene, a solvent, is commonly used in dry cleaning. It has been linked to Parkinson's in small studies.

Head injury is associated with Parkinson's in some but not all studies. Recall bias is a problem and prodromal Parkinson's may increase the risk of falling; this may explain the increased occurrence of falls in the year preceding a diagnosis of Parkinson's (reverse causality).

Stress has been linked to Parkinson's. A diagnosis of posttraumatic stress disorder or an adjustment disorder has been linked with Parkinson's in separate studies (Marras et al., 2019).

Genetics

Parkinson's is usually a sporadic disorder. As a rule of thumb, Parkinson's in a first-degree relative doubles a person's risk for developing Parkinson's. Occasionally, however, Parkinson's runs very strongly in families. In Italy, close study of one such extended family, the Contursi kindred, in 1997 led to the discovery of an autosomal dominantly inherited genetic mutation causing familial Parkinson's. In this family, the age of onset was a few years younger than that in the general Parkinson's population; but as in others with Parkinson's, Lewy bodies were found in the dopaminergic neurons and clinical heterogeneity was noted. The genetic abnormality was located on the fourth chromosome (4q21-q23). The gene SNCA, encoding for α-synuclein, the major constituent of Lewy bodies, is found in this area. In the Contursi kindred, a single-base-pair change in SNCA (PARK1) was found to be responsible for Parkinson's. Inheritance was autosomal dominant with high penetrance. In other words, most of those with the mutation developed the disease.

To date, 19 rare monogenic forms of Parkinson's have been described, the most common of which is PARK8, a mutation in the LRRK2 gene encoding for leucine–rich repeat kinase (Reed et al., 2019). Parkin (PARK2) and PINK1

(PARK6) are the most common autosomal recessive genes causing Parkinson's. Together, all monogenic forms of Parkinson's account for less than 5% of the cases of Parkinson's in the UK.

The Tracking Parkinson's study looked for mutations in four Parkinson's genes: SNCA, LRRK2, Parkin, and PINK1. This UK study comprised 2261 people with Parkinson's and included 424 with young-onset Parkinson's (age of onset less than or equal to 50 years). The study reported pathogenic mutations in 29 (1.4%) participants. Among the young-onset individuals, 3.3% had pathogenic mutations of Parkin or PINK1 and 2.2% had mutations in LRRK2. Among late-onset (> 50 years) patients, mutations in LRRK2 occurred in 0.5% and pathogenic duplications of SNCA in 0.06%. The authors estimated that 1000 people in the United Kingdom have genetic mutations in these genes. It was optimistically concluded that therapies, for example LRRK2 inhibitors, could be developed to target these genetic anomalies (Tan et al., 2019).

Genomewide association studies (GWAS) have identified over 40 common genetic variants (single-nucleotide polymorphisms) that, in the general population, increase risk for developing Parkinson's. Genetic variants identified by GWAS should be considered risk factors for the development of Parkinson's rather than genetic causes of Parkinson's. Typically, they increase the risk for Parkinson's less than twofold. For example, variations in the genes MAPT (encoding microtubule associated protein Tau) and GBA (encoding glucocerobrosidase) are associated with increased risk of Parkinson's. Homozygous mutations in GBA can cause Gaucher's disease, whereas heterozygous mutations increase the risk for Parkinson's fivefold and the risk for dementia with Lewy bodies eightfold. Heterozygote GBA mutations are found in about 3% of people with Parkinson's; hence they constitute the most common genetic risk factor for Parkinson's. Among those with Parkinson's, GBA carriers present 3 to 6 years earlier than those without GBA mutations, and they have a greater incidence of dementia. Although enzyme replacement treatment for the systemic features of Gaucher's disease is available, it does not cross the blood-brain barrier so it is ineffective for the neurologic manifestations of Gaucher's and for GBA-associated Parkinson's.

A potential gene therapy for GBA-associated Parkinson's, PR001 (Prevail Therapeutics New York, New York), is in early-stage trials in the United States. The gene would be introduced using a harmless version of an adenovirus. It is hoped that this treatment will improve lysosomal function and the clearance of abnormal proteins. If such approaches are shown to be safe and effective, testing for GBA mutations will become routine in clinical practice.

Genetics and the multidisciplinary team

Genetic screening tests are available commercially to the public. For example, in the United Kingdom, 23andMe offer screening for 150 gene variants associated with a variety of conditions including GBA, LRRK2 and the ε4 variant of APOE (the gene encoding apolipoprotein E) for around £150 (23andMe, 2020). There are many variants of LRRK2 but only two are tested.

Genetic testing is not currently part of mainstream clinical practice in the United Kingdom and specific treatments for genetic variants of Parkinson's are not yet available. If that changes, inclusion of a clinical geneticist in the multidisciplinary team (MDT) may become necessary.

Pathology and etiology

When one is considering the pathology of Parkinson's, it is helpful to think about both structural and biochemical abnormalities. A full discussion of etiology is outside the scope of this chapter, but a brief review of pathological mechanisms follows. The clinical relevance of these processes is highlighted.

Structural pathology

Parkinson's is characterised by the loss of pigmented dopamine neurons in the substantia nigra pars compacta (SNc) of the midbrain. By the time of diagnosis, more than 50% of the dopamine neurons have already been lost and the dopamine content of this part of the brain has been reduced by 80%. At postmortem, the loss of pigment in the SNc is apparent to the naked eye. Lewy bodies, seen as eosinophilic (pink-staining) collections, are found on standard microscopy. They contain proteins, mainly α-synuclein, but also ubiquitin and parkin. Progressive loss of striatal dopaminergic function with time matches clinical deterioration and worsening motor symptoms. In parallel with the loss of neurons, there is an increase in glial cells (gliosis). These cells are non-neuronal and involved in repair and inflammation.

In summary, the pathological hallmarks of Parkinson's are as follows:

- Neuronal loss in the SNc
- Depigmentation of the SNc
- The presence of Lewy bodies in neurons
- Gliosis

Loss of neurons and the formation of Lewy bodies are not confined to the SNc. Work by Braak and colleagues suggests that the pathology in Parkinson's starts in the olfactory bulb and the dorsal motor nucleus of the vagus nerve (DMVN). The nucleus basalis of Meynert, raphe nuclei, locus coeruleus, autonomic ganglia, and peripheral nerves are also involved. Pathology spreads upward to involve the SNc and finally the cerebral cortex. This theory of the development of Parkinson's pathology in the brain is called the Braak hypothesis, and it explains some clinical features. For example, it is known that olfactory loss often precedes motor symptoms, which usually precede dementia. The main motor pathway involved is the nigrostriatal tract. There are also dopaminergic projections from the tegmentum to the limbic system. Loss of neurons here may account for the increased incidence of depression seen in Parkinson's.

Biochemical pathology

In Parkinson's, the levels of dopamine in the SNc, putamen and caudate are low. Serotonin levels are low in the nigrostriatal tract and the raphe nuclei. Noradrenaline levels are low in the locus coeruleus, which projects widely. Loss of noradrenaline and serotonin at these sites is thought to contribute to sleep disturbance, anxiety, and depression. In the SNc, noradrenaline levels in the caudate and putamen are about 50% those of controls (Espay et al., 2014). Loss of catecholamine function in the postganglionic fibers to the heart leads to abnormalities in cardiac scanning with radiolabeled metaiodobenzylguanidine (MIBG) single photon emission computed tomography. Abnormal MIBG scans have been earmarked as potential biomarkers for Parkinson's, but the scans may be less reliable in the elderly. Aside from the monoamines (dopamine, noradrenaline and serotonin), there are changes in glutamate and acetylcholine. The nucleus basalis, a cholinergic nucleus, shows a marked cholinergic deficit, which is also seen elsewhere in the brain and is linked to cognitive decline and falls. Cholinesterase inhibitors boost the availability of acetylcholine and are effective in the treatment of Parkinson's dementia and dementia with Lewy bodies (see Chapter 9). A phase 2 trial of rivastigmine in people with Parkinson's who fall showed reduced stride-length variability (Henderson et al., 2016), and a phase 3 trial of rivastigmine for the prevention of falls in Parkinson's is underway (see Chapter 10).

Pathological mechanisms

Fortunately, a detailed knowledge of molecular processes leading to cell death in Parkinson's is not required for the clinician. Key mechanisms are as follows:

- Oxidative stress
- Mitochondrial dysfunction
- Dysfunction of the proteosome-ubiquitin system and lysosomes
- Inflammation
- Prion-like mechanisms

These mechanisms and the role of the gut are described briefly in this section. The reader is referred to published reviews for more detail (Przedborski, 2015).

Efforts to understand pathological mechanisms have focused on the dopamine nerves of the SNc and their projections. Some of these mechanisms may also apply to other brain areas and neurotransmitter systems. Late-stage Parkinson's is dominated by non-motor symptoms that are unresponsive to L-dopa; a thorough understanding of the mechanisms leading to the full spectrum of neurological deficits is needed if rational treatments are to be developed. The accumulation of abnormal proteins within neurons seems to be key to an explanation of how they are damaged.

Oxidative stress

In health, the body uses energy to drive cell processes and repair cellular damage. Mitochondria, the cells' power plants, use oxygen to generate adenosine triphosphate (ATP—the cells' energy currency), but in the process they generate reactive oxygen species (ROS), which can damage proteins. ROS may oxidise proteins, leading to misfolding or changes in binding sites and to loss of function. In Parkinson's, the accumulation of abnormal proteins in cells contributes to the formation of Lewy bodies. A pilot trial of the antioxidant vitamins C and E for early Parkinson's showed promise, but a larger trial of α–tocopherol (a component of vitamin E) showed no benefit in improving symptoms or slowing disease progression (Fahn, 1992, Parkinson Study Group, 1993).

Mitochondrial dysfunction

MPTP, a toxin known to cause parkinsonism, interferes with the normal functioning of complex 1 in mitochondria. This contributes to oxidative stress and also impedes energy-dependent clearance of damaged proteins. Abnormal or worn-out mitochondria are tagged by parkin and marked for destruction, a process known as mitophagy. Homozygous Parkin mutations prevent normal mitophagy and cause familial Parkinson's. Faulty clearance of abnormal mitochondria may contribute to cell death in sporadic Parkinson's, but it is doubtful that mitochondrial dysfunction has a primary causative role because known mitochondrial diseases rarely cause significant parkinsonism. Coenzyme Q_{10} is an antioxidant and part of the electron transport chain in mitochondria; sadly, however, it is ineffective in slowing disease progression.

Dysfunction of the proteosome-ubiquitin system and lysosomes

Cellular mechanisms dealing with protein damage include degradation of the damaged protein by the proteasome-ubiquitin system and breakdown of protein by the autophagy-lysosome system. If proteins cannot be repaired, they may be tagged with ubiquitin and marked for destruction. Polyubiquinated proteins are processed in proteosomes. If misfolded proteins are too large for proteosomal degradation, they may be enclosed in a double membrane, a process called autophagocytosis, and transported to a lysosome, where the proteins can be broken down. Failure of this protein clearance system may contribute to a buildup of abnormal proteins, and mutations in genes involved in this system have been linked to Parkinson's.

Inflammation

Inflammation is probably a late response to processes that have already caused significant cell damage. Inflammatory processes may contribute to further cell loss, but the use of NSAIDs has not been shown to reduce the risk of Parkinson's.

Prion-like mechanisms

Could Parkinson's pathology spread from cell to cell? Two observations suggest that it can. First, there is the Braak hypothesis regarding the upward progression of Lewy body pathology; second, there is the discovery of Lewy bodies in tissues transplanted from unaffected fetuses to individuals with Parkinson's. There are some similarities between α–synuclein biology and prion diseases (Ma et al., 2019). In particular, these include the following:

- Both α–synuclein and prion protein can misfold so that they are rich in platelike structures (β sheets).
- Misfolded protein leads to the accumulation of normal protein and acts as a template for misfolding of further protein (permissive templating).
- Misfolded protein can be taken up by other cells.

In the case of α–synuclein, the secretion of misfolded protein by affected cells and uptake by unaffected cells has been demonstrated in vitro. Unlike the case with prions, person-to-person spread of α–synuclein has not been described.

Role of the gut in the pathogenesis of Parkinson's

Evidence is building for a gut-to-brain theory of Parkinson's (Scheperjans et al., 2018). "Torpid" bowels were mentioned by James Parkinson in his original description of the "shaking palsy." Constipation is known to occur years before the motor symptoms of Parkinson's become obvious. Braak noted early involvement of the DMVN, which supplies the gut. Vagotomy and appendicectomy are associated with a lower incidence of Parkinson's (Breen et al., 2019). Small bowel bacterial overgrowth is common in Parkinson's, and α–synuclein is found in the enteric nervous system. Indeed, archived bowel biopsy specimens in subjects subsequently shown to have Parkinson's show α–synuclein pathology more frequently than biopsies from controls. Furthermore, the gut microbiota differs in people with Parkinson's compared with controls, with the former showing a relative abundance of *Akkermansia*, *Bifidobacterium*, and *Lactobacillus* and less *Prevotella* and *Faecalibacterium*.

A landmark study (see Fig. 2.3) showed that mice genetically modified to overexpress α–synuclein (ASO mice) developed Parkinson's-type motor signs. When ASO mice were reared in a germ-free environment, they had much reduced motor signs; however, if these germ-free mice were fed short-chain fatty acids (microbial metabolites), they did develop motor signs. If ASO mice were colonised with gut flora from humans with Parkinson's they developed a more severe motor syndrome than those with normal mouse gut flora. The results imply that:

ASO mouse – a mouse model of Parkinson's genetically modified to overexpress α-synuclein
– developed motor signs like Parkinson's

 ASO mouse with germ-free bowel
– reduced motor Parkinson's signs

 Germ free ASO mouse
- fed specific microbial metabolites (short chain fatty acids)
- developed motor signs like Parkinson's

 ASO mouse colonised with flora from humans with Parkinson's
Developed worse Parkinson's signs

FIGURE 2.3   The effects of manipulating the gut flora in mice genetically predisposed to developing Parkinson's.

- There is an interaction between genetic predisposition and environmental exposure.
- Variation in the microbial environment may influence disease expression.
- The changes in the brain could be mediated via metabolites, specifically short-chain fatty acids (Sampson et al., 2016).

Function of the basal ganglia

The basal ganglia (nuclei) are collections of neurons deep in the forebrain and midbrain. They are involved in the regulation or modulation of voluntary movement, procedural learning and emotions. The motor circuit of the thalamocortical-basal ganglia is shown in Figure 2.4.

The substantia nigra (SNc) can be compared to the accelerator of a car and the subthalamic nucleus (STN) to the brake. Damage to the SNc in Parkinson's leads to slowing of movement. Surgical lesions of the STN—for example, subthalamotomy or STN deep brain stimulation—reduce the inhibitory output from the basal ganglia, thus allowing more movement. The direct (inner) pathway generally facilitates movement, and the indirect (outer) pathway inhibits movement. The motor pathways are the best understood, but there are parallel circuits for the eyes, for executive function and for the limbic system. The circuit shown is a simplified version of reality based on the classic pathway described by deLong and others. However, it includes a more recently described hyperdirect pathway and connections to the PPN, which appears to be important in regulating gait (Wichmann, 2019). Although there is debate about the exact functions and functioning of the basal ganglia, there is some evidence for the following:

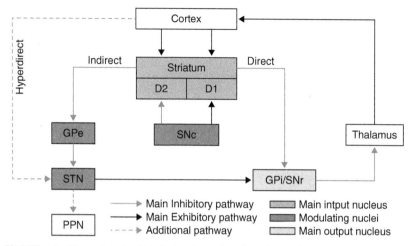

FIGURE 2.4   The motor circuit of the basal ganglia. The main input to the basal ganglia is from the cerebral cortex and is excitatory. The main output from the basal ganglia is to the thalamus and is inhibitory. The SNc, GPe, and STN are regulatory or modulating nuclei. The nigrostriatal pathway uses dopamine as the main neurotransmitter; it stimulates the direct pathway via D1 dopamine receptors while inhibiting the indirect pathway via D2 dopamine receptors. Other excitatory pathways mainly use glutamate as the neurotransmitter, whereas inhibitory pathways mainly use γ–aminobutyric acid (GABA) as the neurotransmitter. **Abbreviations.** SNc: substantia nigra, compact part; GPe: globus pallidus, external part; STN: subthalamic nucleus; GPi: globus pallidus, internal part; SNr: substantia nigra, reticular part; PPN: peduncular pontine nucleus; D1 and D2: striatal dopamine receptors.

1. *Scaling of movement.* The basal ganglia are involved in regulating the speed and size of movement. In Parkinson's, movements are typically underscaled, leading, for example, to handwriting that gets smaller as more is written or to poor preparation for sitting, whereby the person with Parkinson's who wants to sit may find that he or she is too far away from the chair and not aligned properly.
2. *Action selection.* Overall, the output of the basal ganglia is inhibitory. The direct pathway facilitates a desired action whereas the indirect pathway inhibits unwanted movements.
3. *Response inhibition.* The basal ganglia may have a role in go/no-go responses. This might explain some of the impulsivity seen in association with dopaminergic therapy.
4. *Procedural learning.* The basal ganglia appear to be involved in procedural learning. People with Parkinson's may have difficulty with previously well-learned motor skills. They may have particular difficulty with sequential movement and with simultaneous movements, including bimanual movement. Awareness of these difficulties may inform the delivery of therapies. For example, when a person with Parkinson's is struggling with a particular

action, the clinician might suggest doing only one thing at a time or avoiding dual tasking. "Stop talking when walking" is also useful advice. Breaking a complex movement into smaller parts sometimes helps.

5. *Reward responses.* The risk for repetitive reward-seeking behavioral in Parkinson's has been estimated to be 17% in those on dopamine agonists (Wichmann, 2013).

A shared understanding of the functioning of the basal ganglia may help with rehabilitation. An appreciation of problems with scaling of movement should lead to the consistent adoption of approaches that reinforce big movements. Problems with reward help to explain deficits in goal-oriented behavioral that may hamper therapy efforts while also alerting staff to the risk for impulsive behavioral in those on dopaminergic therapy. Finally, issues with sequencing and simultaneous tasks must be borne in mind when person-centred therapies are being developed.

The heterogeneity of Parkinson's

The adage that no two people are alike is especially true in Parkinson's. Indeed, some have suggested that Parkinson's is not a single condition but a syndrome with disparate causes and different outcomes. This might explain why more than 15 disease-modifying drug trials in Parkinson's have failed.

Subtypes of Parkinson's are identifiable. Two motor subtypes have been described: tremor-dominant disease and postural instability gait disorder. The former has a benign course whereas the latter is associated with rapid progression and cognitive decline. Non-motor subtypes have also been described. Using cluster analysis, subtypes that combined motor and non-motor features have been described (Lawton et al., 2018).

Proposed subtyping based on neurotransmitter deficits include the following:

- *Cholinergic deficit*—freezing of gait, dementia
- *Noradrenalin deficit*—akinetic-rigid, dyskinetic, depression, anxiety, apathy, postural hypotension
- *Serotonin deficit*—dyskinesis, fatigue, sleep disturbance, depression, anxiety
- *Dopamine deficit*—classic Parkinson's (Titova et al., 2017)

Subtyping based on neurotransmitter deficits is attractive because it suggests pharmacological interventions. However, there is likely to be substantial overlap between groups, and so far there is no universally accepted system for subtyping.

Conclusion

Parkinson's is the second most common neurodegenerative condition. It is characterised clinically by bradykinesia, rigidity and tremor, and pathologically by Lewy bodies in the substantia nigra. In fact, many parts of the brain are affected and multiple neurotransmitter systems are altered. Therefore people with Parkinson's have a huge variety of symptoms. Many symptoms are currently not responsive to medications so non-drug therapies delivered through coordinated multidisciplinary care is important. The role of the MDT in the treatment of individuals with motor and non-motor symptoms of Parkinson's is described in the following chapters.

Top tips for the multidisciplinary team

1. The cardinal motor features of Parkinson's are bradykinesia, rigidity, and tremor at rest.
2. Parkinson's causes many non-motor symptoms, and some—including constipation, depression, anosmia, and REM sleep behavioral disorder—develop before the motor symptoms.
3. Although Parkinson's is much more common in older people, the MDT should be aware of the differing needs of older and younger people with Parkinson's.
4. Causation is multifactorial: it is likely that in many cases genetic and environmental factors interact to cause Parkinson's.
5. The key pathological hallmarks of Parkinson's are loss of dopaminergic neurons in the substantia nigra and the appearance of Lewy bodies.
6. Multiple brain areas and neurotransmitters—not just the substantia nigra and the dopamine system—are affected in Parkinson's. This helps to explain the plethora of non-motor symptoms and why not all Parkinson's symptoms respond to dopamine treatments.
7. A variety of pathological processes can lead to the buildup of abnormal proteins such as α-synuclein within neurons.
8. The basal ganglia modulate motor activity: the substantia nigra promotes movement and the subthalamic nucleus reduces movement.
9. The basal ganglia are involved in the scaling of movement, action selection, response inhibition, procedural learning, and reward responses.
10. The MDT should encourage large movements.
11. The MDT should be aware that lack of dopamine can lead to apathy and failure to engage in goal-directed behavioral. Dopaminergic treatments can also cause impulsive behavioral.

References

23andMe. Retrieved January 28, 2020, from www.23andme.com/en-gb.

Bauso, D. J., Tartari, J. P., Stefani, C. V., Rojas, J. L., Giunta, D. H., & Cristiano, E. (2012). Incidence and prevalence of Parkinson's disease in Buenos Aires City, Argentina. *European Journal of Neurology*, *19*(8), 1108–1113.

Breen, D. P., Halliday, G. M., & Lang, A. E. (2019). Gut-brain axis and the spread of alpha-synuclein pathology: vagal highway or dead end? *Movement Disorders*, *34*(3), 307–316.

Caslake, R., Taylor, K., Scott, N., Gordon, J., Harris, C., Wilde, K., et al. (2013). Age-, gender-, and socioeconomic status-specific incidence of Parkinson's disease and parkinsonism in northeast Scotland: the PINE study. *Parkinsonism and Related Disorders*, *19*(5), 515–521.

Espay, A. J., LeWitt, P. A., & Kaufmann, H. (2014). Norepinephrine deficiency in Parkinson's disease: the case for noradrenergic enhancement. *Movement Disorders*, *29*(14), 1710–1719.

Fahn, S. (1992). A pilot trial of high-dose alpha-tocopherol and ascorbate in early Parkinson's disease. *Annals of Neurology*, *32*(Suppl), S128–132.

Fielding, S., Macleod, A. D., & Counsell, C. E. (2016). Medium-term prognosis of an incident cohort of parkinsonian patients compared to controls. *Parkinsonism and Related Disorders*, *32*, 36–41.

Henderson, E. J., Lord, S. R., Brodie, M. A., Gaunt, D. M., Lawrence, A. D., Close, J. C., et al. (2016). Rivastigmine for gait stability in patients with Parkinson's disease (ReSPonD): a randomised, double-blind, placebo-controlled, phase 2 trial. *Lancet Neurology*, *15*(3), 249–258.

Kempster, P. A., O'Sullivan, S. S., Holton, J. L., Revesz, T., & Lees, A. J. (2010). Relationships between age and late progression of Parkinson's disease: a clinico-pathological study. *Brain*, *133*(Pt 6), 1755–1762.

Lawton, M., Ben-Shlomo, Y., May, M. T., Baig, F., Barber, T. R., Klein, J. C., et al. (2018). Developing and validating Parkinson's disease subtypes and their motor and cognitive progression. *Journal of Neurology, Neurosurgery, and Psychiatry*, *89*(12), 1279–1287.

Ma, J., Gao, J., Wang, J., & Xie, A. (2019). Prion-like mechanisms in Parkinson's disease. *Frontiers in Neuroscience*, *13*, 552.

Macleod, A. D., Henery, R., Nwajiugo, P. C., Scott, N. W., Caslake, R., & Counsell, C. E. (2018). Age-related selection bias in Parkinson's disease research: are we recruiting the right participants? *Parkinsonism and Related Disorders*, *55*, 128–133.

Maraki, M. I., Yannakoulia, M., Stamelou, M., Stefanis, L., Xiromerisiou, G., Kosmidis, H. H., et al. (2019). Mediterranean diet adherence is related to reduced probability of prodromal Parkinson's disease. *Movement Disorders*, *34*(1), 48–57.

Marras, C., Canning, C. G., & Goldman, S. M. (2019). Environment, lifestyle, and Parkinson's disease: implications for prevention in the next decade. *Movement Disorders*, *34*(6), 801–811.

Oertel, W., Müller, H., Schade-Brittinger, C., Kemp, C., Balthasar, K., Articus, K., et al. (2018). The NIC-PD-study—a randomised, placebo-controlled, double-blind, multi-centre trial to assess the disease-modifying potential of transdermal nicotine in early Parkinson's disease in Germany and N. America [abstract]. *Movement Disorders*, *33*(Suppl 2.), 358.

Parkinson Study Group. (1993). Effects of tocopherol and deprenyl on the progression of disability in early Parkinson's disease. *New England Journal of Medicine*, *328*(3), 176–183.

Parkinson's UK (2017). The prevalance and incidence of Parkinson's in the UK. Results from the Clinical Practice Research Datalink Reference Report. London, UK.

Paul, K. C., Chuang, Y. H., Shih, I. F., Keener, A., Bordelon, Y., Bronstein, J. M., et al. (2019). The association between lifestyle factors and Parkinson's disease progression and mortality. *Movement Disorders*, *34*(1), 58–66.

Picillo, M., Nicoletti, A., Fetoni, V., Garavaglia, B., Barone, P., Pellecchia, M. T., et al. (2017). The relevance of gender in Parkinson's disease: a review. *Journal of Neurology*, *264*(8), 1583–1607.

Przedborski, S. (2015). Etiology and pathogenesis of Parkinson's disease. In J. Jankovic, & E. Tolosa (Eds.), *Parkinson's Disease and Movement Disorders* (pp. 51–64). Wolters Kluwer.

Reed, X., Bandres-Ciga, S., Blauwendraat, C., & Cookson, M. R. (2019). The role of monogenic genes in idiopathic Parkinson's disease. *Neurobiology of Disease*, *124*, 230–239.

Sampson, T. R., Debelius, J. W., Thron, T., Janssen, S., Shastri, G. G., Ilhan, Z. E., et al. (2016). Gut microbiota regulate motor deficits and neuroinflammation in a model of Parkinson's disease. *Cell*, *167*(6), 1469–1480. e1412.

Scheperjans, F., Derkinderen, P., & Borghammer, P. (2018). The gut and Parkinson's disease: hype or Hope? *Journal of Parkinson's Disease*, *8*(Suppl 1), S31–S39.

Szewczyk-Krolikowski, K., Tomlinson, P., Nithi, K., Wade-Martins, R., Talbot, K., Ben-Shlomo, Y., et al. (2014). The influence of age and gender on motor and non-motor features of early Parkinson's disease: initial findings from the Oxford Parkinson Disease Centre (OPDC) discovery cohort. *Parkinsonism and Related Disorders*, *20*(1), 99–105.

Tan, M. M. X., Malek, N., Lawton, M. A., Hubbard, L., Pittman, A. M., Joseph, T., et al. (2019). Genetic analysis of Mendelian mutations in a large UK population-based Parkinson's disease study. *Brain*, *142*(9), 2828–2844.

The Parkinson's Study Group SURE-PD investigators. Study of Urate Elevation in Parkinson's Disease Phase 3 (SURE-PD3). Retrieved February 14, 2020, from https://www.ninds.nih.gov/Disorders/Clinical-Trials/Study-Urate-Elevation-Parkinsons-Disease-Phase-3-SURE-PD3.

Titova, N., Padmakumar, C., Lewis, S. J. G., & Chaudhuri, K. R. (2017). Parkinson's: a syndrome rather than a disease? *Journal of Neural Transmission (Vienna)*, *124*(8), 907–914.

Van Den Eeden, S. K., Tanner, C. M., Bernstein, A. L., Fross, R. D., Leimpeter, A., Bloch, D. A., et al. (2003). Incidence of Parkinson's disease: variation by age, gender, and race/ethnicity. *American Journal of Epidemiology*, *157*(11), 1015–1022.

Wichmann, T. (2013). Functional aspects of the basal ganglia. In D. Burn (Ed.), *Oxford Textbook of Movement Disorders* (pp. 21–31). Oxford, UK: Oxford University Press.

Wichmann, T. (2019). Changing views of the pathophysiology of Parkinsonism. *Movement Disorders*, *34*(8), 1130–1143.

Williams-Gray, C. H., Mason, S. L., Evans, J. R., Foltynie, T., Brayne, C., Robbins, T. W., et al. (2013). The CamPaIGN study of Parkinson's disease: 10-year outlook in an incident population-based cohort. *Journal of Neurology, Neurosurgery, and Psychiatry*, *84*(11), 1258–1264.

Chapter 3

The multidisciplinary team working with Parkinson's patients

Chandler Gill, Serena Hess, Erica Myrick, Rob Skelly, Fiona Lindop, Tom Mace and Jori Fleisher

Chapter outline

Introduction

The introduction of levodopa (L-dopa) in the 1960s was a breakthrough in the treatment of Parkinson's, but pharmacologic treatment still has limitations. On-period freezing of gait and falls are poorly responsive to dopaminergic treatments, as are many non-motor symptoms (NMSs). Indeed, some NMSs, such as hallucinations and orthostatic hypotension, worsen after dopaminergic treatment. Moreover, NMSs may have a greater effect on quality of life (QoL) than do the dopamine-responsive motor symptoms. Other approaches are needed.

Interventions by allied health professionals are effective at improving mobility, speech and functional independence. The members of the multidisciplinary team (MDT) work together to provide comprehensive care and thus to meet the physical and psychosocial needs of people with Parkinson's; this is their fundamental mission (Mitchell et al., 2008). The synergy of teamwork provides holistic benefits that are greater than those resulting from treatments offered by individual clinicians; that is, the team is more than sum of its parts. When the team is closely integrated and coordinated and there is good (ideally face-to-face) communication between team members, MDT work is sometimes said to be interdisciplinary. The work of the MDT may also involve some blurring of disciplinary boundaries (Choi & Pak, 2006). An integrated multidisciplinary approach with specialist staffing across the care pathway is recognised as the optimal model to ensure that people with Parkinson's receive the highest standard of care (NHS Rightcare, 2019).

This chapter includes the following:

- A review of the roles of MDT members
- A summary of the principles of the MDT's work
- An exploration of different models of MDT work
- Suggestions on how to build or develop a Parkinson's MDT

Members of the multidisciplinary team

The individual with Parkinson's should always be at the centre of care. The core MDT around that person should include a consultant with a special interest in movement disorders, a Parkinson's disease nurse specialist (PDNS) who is also a prescriber, a neurological physiotherapist, an occupational therapist (OT) and a speech and language therapist (SLT). Therapists in a Parkinson's MDT should ideally have a specialist interest and expertise in Parkinson's (NICE, 2018, Ypinga et al., 2018). Many other health professionals may be part of the team, including a dietitian, neuropsychologist, psychiatrist, palliative care consultant, social worker, sex therapist and pharmacist. Different members of the team may be involved to a greater or lesser extent at different times according to the needs of the individual. In practice, different health systems and geographic challenges (for example, rural or urban) determine the model of MDT work, such as whether care is delivered in an acute care or community setting. Video-conferencing can improve access to expertise for ongoing care (Pretzer-Aboff & Prettyman, 2015).

Even a small team can improve outcomes for people with Parkinson's. When it was compared with general neurological care, MDT care consisting of a movement disorder neurologist, PDNS and a social worker achieved more meaningful improvements in QoL as measured by the Parkinson's Disease Questionnaire (PDQ-39) (van der Marck et al., 2013a). Likewise, an enhanced MDT that included a nutritionist, pharmacist, psychologist and music therapist as well as standard MDT members (neurologist, physiatrist [rehabilitation medicine specialist], OT, physiotherapist, SLT and medical social worker) achieved greater improvement in QoL, motor function and depression than care from a standard six-member team (Marumoto et al., 2019). A case has been made for including urologists, gastroenterologists and vascular medicine specialists in the team (Radder et al., 2019). Although these specialists may have something to offer individuals with Parkinson's, they are unlikely to join face-to-face MDT meetings.

Roles of team members

Geriatrician or neurologist

In the United States and many European countries, a movement disorders specialist is a neurologist who has completed a formal one- to two-year fellowship or other additional training in movement disorders. The United Kingdom is unusual in that many specialist Parkinson's services are led by geriatricians. The neurologist or geriatrician assesses the individual, arranges investigations if necessary and makes the diagnosis, which must be delivered sensitively and empathically. Positive aspects of diagnosis, such as access to drug therapy and to the MDT, can be emphasised. The neurologist or geriatrician has a role in monitoring the person with Parkinson's for progression of symptoms and medication side effects. He or she adjusts medication, advises on advanced treatments, makes referrals to other teams and facilitates the planning of future care. Research supports that both morbidity and mortality benefits result from seeing a neurologist for Parkinson's compared with seeing a primary care provider (Willis et al., 2012). Physicians are well placed to lead the MDT, although other team members such as the PDNS can also take on this role.

Parkinson's disease nurse specialist

The role of the PDNS differs around the world. However, the coordination of care for the person with Parkinson's is always a crucial part of the job. Other duties may include

- Carrying out postdiagnosis counselling
- Providing regular reviews assessing motor and non-motor symptoms
- Reviewing the medications being taken, including whether they are being prescribed and are taken correctly
- Monitoring medication-related side effects

Many PDNSs are independent prescribers and, following discussion of risks and benefits, adjust medication in order to optimise symptom control and maximise

QoL. The PDNS usually acts as the main point of contact for the person with Parkinson's, providing telephone advice and support as needed, appropriate referral to MDT members and signposting to external support organisations. Hospital-based PDNSs have a key role in supporting the management of people with Parkinson's who are admitted to hospital.

Physiotherapist

The physiotherapist offers advice, education and intervention with an emphasis on self-management. This includes encouraging physical activity and exercise, aiming to avoid deconditioning, improving physical capacity and maintaining independence. The importance of exercise in Parkinson's is further discussed in Chapter 11. Specific assessments and interventions for gait disturbance, balance problems, falls, transfers (e.g., rising from a chair) and functional activities are carried out at all stages of the condition. Pain and postural abnormalities are assessed and treatments offered.

Occupational therapist

The role of the OT includes assessment and intervention for activities of daily living (ADLs), transfers, sleep problems, fatigue, mood disturbance and executive dysfunction. OTs promote self-management through education and may teach cognitive behavioural therapy (CBT) techniques. They advise about assistive devices and equipment; promote independence and participation; and contribute, along with other members of the MDT, to shared goal setting.

Speech and language therapist

The SLT assesses voice volume and quality, speech rate, initiation, fluency, intonation (pitch) and intelligibility. Language processing skills are analyzed. Referral to speech therapy should be made when changes to voice, communication, or swallowing skills affect health and social interactions. The SLT also advises on saliva management, including posture, swallow retraining and lip-seal exercises. Interventions include traditional voice therapy techniques along with more specialised programmes such as Lee Silverman Capitalize Voice Therapy (LSVT). The use of high- and low-technology aids can target pacing of speech, communication support and self-directed therapeutic exercise.

Nurse/continence adviser

In addition to the PDNS, general nursing staff can make a significant contribution to the MDT and to the care of the person with Parkinson's. The role of this individual may include measuring weight and blood pressure (lying and standing), continence promotion, advising on constipation, educating about good sleep hygiene, assessing bone health and supporting caregivers.

The extended team includes members who contribute to the care of selected individuals and who may or may not attend MDT meetings.

Pharmacist

Pharmacists in primary care have a vital role to play in ensuring the safe prescribing and dispensing of Parkinson's medications, which are often complex, involving multiple preparations and frequent dosing. They are the safety net to ensure that the general practitioner has prescribed the correct preparation as recommended by the specialist. They check for potential interactions with other medications and ensure that any new medications for other problems are not contraindicated for the individual with Parkinson's. The community pharmacist is often the last healthcare professional the individual sees before taking a new medication, so he or she is well placed to help patients understand their medications and how they should be taken. The pharmacist can also support adherence to the prescribed regimen by providing compliance aids such as blister packs.

Dietitian

The dietary needs of people with Parkinson's can be influenced by factors such as stage of condition, treatment prescribed and the presence of certain non-motor features or medical comorbidities. It is important for everyone to maintain a balanced, nutritious diet so as to maintain overall good health and a healthy weight and to prevent illnesses such as diabetes and cardiovascular disease. Eating the right foods can also positively affect various NMSs of Parkinson's. For instance, an increased intake of water and high-fiber foods may ease constipation; also, limiting the intake of sugar, alcohol and caffeine before bed can improve the quantity and quality of sleep.

Dietary protein may compete with L-dopa for absorption. Once L-dopa is introduced, and particularly when it is administered frequently according to complex regimens, it can be difficult to maintain adequate nutrition whilst also spacing food apart from medications. Protein redistribution diets are not usually needed; however, if such a diet is recommended by a physician, it should always be supervised by a dietitian. Furthermore, in the more advanced stages of Parkinson's, weight loss is common. This can arise from the difficulty in swallowing, nausea from medications, or motor symptoms that limit the ability to feed oneself. All these issues can be complex and interrelated; thus dietitians represent valuable members of many person-centred MDTs (Bloem et al., 2017; Giladi et al., 2014).

Social worker

The social worker's role in the realm of interdisciplinary care is very important (Giladi et al., 2014; Taberna et al., 2020 Giladi et al., 2014; Taberna et al., 2020), especially for persons with advanced Parkinson's. A sense of isolation and detachment from the world is a unifying theme for many. A social worker who is in touch with the physical, mental and emotional symptoms that may occur in the later stages of Parkinson's is a key component of the team, as she or he can guide the individual and caregiver through such needs as in-home psychotherapy, local services and inexpensive accessible transportation. Social workers can also initiate conversations regarding end-of-life needs, including making a will and assigning a power of attorney. In the United Kingdom, the social worker's role may be confined to advising on benefits and coordinating social care.

Clinical neuropsychologist

Cognitive screening is important at any stage of Parkinson's and is often carried out by the OT. However, some individuals require more detailed assessment, particularly those who are high functioning or still working. In these cases, detailed neuropsychological assessment establishes the individual's cognitive profile and may identify deficits relevant to his or her work life. Alongside assessments from other MDT members, the neuropsychological assessment can be used to help both individual and employer understand the impact of Parkinson's and, where appropriate, can enable the employer to make reasonable adjustments. Psychological therapy can also be offered to support those struggling to come to terms with their diagnosis (and therefore starting to engage in rehabilitation) or those with mood issues and suicidal ideation.

Psychiatrist

Psychiatric disorders including depression, anxiety and psychosis are among the most prevalent non-motor features of Parkinson's (Grover et al., 2015). Sleep disturbances, cognitive impairment, faulty impulse control and apathy also commonly occur. Psychiatric comorbidity has been associated with lower health-related QoL and higher levels of dependence, caregiver strain and nursing home placement in people with Parkinson's (Grover et al., 2015). Furthermore, medications for Parkinsonism can worsen or trigger psychiatric symptoms, and some psychiatric medications can exacerbate Parkinsonism (e.g., dopamine blockers for Parkinson's psychosis) or increase the risk of falls (e.g., benzodiazepines for anxiety). Because the inappropriate medical management of Parkinson's-related psychiatric symptoms can have devastating consequences for both the person with Parkinson's and caregivers, it is important that the MDT include a psychiatrist with expertise and experience in managing movement disorders. The role of the psychiatrist varies based on the MDT model and can range from purely consultative to core membership with attendance at all regular team meetings (Bloem et al., 2017; Giladi et al., 2014; Grover et al., 2015). Management involves identifying comorbidities or medication side effects that could be contributing to psychiatric symptoms and developing a management plan. Symptomatic therapy is highly individualised and may include medications, CBT, or electroconvulsive therapy in severe cases. The psychiatrist may also be able to assist in managing a clozapine service for psychosis in the context of Parkinson's disease. Treatment options are described in greater detail in subsequent chapters.

Palliative medicine specialist

The palliative medicine specialist's role is holistic, addressing the physical, psychological, social and spiritual needs of individuals and their loved ones. Advice and intervention can be offered for the complex symptoms that individuals in the later stages of Parkinson's may experience, such as pain and loss of appetite. The palliative medicine specialist supports the person with Parkinson's in making advanced care planning decisions, ideally building on earlier discussions. Issues for consideration might include preferred place of care for final illness, resuscitation and tube feeding. The palliative medicine specialist ensures that the individual's wishes are clearly documented and communicated to the MDT and the primary care team which includes the GP and other health care professionals who are not working in the acute hospital setting. The role also includes educating and supporting the MDT in addressing the planning of future care throughout the Parkinson's journey.

Competencies in Parkinson's for professionals

Competencies in Parkinson's for different grade levels of allied health professionals in the United Kingdom have been published; Table 3.1 lists the currently available guidelines and competency statements.

TABLE 3.1 Professional guidelines for Parkinson's

Discipline	Guideline/ Competency title
Physiotherapy	European Guidelines for Physiotherapy in Parkinson's Disease (Keus et al., 2014)
Occupational therapy	Occupational therapy for people with Parkinson's (Aragon & Kings, 2018)
Speech and language therapy	Guidelines for speech-language therapy in Parkinson's disease (Kalf et al., 2011) Royal College of Speech and Language Therapists in collaboration with Parkinson's UK (Royal College of Speech and Language Therapists, n.d.)
Dietetics	Best practice guidance for dietitians on the nutritional management of Parkinson's (British Dietetics Association and Parkinson's UK, 2021)
Allied health professionals (dietitians, OTs, physiotherapists, SLTs)	Allied Health Professionals' competency framework for progressive neurological conditions (Parkinson's UK, 2019)
Parkinson's disease nurse specialist	A competency framework for nurses working in Parkinson's disease management (Royal College of Nursing, 2017)

Principles of the multidisciplinary team

The principal tools that an effective MDT will employ include effective communication with the person with Parkinson's and between team members; the sharing of knowledge, skills and expertise among team members; and a focus on empowering individuals with Parkinson's to self-manage their condition as much as possible.

Shared goal setting is a key MDT task. It is important for the team to have a shared understanding of the basal ganglia and their dysfunction in Parkinson's (see Chapter 2) to deliver a consistent approach to rehabilitation (Skelly et al., 2012). Where possible, regular face-to-face meetings should take place to aid in the delivery of effective, integrated care and ensure that shared goals can be met. Such meetings also help to develop rapport and respect among team members, make team members more aware of the roles and potentials of other disciplines, and avoid the duplication of effort (Skelly et al., 2012). Trust and respect among team members is fundamental to effective teamwork. Key principles of multidisciplinary rehabilitation in Parkinson's are outlined in Table 3.2.

Person-centred care

The person with Parkinson's should be at the centre of the care process. Parkinson's is a heterogeneous condition with identifiable subtypes (Lawton et al., 2018), and individuals have different needs according to the stage of their Parkinson's and their specific symptoms. Clinicians and people with Parkinson's often have different views on the most important symptoms. Whereas the clinician may focus on easily measured, dopamine-responsive motor symptoms, those with Parkinson's have other important concerns: fatigue, handwriting problems, excessive daytime sleepiness, mood disturbance and drooling, as well as slowness, tremor, cramps and response fluctuations (Mischley et al., 2017; Politis et al., 2010). Today, people with Parkinson's want to have an active role in managing their condition. They have access to health information via the internet and use online communities for support and advice. Collaborative person-centred care involves listening to what people say they need and respecting their values and perspectives. Person-centredness is multifaceted and involves accessibility, empathy, continuity, emotional support, involving individuals in decision making, sharing information. It also involves sign-posting individuals to resources, collaborating with the individual and other professionals as well as co-ordinating care (van der Eijk et al., 2013). This type of care provides a better experience for the individual, improves concordance with treatment plans and reduces costs. MDTs are well placed to deliver collaborative person-centred care, and PDNSs may coordinate care. Old age and cognitive impairment may be barriers to shared decision-making and it is important to consider the views of caregivers (van der Eijk et al., 2013).

TABLE 3.2 Key principles of multidisciplinary rehabilitation in Parkinson's

1. **A holistic, person-centred approach.** The person with Parkinson's is the focus of care and his or her priorities, perspectives and values are respected. The MDT should be aware of the links between mental and physical health and of the importance of contextual factors such as social support and living conditions.

2. **Shared goals.** Goals help focus the efforts of the person with Parkinson's and the MDT. They should be specific, measurable, achievable, relevant and time-bound (SMART). Goals should be set, and treatment plans made collaboratively. Standardized outcome measures should be used to assess the efficacy of interventions. A mix of objective outcome measures, such as Timed Up and Go, and subjective person-reported experience measures, such as the Parkinson's disease questionnaire (PDQ-39), may be appropriate.

3. **One thing at a time.** Parkinson's results in reduced automaticity of learned motor skills. Well-functioning basal ganglia enable the completion of complex motor tasks (such as walking) while attention is focused elsewhere (such as talking). If a person with Parkinson's is struggling with walking, reducing the distractions may help. On the other hand, it is recognised that in real-life situations people with Parkinson's have to multitask, so there is increased recognition of the need for dual-task training (Mirelman et al., 2016).

4. **Breaking down complex tasks into simple steps.** Daily complex tasks such as getting out of a chair are affected by the loss of automaticity of movements, but the physical ability to carry out the task is still present. Breaking down the task into separate steps can facilitate its execution.

5. **Cognitive behavioural therapy techniques**. Parkinson's remains an incurable progressive condition. Disease progression is outside the control of persons with Parkinson's, but their reactions and responses are not. Learning to behave and think differently about a situation can improve how such a person feels.

6. **Cues and strategies** (see Chapters 6 and 7)

7. **Size matters.** The tendency of people with Parkinson's to underscale movement should be countered by practicing big movements (and loud speech). Biofeedback may be helpful.

8. **Exercise and physical activity are beneficial** (see Chapter 11)

Self-management is a key principle in dealing with chronic disease. People with Parkinson's may spend an hour or two with a Parkinson's professional during some weeks and have no professional contact at all in other weeks. Most of their time is spent without professional support, so self-management skills are important. Self-management involves having knowledge; solving problems and making decisions; regulating thoughts, emotions and behaviours; interacting with health services; and being an active participant. MDTs can contribute to teaching self-management skills through education courses for the newly diagnosed (Table 3.3 offers an example). Charities also run self-management courses; for example, "A path through Parkinson's;" which is available through the Parkinson's UK website (www.parkinsons.org.uk).

TABLE 3.3 Example of an education and exercise group for those recently diagnosed

Week	Education topic	Exercise	Relaxation	Survey/Carers
1	Parkinson's symptoms	Importance of exercise	Breathing for relaxation	Baseline survey
2	Medication	Upper body	Hold/relax technique	Carer Support Group
3	Diet, bladder and bowels	Chair hockey	Fantasy journey	
4	Cognition, sleep, driving	Wii Fit	Hold/relax Fantasy journey	
5	Speech and swallowing	Singing	Hold/relax Fantasy journey	Carer support Group
6	Will and power of attorney	Group games, transfers		Feedback survey

Documentation

Depending on the composition and setting of the MDT, numerous tools can be adapted or created to streamline documentation. Particularly within the electronic medical record, templates can be created and shared for use and editing by members of the team. Such templates are helpful for delineating each individual team member's role in gathering information and can facilitate easier interprofessional communication. In establishing workflows, MDTs may consider pre-visit screening phone calls to identify key concerns and the most relevant team members needed for that visit. Additional templates may be used to standardise a person-centred MDT after-visit summary of team-member recommendations and to encourage therapeutic adherence (Federman et al., 2018).

The efficacy of multidisciplinary work in Parkinson's

Several trials (Carne et al., 2005; Ellis et al., 2008; Ferrazzoli et al., 2018; Guo et al., 2009; Marumoto et al., 2019; Monticone et al., 2015; Ritter & Bonsaksen, 2019; Tickle-Degnen et al., 2010), but not all (van der Marck et al., 2013b; Wade et al., 2003) have shown the benefits of multidisciplinary care in Parkinson's. Trials differ in design (observational trials, randomised controlled trials [RCTs], setting (inpatient, clinic, home), study population, professionals involved (as few as three disciplines to as many as twelve), intensity of intervention (up to 17 hours per week for 8 weeks) (Marumoto et al., 2019), outcome measures and length of follow up. In an RCT of outpatient self-management rehabilitation consisting of OT, physiotherapy and SLT for 3 to 4.5 hours per week (for 6 weeks), QoL as measured by the PDQ-39 improved immediately after the intervention (Tickle-Degnen et al., 2010). Self-management training included group discussions about, for example, barriers to exercise, strategies to improve walking, stress management and talking on the phone. The researchers hoped skills learned on the programme would have lasting benefits, and this proved to be the case, with improvements in the PDQ-39 still present at follow up 6 months after the intervention. Impairments specifically targeted by the intervention (mobility and communication) improved more than non-targeted domains, such as stigma. Individuals with greater impairments of mobility and communication at baseline improved more than those with milder impairments.

Published studies have focused on multidisciplinary rehabilitation, but MDTs can also provide effective crisis intervention. A clinic-based Parkinson's advanced symptom unit—including a movement disorder neurologist, OT, physiotherapist, SLT, PDNS and community psychiatric nurse—was able to see individuals with psychosis, falls or declining mobility promptly. Hospital and care-home admissions were averted, hip fractures cut and costs reduced (Archibald, 2018).

Professionals also benefit from interdisciplinary work. Teamwork fosters creativity and healthy risk taking. Team membership brings greater job satisfaction, role clarity and enhanced well-being (Mickan, 2005). MDT members develop conflict-resolution skills and learn from one another.

Models of multidisciplinary teams

ParkinsonNet

ParkinsonNet is a novel model of integrated care established in the Netherlands by Bloem and Munneke in 2004. Initially beginning with 37 physical, occupational and speech therapists, this model was designed to improve the efficiency and efficacy of treatment for Parkinson's by establishing regional networks of motivated specialists. Each person with Parkinson's is assessed initially by a team of university-based experts; individualised treatment recommendations then are made. Referrals to regional specialists in the network are provided so that people can receive specialised Parkinson's care locally (Bloem & Munneke, 2014). ParkinsonNet has expanded to include neurologists, nursing home physicians, rehabilitation specialists, psychiatrists, psychologists, pharmacists, PDNSs, dieticians, social workers and sex therapists. It now provides nationwide coverage through 70 regional networks comprising 3000 specialists from 12 disciplines (Bloem et al., 2017). The primary goals of ParkinsonNet include standardising and integrating the delivery of care, ensuring delivery of evidence-based care by specialists, and creating infrastructure for clinical trials. These goals are accomplished by:

1. The selection of a restricted number of motivated healthcare providers who agree to provide Parkinson's care according to evidence-based guidelines
2. The development and implementation of guidelines (both monodisciplinary and multidisciplinary)
3. Transparency about the quality of services and outcomes through publication in a directory called the Parkinson's Atlas.

Education is a central tenet and all member providers receive mandatory education in the form of 4-day training on treatment guidelines at baseline, annual attendance at national and regional conferences and augmented on-the-job learning by seeing an enriched Parkinson's population through participation in the network. Information technology plays a key role in education for both providers and service users; initiatives developed thus far include an informational website, a healthcare search engine, web-based communities for both service users and providers, an electronic health record with decision support and telehealth specialist consultations. Finally, person-centredness is another important objective that is achieved through creation of person-focused guidelines, online communities and other initiatives.

ParkinsonTV is one noteworthy component of ParkinsonNet's educational initiatives. Each of the more than forty web-based TV episodes features a neurologist, a topic expert and an individual with Parkinson's as they discuss a particular issue. In 2017, a successful English-language version was launched in partnership with the University of Rochester. The second season, filmed in 2018, was themed "Mental Health and PD." To date, the content has been shown more than 2 million times and watched for more than 650,000 minutes (data from https://parkinsontv.org).

Along with the expected increase in Parkinson's referrals and awareness of fellow specialists among network providers, ParkinsonNet has been linked to improved quality of care, better adherence to evidence-based guidelines and substantial cost savings, ranging from $439 to $1675 per individual annually (Bloem et al., 2017). Although the early clinical trials did not show improved outcomes for individuals with Parkinson's, these studies may reflect the limitations of a newly established and therefore inexperienced network and incomplete implementation of ParkinsonNet recommendations (Munneke et al., 2010; van der Marck et al., 2013b). Analyses of health outcomes based on observational studies and analyses of insurance claims demonstrated significant reductions in hip fractures, inpatient admissions and mortality (Bloem et al., 2017; Ypinga et al., 2018). The impact is expected to increase over time as networks mature and provider experience grows (Bloem et al., 2017), with additional research underway. The cost of ParkinsonNet in the Netherlands is currently supported through health innovation grants and an annual membership fee paid by participating network providers (Bloem et al., 2017).

The outpatient hospital–based multidisciplinary team in Derby, UK

The Parkinson's service in Derby is an example of a hospital-based, integrated, holistic, multidisciplinary service (Skelly et al., 2012). It is recognised as a Centre of Excellence by the Parkinson's Foundation largely because of its model of multidisciplinary work. It comprises a movement disorder neurologist, geriatrician, PDNS, clinical psychologist, old-age psychiatrist, physiotherapist, OT, SLT, dietitian, continence nurse and general nurse. A palliative consultant joins the clinic once a month.

Following a diagnosis of Parkinson's, the PDNS contacts the individual by telephone to offer postdiagnostic counselling. The PDNS is the key contact for the individual throughout the journey with Parkinson's. The diagnosing clinician or PDNS offers early therapy referral for assessment, advice and education according to need. Even those in the early stages of Parkinson's are likely to benefit from physiotherapy, and that hypothesis is being tested in a clinical trial. Gait and posture abnormalities can be identified and remedial action taken at an early stage. Also, advice on physical activity and exercise may have greater impact if adopted at an early stage. Early OT assessment is usually offered. Assessment of ADLs by the OT often uncovers problems not identified by the doctor or PDNS. The OT screens for cognitive impairment and for anxiety and depression using standardised assessment tools. Those of working age also benefit from OT assessment and advice.

A 6-week education, exercise and relaxation group is available to help the individual and caregiver understand and manage this condition (see Table 3.3).

The information needs of people with Parkinson's vary as time passes. There is an annual symposium covering a variety of issues of interest to people with Parkinson's and their caregivers as well as outreach (e.g., speaker provision) to local Parkinson's support groups.

Central to the functioning of the multidisciplinary Parkinson's service is the weekly multidisciplinary clinic and MDT meeting (Skelly et al., 2012). Individuals attending this clinic may be frail older adults with comorbidities or may have complex symptoms. Assessment is tailored to the individual, but a comprehensive assessment is offered least once a year. This includes

1. Physiotherapist assessment of gait and bed mobility using the Lindop Parkinson's Assessment Scale (Pearson et al., 2009)
2. OT assessment of ADLs, cognition and mood and consideration of caregiver strain and need for social support
3. Nursing assessment including measurement of weight, postural blood pressure, falls inquiry, bowel and bladder symptoms, and fracture risk assessment (every 3 years or yearly in those who fall)

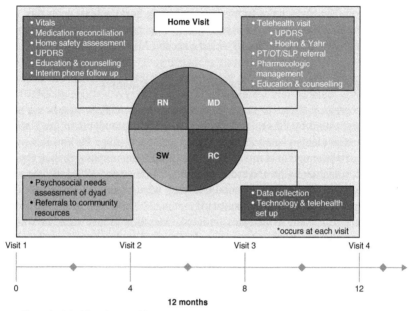

FIGURE 3.1   Activities and assessments conducted by members of the multidisciplinary team at home visits for individuals with advanced Parkinson's.

Outpatient palliative multidisciplinary care

Miyasaki and colleagues have described additional models of MDT for more advanced stages of Parkinson's and related disorders with a focus on incorporating palliative care (Boersma et al., 2016; Kluger et al., 2019, 2020; Miyasaki et al., 2012). In these models, individuals are typically cared for by a team led by a neurologist (with formal or informal palliative care training) with additional involvement of nursing, social work and chaplaincy. Caregivers and people with Parkinson's seen in these clinics have expressed a high degree of unmet need, which such models can more effectively address (Boersma et al., 2016, 2017). Kluger et al. (2020) have published the results of a multicenter randomised pragmatic comparative effectiveness clinical trial in which individuals and caregivers were randomly allocated to one of three different models of integrated/ MDT palliative care for Parkinson's or to standard care with a primary care physician and neurologist. Those receiving integrated care for Parkinson's had a better QoL after 6 months compared with those receiving standard care. In secondary outcomes measured at 12 months, both motor and non-motor symptom severity, caregiver burden and completion of advance directives all favored MDT versus standard care. The pragmatic design of this trial allowed for varying composition of the MDT team and visit logistics, yet all demonstrated superiority over standard care.

Home hospice/palliative care

Incorporating palliative care into Parkinson's treatment is an important and often overlooked step. Palliative care aims to alleviate the burden of chronic illness through the improvement of QoL, initiating communication pathways between disciplines and attempting to address gaps in symptom management (Finn & Malhotra, 2019). Although palliative care and hospice are often conflated, hospice is a smaller component of palliative care. In the United States, hospice is restricted to "care and support of people who are terminally ill with a life expectancy of 6 months or less" (US Department of Health and Human Services, 2020). Many individuals with Parkinson's and their caregivers are unaware that home hospice offers wraparound support with such benefits as the following:

- An on-call nurse or physician 24 hours a day
- Provision and billing of medical equipment and supplies (wheelchairs, hospital beds, toileting needs, etc.)
- Hospice aides/homemaker services
- Short-term respite care

Hospice will not cover curative treatments, inpatient or outpatient hospital services or emergency room/ambulance services. Often in Parkinson's, palliative care is introduced only in the setting of rapid functional decline. However, a growing body of Parkinson's-specific research indicates that when palliative care is introduced earlier in the course of the condition, the caregiver and person with Parkinson's both benefit from improved end-of-life experiences and have more meaningful interactions (Boersma et al., 2016, 2017; Kluger et al., 2020).

Elective inpatient services

Trials of inpatient rehabilitation for Parkinson's have had consistently impressive results (Ferrazzoli et al., 2018; Marumoto et al., 2019; Monticone et al., 2015, Ritter & Bonsaksen, 2019). In Italy, Monticone et al. (2015) targeted individuals who had had Parkinson's for at least 10 years, were at Hoehn-Yahr stage 2.5-4, and who were having falls, declines in mobility or difficulty with transfers. In this randomised controlled trial, participants were randomly allocated to 8 weeks of inpatient task-oriented exercise, OT, CBT and Parkinson's education or to a control intervention of general physiotherapy. The intensity of the intervention was 90 minutes of physiotherapy per day, 30 minutes of psychologist-led CBT twice a week, and 30 minutes of OT per week, amounting to a total of 9 hours of therapy per week. Both groups saw improvements in the UPDRS motor score, Berg balance score, functional independence measure

(ADLs) and QoL (PDQ-39). Those receiving the multidisciplinary intervention had significantly greater improvements in all these measures at the end of the trial, and improvements were still evident when participants were followed up after 12 months. The improvements were clinically meaningful. For example, the UPDRS motor scale improved by 25 points more and PDQ-39 total score improved by 14 points more in the multidisciplinary care group. To put the scale of these improvements in context, a major trial of deep brain stimulation for Parkinson's showed a 19-point improvement in the UPDRS motor score and 9-point improvement in the PDQ-39 (Deuschl et al., 2006). The authors felt that the following factors were important to the success of the programme: daily practice, individualised rather than group therapy and task-oriented principles. The cost of treatment was estimated at €20,000 (approximately $25,200 US dollars in 2006) per person. Another Italian group studied a 4-week programme of inpatient multidisciplinary intensive rehabilitation therapy (Ferrazzoli et al., 2018). Participants were at Hoehn-Yahr stages 2 to 4 (median 2.6), of median age 66 years, and had a median duration of Parkinson's of 7.5 years. The intervention was goal-oriented and included the following:

- Aerobic exercise (up to 15 minutes treadmill exercise twice a day)
- Exercises for posture, balance and range of motion
- Daily OT for work on ADLs, handwriting and dexterity
- Daily SLT
- Use of CBT and self-management principles
- Hydrotherapy and psychologist input for selected participants

There were weekly MDT meetings. Significant improvements were seen in UPDRS motor score (12 points) and PDQ-39 (8 points), and L-dopa requirements were reduced at the end of the intervention. Improvements in PDQ-39 were largely maintained at 4-month follow up.

In Japan, Marumoto et al. (2019) investigated the effects of an 8-week inpatient enhanced multidisciplinary rehabilitation programme. Participants had a mean age of 69 years and mean Parkinson's duration 10.6 years. Intensity was 17 hours per week and the intervention included daily individual OT, physiotherapy and SLT as well as group exercise and education about Parkinson's. The mean UPDRS motor score had improved by 3 points and PDQ-39 by 19 points at the end of the intervention. Depression also improved. Long-term follow-up was not reported. So far there has been no direct comparison of inpatient and outpatient multidisciplinary care for Parkinson's. Although inpatient rehabilitation can be intensive, it is also expensive. Other expensive treatments such as deep brain stimulation and L-dopa–carbidopa intestinal gel are funded in many health services, and a case can be made for funding inpatient multidisciplinary rehabilitation. In the United Kingdom and the United States, inpatient rehabilitation is currently available only following emergency admission to an acute-care hospital and typically would last only until the individual's discharge.

Commissioning and funding multidisciplinary teams

Funding MDT clinics and team members is highly variable internationally. In the United Kingdom, the National Health Service (NHS) provides comprehensive health care, free at the point of delivery and funded through general taxation. The NHS has a provider arm (e.g., hospitals) and a commissioning arm (e.g., clinical commissioning groups). Commissioners control the health budget for the local population and are guided from the centre (e.g., NHS England, NHS Scotland, NHS Wales, Health and Social Care [Northern Ireland]) and by the National Institute for Health and Care Excellence (NICE).

Within the United States, for example, there are specific billing codes for direct and non-direct prolonged durations of service (i.e., codes for face-to-face services versus non–face-to-face services, counselling regarding advance directives, etc.). Despite their existence, these codes are largely underutilised, require additional documentation and may be subject to institutional policies and payer-specific guidelines; if the individual with Parkinson's has insurance at all, reimbursements are relatively low.

Alternative means of support for MDT clinics and staff may include institutional support and philanthropic support, either directly from individual donors or from foundations in the form of support for centres of excellence or grants directed toward clinical care, research, education, outreach or a combination of these. Similarly, novel models of care, or adaptations of established MDT models introduced to new patient populations, may be supported via research funding from federal, foundation or private sources.

How to build a team

Owing to the complexity of Parkinson's, utilizing the knowledge and skills of experts from different healthcare professions provides a more personalized and efficient approach to the management of Parkinson's symptoms. Building an MDT begins with identifying members who will be part of the core team from among the specialties described earlier in this chapter. The core MDT team may also want to develop a list of frequently consulted disciplines or specific local healthcare professionals who are not part of the individual MDT but have demonstrated willingness to care for individuals with Parkinson's. This might include dentists, urologists, gastroenterologists, neuro-ophthalmologists, sexologists, neuropsychologists and dietitians (Giladi et al., 2014; van der Marck & Bloem, 2014). This not only streamlines referrals in the future but also allows the core MDT team to focus on the issues they can best address individually rather than trying to subsume other specialists' roles or duplicating efforts. Ultimately, each team member will have specialty-specific objectives while working toward the MDT's combined goal of maintaining and increasing the QoL of people with Parkinson's and their caregivers. Seeking guidance from an established MDT or interdisciplinary clinic may be beneficial in determining logistics. Critical, too, is garnering early support from administration to assist with finding designated time and space for the MDT.

Once the team members have been identified, training may be twofold: first, training in discipline-specific approaches to Parkinson's, and second, training in how the team and clinical services will function together. For the former, training may include reading pertinent articles and textbooks, shadowing another clinician, or attending relevant conferences or workshops (Kluger et al., 2018). The Allied Team Training for Parkinson's (ATTP) interprofessional education programme demonstrates the value of formal training. Cohen and colleagues compared knowledge about Parkinson's along with validated measures of attitudes toward team-based care among 1468 ATTP trainees compared with 100 healthcare professionals serving as controls (Cohen et al., 2016). ATTP trainees demonstrated significant improvements in objective knowledge and in attitudes towards team-based care, both of which were sustained 6 months after the training ended.

The heterogeneity of Parkinson's symptoms calls for interventions to be tailored to the specific needs of the individual. However, such an individualised approach can pose difficulties for teams. Through training, setting expectations and keeping lines of communication clear and open, MDTs may alleviate some of these challenges. Once the various members have been trained, the team must determine the best structure for clinical visits. Options include having multiple clinicians in the visit simultaneously, clinicians rotating in series with the individual, some clinicians seeing the individual in subsequent visits only if a need is established, or some combination of these. The team must also establish and adapt routes of communication. These will include intra-visit communication, sharing with either the whole team, or with just one or two relevant team members, the needs of the person with Parkinson's that one clinician has identified. The team members can then tackle that need. Team communication will also include deciding how to share pre- and post-visit findings in a unified manner with other members of the team. The team should establish whether some form of pre- or postclinic team meeting or huddle will take place, whether all individuals are to be discussed or only those meeting certain criteria, and whether a unified presentation style will be used to streamline communication. Finally, Kluger and colleagues highlight key opportunities for MDT self-care (Kluger et al., 2018). Box 3.1 gives an example of building an MDT.

One key component of Fleisher and colleagues' home visit model is education for both the person with Parkinson's and the caregiver (Fleisher et al., 2020), which can be incorporated into outpatient MDTs. Curated, health literacy–friendly reading material from the Parkinson's Foundation, Parkinson's UK, and other resources can be compiled into a binder to educate individuals on Parkinson's medications and caregiver support. The MDT may also add various published or homegrown tip sheets covering common issues such as constipation, orthostatic hypotension, swallowing, excess saliva, dry mouth, cough and cold, medication management and a fall-prevention checklist. If caregivers are struggling with one of these issues at or between visits, the MDT members can easily reference the tip sheets and binder, empowering families to solve some of these regularly occurring problems.

BOX 3.1 Example of building a service

The Hull Parkinson's Hub

Hull Clinical Commissioning Group (CCG) has developed an integrated care service for individuals living with frailty. Proactive comprehensive geriatric assessments (CGA) are performed at a bespoke building. As part of this, a 'Parkinson's Hub' was created in November 2019 using principles of integrated care for people with Parkinson's and moderate to severe frailty or multiple troublesome symptoms (Mace & Peel, 2020). The hospital's Parkinson's and community frailty teams are the main source of referrals, and criteria are loose. The service utilises wide-ranging local health expertise and voluntary sector support, including Parkinson's UK.

Working tightly with commissioners and transformation leads who encourage innovation and acknowledge that traditional models do not often meet all the needs of people with Parkinson's, barriers were broken down to create a "one team" culture regardless of employer. Governance issues were overcome by flexibility and using detailed service specification and standard-operation-procedure documents.

The "core" team consists of a consultant physician, PDNS, specialist physiotherapists, OT, therapy assistant, MDT coordinator, pharmacy technicians and clinical support workers. Relationships have developed, with a community psychiatric nurse, SLT, the district nursing team, "talk" therapies, and palliative care services, among others.

The MDT coordinator role is essential. It relies on good people as well as administrative and troubleshooting skills. MDT coordinators develop relationships with individuals as a single point of contact and can refer queries to the correct colleague. They organise appointments, provide transport and ensure that the clinic's capacity is fully utilised. They welcome the individual on arrival to the centre and offer a beverage and snack. During each MDT meeting, they create individualised plans, assign tasks and complete referrals. They liaise with colleagues to ensure the timely completion of tasks, thus easing the strain on people with Parkinson's and their caregivers.

The initial assessment, performed by a specialist physiotherapist, begins at the individual's home and includes a modified non-motor questionnaire. A rapid domiciliary OT and social services review (within 2-24 hours) can be triggered if required. Assessments follow a "trusted assessor" model to avoid repetition. Each individual is placed into the category of "stable," "precrisis" "crisis" or "end-of-life care" so as to aid resource allocation.

Tom Mace, Consultant Physician

Telehealth

Telehealth plays an increasing role in the delivery of healthcare worldwide, connecting people with Parkinson's and caregivers to their healthcare providers at a distance. The value and acceptability of telehealth in Parkinson's has been demonstrated by Dorsey and colleagues (Beck et al., 2017; Dorsey et al., 2012, 2016). However, to date, telehealth has been delivered as largely one-on-one visits between the individual and clinician. Although telehealth capability is dependent on users having compatible devices, technologic savvy and a willingness to use telehealth, additional technical challenges arise when this service also involves MDTs. Fleisher and colleagues describe a hybrid approach to telehealth home visits, with some team members physically present at the individual's home and others located remotely yet participating in synchronous telehealth (Fleisher et al., 2020). Beyond Parkinson's, both synchronous and asynchronous models of MDT telehealth have been studied in amyotrophic lateral sclerosis and other neuromuscular disorders (Haulman et al., 2020) and in palliative care (Watanabe et al., 2013), although long-term data on feasibility and cost-effectiveness will be critical to adaptation and broader implementation for the Parkinson's population. During the COVID-19 pandemic, many Parkinson's services had to quickly learn telehealth skills. Going forward, it is likely that people with Parkinson's will want to have the option of remote consultations, and telehealth will become increasingly important.

Conclusion

Many people with Parkinson's can benefit from multidisciplinary care. Those with moderate disability and good cognition clearly benefit. Those with cognitive decline may benefit less from interventions that rely on implementing newly learned strategies at home, but they can benefit from judicious medication review, advice about management of the daily routine and cognitive stimulation therapy. Those with advanced Parkinson's can benefit from interdisciplinary home visits. Integrated palliative services have clear benefits, and not just for those near the end of life. People need support throughout their journey with Parkinson's, and we strongly believe that a Parkinson's service should provide comprehensive care from diagnosis to death. Various chapters in this book are dedicated to service considerations at different stages of the journey.

Top tips on how to develop a Parkinson's multidisciplinary team	
Component	**Suggestion**
The core Parkinson's MDT	• Geriatrician or neurologist specialising in movement disorders • Nurse specialist with prescribing privileges • Neurology-focused physiotherapist or physical therapist • Occupational therapist • Speech therapist • Others: social worker, mental health specialists, dietician, palliative or hospice care workers
MDT principles	• Holistic and person-centred approach with self-management • Shared goals (specific, measurable, achievable, relevant and time bound) • Emphasis on doing "one thing at a time" • Complex tasks broken down into simple steps • Possibly of use: CBT techniques, "cues and strategies," big movements and exercise

Component	Suggestion
MDT models	• ParkinsonNet MDT: train and motivate providers to give Parkinson's care, follow evidence-based guidelines, and publish results in the Parkinson Atlas • Outpatient hospital-based (Derby, UK): "one-stop shop" where people with Parkinson's are treated by the entire MDT within a single day, culminating in a comprehensive MDT treatment plan • Interdisciplinary home care for advanced Parkinson's can involve the following: • RN, SW and MD (via video) the assess the individual at home; the visit ends with a person-centred plan incorporating all disciplines and providing referrals when applicable
Funding for an MDT	• Government (in the United Kingdom) • Specialised billing codes, insurance coverage (in the United States) • Institutional and/or philanthropic support
Building an MDT	• Identify population for treatment (i.e., moderate disability and good cognition for outpatient; those with advanced disease may benefit more from interdisciplinary home visits) • Identify members who will constitute the core team • Train the team in Parkinson's-specific approaches and show them how team will work together • Determine the structure for visits: pre- and/or postvisit huddles, common templates for charting, providing Parkinson-specific symptom-management tip sheets, etc. • Discuss the role of telehealth

Abbreviations: CBT, cognitive behavioural therapy; MD, medical doctor; RN, registered nurse; SW, social worker

References

Aragon, A., & Kings, J. (2018). Occupational therapy for people with Parkinson's. Royal College of Occupational Therapists. Retrieved November 19, 2020, from https://www.rcot.co.uk/occupational-therapy-people-parkinsons.

Archibald, N. (2018). *Parkinson's Advanced Symptoms Unit (PASU) Business Case 2017/18:* South Tees Hospitals NHS Foundation Trust. Available at https://multiplesclerosisacademy.org/wp-content/uploads/sites/2/2019/07/PASU-business-case-2017.18.pdf.

Beck, C. A., Beran, D. B., Biglan, K. M., Boyd, C. M., Dorsey, E. R., Schmidt, P. N., et al. (2017). National randomised controlled trial of virtual house calls for Parkinson's disease. *Neurology*, 89(11), 1152–1161.

Bloem, B. R., & Munneke, M. (2014). Revolutionising management of chronic disease: the ParkinsonNet approach. *British Journal of Medicine*, 2014, Mar 19; 348: 1838.

Bloem, B. R., Rompen, L., Vries, N. M., Klink, A., Munneke, M., & Jeurissen, P. (2017). ParkinsonNet: a low-cost health care innovation with a systems approach from The Netherlands. *Health Affairs (Millwood)*, 36(11), 1987–1996.

Boersma, I., Jones, J., Carter, J., Bekelman, D., Miyasaki, J., Kutner, J., et al. (2016). Parkinson disease patients' perspectives on palliative care needs: what are they telling us? *Neurology Clinical Practice*, 6(3), 209–219.

Boersma, I., Jones, J., Coughlan, C., Carter, J., Bekelman, D., Miyasaki, J., et al. (2017). Palliative care and Parkinson's disease: caregiver perspectives. *Journal of Palliative Medicine*, *20*(9), 930–938.

British Dietetics Association and Parkinson's UK (2021). Best practice guidance for dietitians on the nutritional management of Parkinson's. Retrieved February 17, 2021, from https://www.parkinsons.org.uk/professionals/resources/best-practice-guidelines-dietitians-management-parkinsons.

Carne, W., Cifu, D. X., Marcinko, P., Baron, M., Pickett, T., Qutubuddin, A., et al. (2005). Efficacy of multidisciplinary treatment programme on long-term outcomes of individuals with Parkinson's disease. *Journal of Rehabiltation Research and Development*, *42*(6), 779–786.

Choi, B. C., & Pak, A. W. (2006). Multidisciplinarity, interdisciplinarity and transdisciplinarity in health research, services, education and policy: 1. Definitions, objectives and evidence of effectiveness. *Clinical and Investigative Medicine*, *29*(6), 351–364.

Cohen, E. V., Hagestuen, R., Gonzalez-Ramos, G., Cohen, H. W., Bassich, C., Book, E., et al. (2016). Interprofessional education increases knowledge, promotes team building, and changes practice in the care of Parkinson's disease. *Parkinsonism and Related Disorders*, Jan *22*, 21–27.

Deuschl, G., Schade-Brittinger, C., Krack, P., Volkmann, J., Schafer, H., Botzel, K., et al. (2006). A randomised trial of deep-brain stimulation for Parkinson's disease. *New England Journal of Medicine*, *355*(9), 896–908.

Dorsey, E. R., Achey, M. A., Beck, C. A., Beran, D. B., Biglan, K. M., Boyd, C. M., et al. (2016). National randomised controlled trial of virtual house calls for people with Parkinson's disease: interest and barriers. *Telemedicine Journal and E-Health*, *22*(7), 590–598.

Dorsey, E. R., George, B. P., Leff, B., & Willis, A. W. (2013). The coming crisis: obtaining care for the growing burden of neurodegenerative conditions. *Neurology*, *80*(21), 1989–1996.

Ellis, T., Katz, D. I., White, D. K., DePiero, T. J., Hohler, A. D., & Saint-Hilaire, M. (2008). Effectiveness of an inpatient multidisciplinary rehabilitation programme for people with Parkinson disease. *Physical Therapy*, *88*(7), 812–819.

Federman, A. D., Jandorf, L., DeLuca, J., Gover, M., Sanchez Munoz, A., Chen, L., et al. (2018). Evaluation of a patient-centred after visit summary in primary care. *Patient Education and Counselling*, *101*(8), 1483–1489.

Ferrazzoli, D., Ortelli, P., Zivi, I., Cian, V., Urso, E., Ghilardi, M. F., et al. (2018). Efficacy of intensive multidisciplinary rehabilitation in Parkinson's disease: a randomised controlled study. *Journal of Neurology, Neurosurgery, and Psychiatry*, *89*(8), 828–835.

Finn, L., & Malhotra, S. (2019). The development of pathways in palliative medicine: definition, models, cost and quality impact. *Healthcare (Basel)*, *7*(1.).

Fleisher, J., Barbosa, W., Sweeney, M. M., Oyler, S. E., Lemen, A. C., Fazl, A., et al. (2018). Interdisciplinary home visits for individuals with advanced Parkinson's disease and related disorders. *Journal of the American Geriatric Society*, *66*(6), 1226–1232.

Fleisher, J. E., Klostermann, E. C., Hess, S. P., Lee, J., Myrick, E., & Chodosh, J. (2020). Interdisciplinary palliative care for people with advanced Parkinson's disease: a view from the home. *Annals of Palliative Medicine*, *9*(Suppl 1), S80–S89.

Giladi, N., Manor, Y., Hilel, A., & Gurevich, T. (2014). Interdisciplinary teamwork for the treatment of people with Parkinson's disease and their families. *Current Neurology and Neuroscience Reports*, *14*(11), 493.

Grover, S., Somaiya, M., Kumar, S., & Avasthi, A. (2015). Psychiatric aspects of Parkinson's disease. *Journal of Neuroscience Rural Practice*, *6*(1), 65–76.

Guo, L., Jiang, Y., Yatsuya, H., Yoshida, Y., & Sakamoto, J. (2009). Group education with personal rehabilitation for idiopathic Parkinson's disease. *Canadian Journal of Neurological Sciences*, *36*(1), 51–59.

Hack, N., Akbar, U., Monari, E. H., Eilers, A., Thompson-Avila, A., Hwynn, N. H., et al. (2015). Person-centred care in the home setting for Parkinson's disease: operation house call quality of care pilot study. *Parkinson's Disease*, 639494. Parkinsons Dis 2015;2015:639494.doi 10.1155/2015/639494. Epub 2015May 19. PMID:26078912;PMCID:PMC4452493.

Haulman, A., Geronimo, A., Chahwala, A., & Simmons, Z. (2020). The use of telehealth to enhance care in ALS and other neuromuscular disorders. *Muscle Nerve* Jun, 61(6):682–691.

Hurwitz, A. (1986). Home visiting by nursing students to patients with Parkinson's disease. *Journal of Neuroscience Nursing*, 18(6), 344–348.

Kalf, H., de Swart, B., Bonnier-Baars, M., Kanters, J., Hofman, M., Kocken, J., et al. (2011). Guidelines for speech-language therapy in Parkinson's disease. ParkinsonNet/National Parkinson Foundation. Retrieved from https://www.parkinsonnet.nl/app/uploads/sites/3/2019/11/dutch_slp_guidelines-final.pdf.

Keus, S.H. J., Munneke, M., Graziano, M., et al. (2014). European physiotherapy guideline for Parkinson's disease. www.parkinsonnet.info.guidelines/parkinsonsKNGF/ParkinsonNet.

Kluger, B. M., Katz, M., Galifianakis, N., Pantilat, S. Z., Kutner, J. S., Sillau, S., et al. (2019). Does outpatient palliative care improve patient-centred outcomes in Parkinson's disease: Rationale, design, and implementation of a pragmatic comparative effectiveness trial. *Contemporary Clinical Trials*, 79, April 2019 28–36 doi:10.1016/j.cct2019.02.005.Epub 2019 Feb 16. PMID 30779960.

Kluger, B. M., Miyasaki, J., Katz, M., Galifianakis, N., Hall, K., Pantilat, S., et al. (2020). Comparison of integrated outpatient palliative care with standard care in patients with Parkinson disease and related disorders: a randomised clinical trial. *JAMA Neurology* 2020 May 1;77(5). 551–560.

Kluger, B. M., Persenaire, M. J., Holden, S. K., Palmer, L. T., Redwine, H., Berk, J., et al. (2018). Implementation issues relevant to outpatient neurology palliative care. *Annals of Palliative Medicine*, 7(3), 339–348.

Lawton, M., Ben-Shlomo, Y., May, M. T., Baig, F., Barber, T. R., Klein, J. C., et al. (2018). Developing and validating Parkinson's disease subtypes and their motor and cognitive progression. *Journal of Neurology, Neurosurgery, and Psychiatry*, 89(12), 1279–1287.

Mace, T., & Peel, C. (2020). Parkinson's hub: an integrated pathway for people with Parkinson's and frailty. *Advances in Clinical Neuroscience and Rehabilitation*, 19(4), 38–41. Available at www.acnr.co.uk/2020/2010/parkinsons-and-frailty.

Marumoto, K., Yokoyama, K., Inoue, T., Yamamoto, H., Kawami, Y., Nakatani, A., et al. (2019). Inpatient enhanced multidisciplinary care effects on the quality of life for Parkinson disease: a quasi-randomised controlled trial. *Journal of Geriatric Psychiatry and Neurology*, 32(4), 186–194.

Mickan, S. M. (2005). Evaluating the effectiveness of health care teams. *Australian Health Review*, 29(2), 211–217.

Mirelman, A., Rochester, L., Maidan, I., Del Din, S., Alcock, L., Nieuwhof, F., et al. (2016). Addition of a non-immersive virtual reality component to treadmill training to reduce fall risk in older adults (V-TIME): a randomised controlled trial. *Lancet*, 388(10050), 1170–1182.

Mischley, L. K., Lau, R. C., & Weiss, N. S. (2017). Use of a self-rating scale of the nature and severity of symptoms in Parkinson's disease (PRO-PD): correlation with quality of life and existing scales of disease severity. *Nature Partner Journals Parkinson's Disease*, 3, 20 2017 Jun 16; 3:20. doi 10.1038/s41531-017-0021-5. e-Collection 2017.

Mitchell, G. K., Tieman, J. J., & Shelby-James, T. M. (2008). Multidisciplinary care planning and teamwork in primary care. *Medical Journal of Australia*, 188(S8), S61–S64.

Miyasaki, J. M., Long, J., Mancini, D., Moro, E., Fox, S. H., Lang, A. E., et al. (2012). Palliative care for advanced Parkinson disease: an interdisciplinary clinic and new scale, the ESAS-PD. *Parkinsonism and Related Disorders*, 18(Suppl 3), S6–S9.

Monticone, M., Ambrosini, E., Laurini, A., Rocca, B., & Foti, C. (2015). In-patient multidisciplinary rehabilitation for Parkinson's disease: a randomised controlled trial. *Movement Disorders*, *30*(8), 1050–1058.

Munneke, M., Nijkrake, M. J., Keus, S. H., Kwakkel, G., Berendse, H. W., Roos, R. A., et al. (2010). Efficacy of community-based physiotherapy networks for patients with Parkinson's disease: a cluster-randomised trial. *Lancet Neurology*, *9*(1), 46–54.

NHS Rightcare (2019). Progressive Neurological Conditions Toolkit. Available at https://www.england.nhs.uk/rightcare/wp-content/uploads/sites/40/2019/08/progressive-neuro-toolkit.pdf.

NICE (2018). Quality Standards for Parkinson's disease. Available at http://www.nice.org.uk/guidance/qs164.

Parkinson's UK. *A Path Through Parkinson's*. Available at https://www.parkinsons.org.uk/sites/default/files/2018-02/Introduction to Path Through Parkinsons.pdf.

Parkinson's UK (2019). Allied Health Professionals' competency framework for progressive neurological conditions. Retrieved November 19, 2020, from https://www.parkinsons.org.uk/sites/default/files/2020-10/FinalAHP competencies-framework-14May19.pdf.

Pearson, M. J., Lindop, F. A., Mockett, S. P., & Saunders, L. (2009). Validity and inter-rater reliability of the Lindop Parkinson's Disease Mobility Assessment: a preliminary study. *Physiotherapy*, *95*(2), 126–133.

Politis, M., Wu, K., Molloy, S., Bain, P. G., Chaudhuri, K. R., & Piccini, P. (2010). Parkinson's disease symptoms: the patient's perspective. *Movement Disorders*, *25*(11), 1646–1651.

Pretzer-Aboff, I., & Prettyman, A. (2015). Implementation of an integrative holistic healthcare model for people living with Parkinson's disease. *Gerontologist*, *55*(Suppl 1), S146–S153.

Radder, D. L. M., de Vries, N. M., Riksen, N. P., Diamond, S. J., Gross, D., Gold, D. R., et al. (2019). Multidisciplinary care for people with Parkinson's disease: the new kids on the block! *Expert Review of Neurotherapy*, *19*(2), 145–157.

Ritter, V. C., & Bonsaksen, T. (2019). Improvement in quality of life following a multidisciplinary rehabilitation programme for patients with Parkinson's disease. *Journal of Multidisciplinary Healthcare*, *12*, 219–227 2019 Mar 20; 12: 219–227.

Royal College of Nursing (2017). A competency framework for nurses working in Parkinson's disease management. Retrieved November 19, 2020, from https://www.parkinsons.org.uk/professionals/resources/competency-framework-nurses-working-parkinsons-disease-management-3rd.

Royal College of Speech and Language Therapists (n.d.). Supporting people attected by Parkinson's. Retrieved July 4, 2020, from https://www.rcslt.org/-/media/Project/RCSLT/rcslt-parkinsons-factsheet.pdf.

Skelly, R., Lindop, F., & Johnson, C. (2012). Multidisciplinary care of patients with Parkinson's disease. *Progress in Neurology and Psychiatry*, *16*(2), 10–14.

Taberna, M., Gil Moncayo, F., Jane-Salas, E., Antonio, M., Arribas, L., Vilajosana, E., et al. (2020). The multidisciplinary team (MDT) approach and quality of care. *Frontiers in Oncology*, 2020 March 20; 10: 85.

Tickle-Degnen, L., Ellis, T., Saint-Hilaire, M. H., Thomas, C. A., & Wagenaar, R. C. (2010). Self-management rehabilitation and health-related quality of life in Parkinson's disease: a randomised controlled trial. *Movement Disorders*, *25*(2), 194–204.

US Department of Health and Human Services. (2020). Medicare hospice benefits. Retrieved April 29, 2020, from https://www.medicare.gov/Pubs/pdf/02154-medicare-hospice-benefits.pdf.

van der Eijk, M., Nijhuis, F. A., Faber, M. J., & Bloem, B. R. (2013). Moving from physician-centered care towards patient-centred care for Parkinson's disease patients. *Parkinsonism and Related Disorders*, *19*(11), 923–927.

van der Marck, M. A., & Bloem, B. R. (2014). How to organise multispecialty care for patients with Parkinson's disease. *Parkinsonism and Related Disorders*, 20(Suppl 1), S167–S173.

van der Marck, M. A., Bloem, B. R., Borm, G. F., Overeem, S., Munneke, M., & Guttman, M. (2013a). Effectiveness of multidisciplinary care for Parkinson's disease: a randomised, controlled trial. *Movement Disorders*, 28(5), 605–611.

van der Marck, M. A., Munneke, M., Mulleners, W., Hoogerwaard, E. M., Borm, G. F., Overeem, S., et al. (2013b). Integrated multidisciplinary care in Parkinson's disease: a non-randomised, controlled trial (IMPACT). *Lancet Neurology*, 10(12), 947–956.

Wade, D. T., Gage, H., Owen, C., Trend, P., Grossmith, C., & Kaye, J. (2003). Multidisciplinary rehabilitation for people with Parkinson's disease: a randomised controlled study. *Journal of Neurology, Neurosurgery, and Psychiatry*, 74(2), 158–162.

Watanabe, S. M., Fairchild, A., Pituskin, E., Borgersen, P., Hanson, J., & Fassbender, K. (2013). Improving access to specialist multidisciplinary palliative care consultation for rural cancer patients by videoconferencing: report of a pilot project. *Supportive Care in Cancer*, 21(4), 1201–1207.

Willis, A. W., Schootman, M., Tran, R., Kung, N., Evanoff, B. A., Perlmutter, J. S., et al. (2012). Neurologist-associated reduction in PD-related hospitalisations and health care expenditures. *Neurology*, 79(17), 1774–1780.

Ypinga, J. H. L., de Vries, N. M., Boonen, L., Koolman, X., Munneke, M., Zwinderman, A. H., et al. (2018). Effectiveness and costs of specialised physiotherapy given via ParkinsonNet: a retrospective analysis of medical claims data. *Lancet Neurology*, 2018 Feb; 17(2):153–161.

Chapter 4

Living with Parkinson's

Brian Greaves and Liz Greaves

Introduction

Until I was diagnosed with Parkinson's at the age of 57, I had lived a very ordinary, uneventful life, and I was happily married to Liz. We had two sons who had grown up and flown the nest; one lived in Canada and the other closer to home. I had worked at Rolls-Royce since leaving school, and although my life had its ups and downs, I was settled. Liz had worked as a nursery nurse all her adult life and was a manager in a private nursery. For several years I had wanted to run my own business. My hobby was woodworking, which I loved, and I had investigated the possibility of owning my own shop. However, this plan had never come to fruition.

In 1998, Liz and I were asked if we would like to take over the franchise for the nursery. This was an ideal opportunity; my ambition to have my own business could be fulfilled and, as life was beginning to get stressful at Rolls-Royce, we decided to take this opportunity. The original idea was that I would stay at Rolls-Royce and Liz would manage the day-to-day running of the nursery. We employed a full-time business manager and I helped with the business side of things in my spare time.

However, in trying to keep my job at Rolls-Royce, which was extremely demanding, while also helping with the nursery, my life became very stressful and I almost had a breakdown. I had to take a lot of stress-related time off from work. As a result, in 2000, we took the decision that I should leave Rolls-Royce and work full time at the nursery.

This turned out to be the best decision I had ever made and life was good and settled. I loved the challenge and Liz and I worked well together. Over the next few years we built up the business and had a great rapport with staff and parents. This job also had its stresses, but I learned to cope.

As time passed, I noticed that I was feeling unwell and symptoms that I did not understand were gradually appearing. My stomach was often churning and I was told that I might have lactose intolerance, so I changed to a lactose-free diet, which seemed to help. Then I started to experience aches and pains in my neck and shoulders and began shuffling around the house, as I could not lift my legs properly. Over a 2-year period I went to see my general practitioner (GP) regularly and was told, every time, that there was nothing wrong with me. I was given no explanation for why I was feeling like this. My neck and shoulders became more painful and my posture more rounded; also, I had no arm swing when walking. Once again, I visited my GP. Once again, he told me there was nothing wrong. I was upset and burst into tears because I knew that I was not well. The GP decided that I was depressed and therefore prescribed antidepressants. However, I was convinced that this was not depression.

I was feeling low and fed up because I felt rough and was getting no answers, but I did not believe that depression was causing the symptoms. After taking the antidepressant tablets, I developed a slight tremor in my hand, so I went back to the surgery. The GP changed the tablets and advised that if this second medication did not work, he would send me to see a neurologist.

Getting the diagnosis

I had no idea what being sent to a neurologist would mean. I went home and asked Liz what a neurologist was and why I would need to see one. Liz suggested that the GP might be considering Parkinson's because of the tremor.

I immediately went upstairs and searched "Parkinson's" on my computer. The answers were all there. I had no sense of smell and no arm swing. My neck and shoulders were stiff. I was shuffling around the house. My writing had become very small and almost illegible. I had lost my smile; Liz had been telling me that I did not smile like I used to, but we had assumed it was because I was worried about things.

Although the tremor seemed to point to Parkinson's, I had not had "the shakes" until I started taking the antidepressant tablets. Indeed, the tremor stopped when I stopped taking them!

I went back to the GP the following day and told him that I was sure I had Parkinson's, and I wanted a second opinion. To get a quick diagnosis, we went to see a neurologist privately. Within two weeks we had it confirmed. It was indeed Parkinson's!

It all felt a bit surreal. On the one hand, at least we now knew that there was an explanation for why I was feeling like this. On the other hand, what would happen now? We came out of the clinic with very mixed feelings and were wondering what all this meant. As it was a private clinic, there was no information or help regarding services that might be available to support us other than the phone number of the local Parkinson's disease specialist nurse.

That was the day our lives changed.

Impact

The diagnosis was a two-edged sword. We had a reason for why I was feeling so bad, but we could have been given a diagnosis that was worse, so we came out of the neurology appointment feeling relieved but also very scared. I was prescribed medication but also told that I would "have 15 years"! What was that supposed to mean? Fifteen years of good living before things got worse or fifteen years before the end of life? We had no idea. We felt rather alone. I was concerned that if the tremor returned, I might have to give up my woodturning hobby. I needed to be able to safely use the power tools and lathe in my workshop. I discussed this with my consultant, who reassured me that he would try hard to ensure that, with the right medication, I could continue for as long as possible.

Although we had the contact details for the Parkinson's nurse, we knew nothing about a Parkinson's multidisciplinary clinic or anything about Parkinson's support in the area.

We were still very heavily involved with work at the nursery and, as my medication had kicked in and was effective, we hid our heads in the sand for a while. We were in this together. Liz gives her perspective of those early days in Box 4.1.

Support from the multidisciplinary team

Two years after being given the diagnosis, we decided to stop seeing the private consultant and switched over to the National Health Service (NHS).

I was signposted to the Parkinson's multidisciplinary team (MDT), where we received amazing support from the outset. We were invited along with six other couples to attend a 6-week Parkinson's education course. This was when our lives changed again.

We learned all about the Parkinson's symptoms and how to deal with them as well as how to confront different situations. We were able to talk to others in a similar position to ours, and we realised that we were not alone.

At the end of the course, all the participants decided to keep in touch with one another and exchanged email addresses. We then met every month in each

BOX 4.1 Liz's perspective

After Brian's diagnosis in 2006, our biggest concern was how it would affect our working life. We had only just begun a new chapter with the nursery business and we loved what we were doing. But how long would Brian be able to cope and continue to work at the nursery? Would we have to make changes, and how soon would things change? All of this was difficult to comprehend and come to terms with.

We felt that it was important for us to tell our family, friends, and colleagues about the diagnosis, because many of them had recognised that there was a problem and they were concerned. For us, this was the right decision. It is difficult to accept that there is a problem that will only progress, but we tried very hard not to go into denial and at the same time not to look too far into the future. As time went on, this was not always easy, and facing the full impact of the future was daunting. Still, we had friends and family to help us on our journey. We did not hide the fact that Brian had Parkinson's and tried to face it head on. However, in those early days we were reluctant to join any local support groups, as we found it difficult to come to terms with the thought of seeing others who were further down the road of the Parkinson's journey.

We continued running the nursery business for another 7 years before our working life became more difficult. Brian was responsible for managing the staff's wages and paying bills. As his concentration declined, he found it increasingly difficult to manage numbers and figures. The staff were very patient and supportive, but when they began having to worry about receiving their correct salaries, they were not so happy! Initially we arranged for an outside company to take over the administration of salaries and hired an accountant to help with the finances that Brian had previously been able to manage. I was already heavily committed to the day-to-day running of the nursery and felt unable to take on this financial burden as well. Therefore we faced a very difficult decision. We had no idea of how long it might be before Brian's condition worsened, and I found it hard to watch him beginning to struggle with things he had managed before. We felt that it was important for us to leave the business while we were still able to enjoy life together. We were able to return the franchise to the original owner and found a new manager to continue the day-to-day operation.

As we began our retirement, we were lucky enough to be able to go on a cruise, which gave us time to think about the future.

We asked ourselves what the future would hold and what would happen next.

other's homes, enjoying tea, cakes and chat. We were a great support to one another. Those with Parkinson's could exchange notes about their medications and how they were feeling, whereas the spouses could talk about how Parkinson's was affecting them.

The members of the MDT were fantastic. The fact that they were all trained in their own disciplines and were also experts in Parkinson's was comforting.

We felt very supported and were able to access specific support from physiotherapy, occupational therapy (OT), speech therapy and the dietitian. To us, the OT was the most valuable in those early days. Both Liz and I were able to ask lots of questions without feeling uncomfortable, and we were given strategies that enabled us to cope with many difficult situations. Over the years, the MDT clinic has become a haven of help and support for us.

The MDT operates a one-stop clinic, and the team members are all based in the same department working together to deliver the best care for each individual. We are extremely lucky to live in Derby, with all the support available to us under one roof. I have access to my consultant and have participated in exercise programs, a relaxation course, a handwriting course and a singing class as well as having one-to-one sessions with the different disciplines when I needed them.

Thirteen years since my diagnosis, I still do some wood turning, although much less than I used to. My workshop has been my haven—a place of normality for me to escape to where I can reflect and work out my feelings.

Challenges of living with Parkinson's

After coming to terms with having Parkinson's, the biggest challenge we faced was early retirement. Liz and I loved the job we were doing and were proud of our achievements. We would not have retired so early if Parkinson's had not presented us with difficulties. I retired when I was 62 and Liz was 63. Liz shares the challenges she has faced as a caregiver in Box 4.2.

BOX 4.2 Liz's perspective as a caregiver

There are challenges and questions for the caregiver when a loved one is diagnosed with Parkinson's. For me, it is a fine balance between offering assistance and encouraging Brian to remain independent.

Our challenges have included these issues:

- Questions about how Parkinson's will affect our life together.
- Questions about how much I should do for Brian. Should I help with putting on a coat or fastening zips and buttons?
- Asking myself "When should I step in to help? Or should I step back in some situations, as in paying a restaurant tab or carrying food to the table?
- It can be difficult to find ways to cope after nights when Brian's sleep has been bad. It is painful having to be aware of his nightmares and hallucinations.
- There is also the question of whether to go to appointments with Brian. A person with Parkinson's needs to have the opportunity and time to talk confidentially, but it is also important for the caregiver to know what is happening, so as to help remember what has been said in a consultation as well as to be aware of what can be done to offer support.

Further challenges that I continue to face are based around remaining independent. They include:

1. *Trying to take money out of my pocket or wallet, especially if I am in a queue.* It is so embarrassing when it drops on the floor and I cannot pick it up. I tend to just pass notes over to the cashier so that I do not have to deal with small change. I find working out coins very difficult, especially under pressure.
2. *Stopping driving.* Having to give up my driver's licence was devastating, and it was difficult adapting to getting around without a car. Going into town on my own on the bus is a challenge. Before setting off, I must work out my route very carefully, going over again and again in my head the times of buses and where I will have to get on and off. I rarely catch the bus now.
3. *Going into cafés and restaurants.* I find that I have to stand and plan a way to and from a table before finding a seat. I do not like places where tables are very close together and where pathways through are very narrow. I become anxious about freezing or stumbling in front of people.
4. *Keeping active.* Unrelated to the Parkinson's, I have problems with arthritis in the top of my foot, and it can be very painful to walk any distance, which makes it challenging to keep active and avoid the problems related to Parkinson's that might arise from being inactive. I was getting to the point of not going out, as it was too much effort to walk very far. I bought a mobility scooter to give me more independence, but I have found driving this to be a huge challenge and I have a lost a lot of confidence in using it. The footpaths are narrow and uneven, and crossing roads is scary. If I am not having a good day but still want to go out fairly far, I have to accept using a wheelchair. My wife tells me that that it is better than staying in!
5. *Remembering passwords on my computer.* I have always enjoyed using my computer, but every day poses the big challenge of remembering passwords to get into the program! By the time I am into the program it is time to close it down!

Members of the MDT have been amazing at helping me with all my challenges: the physiotherapist for mobility and exercises, the speech therapist for speech problems, and the OT for boosting my confidence and giving me strategies for coping with all aspects of my life. The OT has also helped with cognitive and dexterity problems. The Parkinson's nurse is always available to talk with about medication issues.

The local branch of Parkinson's UK

Support for those newly diagnosed

After meeting others in the education course, we recognised that there were many other individuals at the same stage of Parkinson's as I was. They were all nice people, and there was nothing to be afraid of in terms of seeing people at a later stage of this condition. At around the same time, I met a gentleman at a Parkinson's information table outside a local supermarket and I began to chat with him. He invited me along to a local Parkinson's UK branch meeting and told me that I would receive a warm welcome. This was the place where Liz and I started to feel comfortable about meeting others. Now that we were retired, we could get involved at a local level and offer to work with the MDT to help support others with Parkinson's.

We went to the monthly branch meetings, and it was not long before I was on the committee. Then Liz followed! In fact, 18 months later, she became chairperson and continued in that role for another 5 years.

At this time branch activities were confined to monthly meetings and, for those who enjoyed exercising in water, branch-sponsored Parkinson's hydrotherapy sessions were held weekly at the hospital.

Soon after we became involved, the branch received a large donation, a legacy, which was to be used over the next 3 years specifically for the benefit of local people with Parkinson's. As it was a substantial amount of money, the branch had to work closely with the Parkinson's UK national office to make sure that the funds were used wisely. We decided that most of the money should be used to set up exercise and activity groups as well as a carers' group.

Singing

In setting up a community singing group, we worked closely with the MDT, which supported us. The speech therapist helped us to find a musical director and then came along to evaluate the sessions and ascertain what difference it made in people's voices. We began with eight people and now, 7 years later, there are more than thirty meeting for the weekly 2-hour "Movers and Shakers" sessions. This is the most popular group currently run by the branch, and many friendships have been formed because of it. For the first and last half hour of each meeting we share tea and biscuits; in fact, most of our groups involve tea and biscuits! This group has been the most beneficial for me. I have gained confidence in using my voice in conversation, and the music lifts my spirits. Disabilities disappear when you are having a good time with others.

Tai chi

In addition to this, because it is known that exercise is good for well-being and movement in Parkinson's, the branch set up a community tai chi group. The physiotherapist supported us, making sure that the tai chi instructor understood the difficulties that can be experienced by people with Parkinson's. The instructor adapted routines to make sure that they were suitable for people at all stages of the condition. People could either sit, stand, or hold the back of a chair while standing. Seven years later, this group, too, is still running and subsidised by the branch. Although it is a popular group, I have found tai chi difficult and stopped attending after a couple of years. I found facing a full-length mirror a bit daunting and did not like to see myself doing the moves. Coordinating at the best of times is difficult, but when you are using a mirror it is even harder to accept what you see!

Dance

Following a pilot 6-week music and movement dance group run by the MDT in its department, the branch set up a weekly community dance group with the same "Dance for Parkinson's" instructor. Dance appealed to me much more that tai chi, and I got such a lot out of this. These dance sessions were more beneficial to me, as I could do the moves sitting down or standing and they were set to lots of different types of music. The moves were "freedom of expression" movements, and I was under no pressure to do moves correctly but rather to express myself in whatever way I wished. This group has continued to meet, moving to online sessions during and after the COVID-19 lockdown restrictions. I know I have benefited from this group and intend to continue attending. For me, the discipline of regular exercise is very fulfilling, and I find it easier to exercise in a group than on my own.

High-intensity exercise and boxing

Following another MDT-based pilot, the branch set up a community high-intensity exercise group. A community Parkinson's boxing group is also running. These are proving popular with many of our members, who are gaining a lot from them, although they are a step too far for me.

Saturday social

The MDT was instrumental in helping the branch set up a new monthly Saturday morning coffee time. We needed a venue close to the town centre that would available by public transport. The MDT suggested that we could use their clinic premises, as they did not use them on Saturdays. Staff volunteered to come in on their day off and open the doors for us, locking up when we finished. By holding this meeting on a Saturday, anyone still working during the week could attend. Initially, I was concerned about the new venue, fearing that some branch members might feel uncomfortable meeting for coffee in a hospital environment. We put the MDT's offer to our members, and one lady replied, "Of course we don't mind; this is our spiritual home." People feel comfortable about being in the clinic environment. The staff know us all by name, welcome us, and make us feel at ease.

Younger age group

I also helped set up a younger-aged Parkinson's support group. I was 57 years old when I was diagnosed and soon realised that other people of my age were also being diagnosed. It was much easier to meet with others of a similar age who were just setting out on the Parkinson's journey. This group continues to meet once a month, even though many of us are not necessarily of a younger age now! We are a discussion group, and members suggest the topics that are relevant to them.

Men's group

As I grew a little older and journeyed further with Parkinson's, I found that men are not always good at talking to each other about their feelings, so I set up a men-only group. We meet once a month in the foyer of a local hotel. We sit and chat over coffee and, although there are not many of us, we enjoy each other's company. It gives our wives time to go off for an hour or so on their own. We have had a couple of meetings at the bowling alley, with hilarious results, and we have also tried footy golf (golf using feet instead of clubs)!

Creative group

A Creative Challenge group has also been formed, which meets weekly in a local hotel. Liz attends this art-and-crafts group.

This is how we filled our time after retirement. We were never meant to sit still! We recognise that no one should face Parkinson's alone, and we have tried very hard to make sure that there are enough different activities for people to become involved in if they so wish.

Working with the multidisciplinary team

From the early days after my diagnosis, I became involved with Parkinson's research programmes and had several brain scans at Nottingham hospital. I also took part in a research programme at Leicester hospital.

A few years after my diagnosis, I was asked by the Derby Parkinson's consultant if I would consider sitting in the waiting area of the Parkinson's clinic so that, as people who were newly diagnosed came in, I would be able to chat with them about the support that was available. I was very eager to do this as, when I was diagnosed outside the NHS, there was no information about where I could get help and support. I felt that it was important for people who were newly diagnosed to be aware of support in the area in addition to what the hospital was able to offer. I wanted to make sure that others were not in the unfortunate position I had been, so I jumped at the chance to do this.

I was given a room in the clinic area so that, if anyone wished to talk, we could have a private space. I continued to do this for 10 years and met many people who were starting out on their Parkinson's journey. I enjoyed being able to give them information regarding what help was available should they need it. Most people found it helpful and, when they came back for follow-up appointments, would enjoy a chat. Many joined the Parkinson's UK local branch group.

Liz and I regularly give presentations at the 6-weekly MDT Parkinson's Education Group, (the one we attended at the start of our journey). We share our story and provide information about the local branch, and we also contact numbers. We try to reassure people that there is still life after Parkinson's and that they need not feel alone. This was another positive step for us; we meet such a lot of lovely people and enjoy being able to work closely with the MDT and with Parkinson's UK.

Conclusion

Parkinson's has definitely changed our lives, but without the help, advice, and support we have received from the MDT team in Derby, my life would have been very different and Liz and I would never have had the confidence to be as involved as we are in helping others with Parkinson's. We would not be the people we are now. We have gained such wonderful friendships with so many people with Parkinson's over the years and we all help to support one another.

I am grateful for the care and support that I and others in Derby receive. It really is a centre of excellence.

Brian and Liz's top tips

1. People with Parkinson's must take their medication on time; therefore performance, such as mobility, at clinic appointments may not be as good as usual if they have not taken their medications as scheduled.
2. People with Parkinson's have "on" and "off" times.
3. Individuals need time to explain their problems, because they may have speech issues, such as a quiet voice, or they may be very anxious.
4. A course for those not so newly diagnosed could be useful. After living with Parkinson's for 13 years, we feel that it would be beneficial to attend a course with others in our situation to see how we move forward positively into the later stages of Parkinson's.
5. People attending multidisciplinary clinics might be offered a snack or beverage before their appointments in order to help them feel calm before they see the health professional. The waiting area can also offer opportunities for people with Parkinson's to network with each other.
6. Multidisciplinary teams should have a dedicated member who can be available for caregivers to talk to, and caregiver groups can provide opportunities for sharing and support.

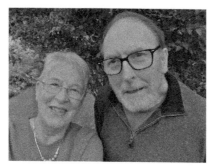

Photo: Brian and Liz

Chapter 5

Diagnostic Stage of Parkinson's

David Gallagher, Lisa Brown, Clare Johnson and Fiona Lindop

Chapter outline

Introduction

In recent decades, the approach to the diagnosis and treatment of Parkinson's has progressed to the point where it is considered a complex multisystemic disorder rather than primarily a motor disorder. Better understanding of its pathophysiology and early symptomatology has demonstrated the importance of non-motor symptoms (NMSs) in the diagnosis, often with input from other specialists. Also, NMSs and non-dopaminergic functional imaging have been incorporated into diagnostic frameworks.

Non-motor symptoms and signs

Parkinson's is a neurodegenerative disorder; pathologically, it is characterised by the presence of alpha synuclein–containing inclusions, Lewy bodies (LBs), and Lewy neurites. The typical motor features of idiopathic Parkinson's—tremor, rigidity, bradykinesia and gait disturbance—result from the degeneration of dopaminergic neurons in the substantia nigra. It is estimated that an approximately 50% loss of nigral dopaminergic neurons is required before motor symptoms become clinically apparent. However, LBs are also found in many extranigral locations in the central and peripheral nervous systems and affect non-dopaminergic neurotransmitters. Braak and colleagues (2006) have proposed, from detailed postmortem studies, a staging of LB pathology in Parkinson's (Fig. 5.1). Stage 1 includes LB pathology in the anterior olfactory structures and the dorsal

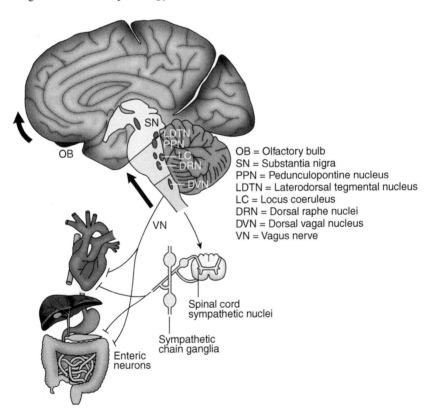

OB = Olfactory bulb
SN = Substantia nigra
PPN = Pedunculopontine nucleus
LDTN = Laterodorsal tegmental nucleus
LC = Locus coeruleus
DRN = Dorsal raphe nuclei
DVN = Dorsal vagal nucleus
VN = Vagus nerve

FIGURE 5.1 Anatomical correlates for prodromal non-motor symptoms in Parkinson's. Lewy bodies first emerge in the olfactory bulb, autonomic nervous system and lower brainstem. Pathology spreads rostrally to involve brainstem nuclei involved in several early non-motor symptoms.

motor nucleus of the glossopharyngeal and vagal nerves as well as peripheral autonomic ganglia. These are, respectively, proposed pathological correlates for hyposmia and autonomic symptoms. At stage 2 there are LBs in various brainstem nuclei, including the reticular formation, noradrenergic locus coeruleus and serotoninergic brainstem raphe nuclei. These anatomic locations are implicated in rapid-eye-movement (REM) sleep behaviour disorder and mood disorders such as depression or anxiety. This staging hypothesis provides an explanation for the observation of NMSs early in the course of Parkinson's and often preceding, sometimes by several years, clinically significant motor signs or symptoms. It has also led to the concept of prodromal Parkinson's. Only in stages 3 to 4, according to this hypothesis, is there significant LB involvement in the substantia nigra. In stages 5 to 6 there is more diffuse neocortical involvement, contributing to cognitive dysfunction, dyspraxia, visuoperceptual disorders and other problems with higher cortical function.

An accurate history of NMSs can provide support for the diagnosis of Parkinson's, both at an early stage when motor symptoms may be equivocal and at later stages, to differentiate it from other extrapyramidal disorders. Loss of smell sensation, REM sleep behaviour disorder, autonomic symptoms and mood disorders are important early NMSs in Parkinson's and should be routinely asked about at the diagnostic stage.

Rapid-eye-movement sleep behaviour disorder

REM sleep is the dreaming component of sleep, characterised by REMs and generalized reduced body tone. Parkinson's and other LB disorders—such as multiple system atrophy and dementia with Lewy bodies (DLB)—are strongly associated with REM sleep behaviour disorder (RBD), in which there is loss of atonia during REM sleep, as manifested by nocturnal vocalisation (talking or shouting during sleep) and dream enactment. The sleeper may be entirely unaware of this; therefore a detailed history from the person's partner, family or caregivers is important. Sometimes the bed partner moves to another room owing to the severity of symptoms, and this is an important diagnostic clue.

On careful assessment, a significant proportion of people presenting to sleep clinics with RBD are found to have an underlying neurological disorder, particularly Parkinson's (Olson et al., 2000). When those with apparently idiopathic RBD are imaged with dopamine transporter scans (DaTSCANs), there is often evidence of dopaminergic loss compared with normal controls. On long-term follow-up, many such individuals progress to clinically defined Parkinson's (Iranzo et al., 2017). RBD can precede diagnosis and definite clinical features of Parkinson's by several years.

Probable diagnosis of RBD can be made from a compelling clinical history. However, a full sleep history and medication list should be acquired. For example, dream enactment can occur in narcolepsy and with antidepressant medications (such as selective serotonin reuptake inhibitors). Otherwise, referral to a dedicated sleep physician may be required to exclude other common sleep disorders, such as obstructive sleep apnoea or non-REM parasomnias. This can be done, for example, by nocturnal pulse oximetry or polysomnography (nocturnal electroencephalography and electromyography).

Olfaction

Loss of smell is an early marker of Parkinson's. Large epidemiological studies have shown that olfactory loss can often precede Parkinson's by several years (Chen et al., 2017; Ross et al., 2008). In idiopathic hyposmia without apparent motor symptoms, some subjects already demonstrate either substantia nigra hyperechogenicity on transcranial sonography or abnormalities on DaTSCAN (Jennings et al., 2014; Sommer et al., 2004) suggestive of prodromal Parkinson's.

Methods of olfactory testing include odour identification, smell discrimination and threshold detection. For example, the 40-item multiple-choice University of Pennsylvania Smell Identification Test has been used extensively in both research and clinical practice.

The reliability of smell identification tests is reduced in those with cognitive impairment (for example, semantic memory) and/or depression and in those who smoke. Also, evidence of previous or current sinus-nasal disease should be sought to exclude conductive olfactory loss.

Mood disorders

There is a high prevalence of mood disorders in early Parkinson's. Systematic reviews of cohort and case control studies have demonstrated that low mood and anxiety can often precede the diagnosis of Parkinson's (Ishihara & Brayne, 2006). It is proposed that early LB involvement of the noradrenergic locus coeruleus and serotoninergic raphe nuclei is important in the development of prodromal psychiatric symptoms.

Autonomic symptoms and signs

Parkinson's has widespread autonomic symptoms affecting gastrointestinal, cardiovascular, genitourinary and thermoregulatory function. There is early LB involvement in the central (lower brainstem) and peripheral (sympathetic and parasympathetic) nervous systems.

Constipation is very common throughout all stages of Parkinson's and can precede the diagnosis by several years and sometimes decades. For example, a meta-analysis of observational epidemiological studies has confirmed that constipation is a risk factor for subsequently developing Parkinson's, increasing the risk approximately twofold. This includes studies assessing constipation 10 or more years before the diagnosis of Parkinson's (Adams-Carr et al., 2016).

Cardiovascular dysfunction is proposed as a premotor feature of Parkinson's. Radionucleotide metaiodobenzylguanidine (MIBG) scans demonstrate cardiac sympathetic degeneration even in early Parkinson's (Palma & Kaufmann, 2014), and cohort studies have suggested a blunted heart rate response during cardiac stress testing in individuals who later develop Parkinson's. Orthostatic hypotension is also a possible premotor feature. Although this has not been confirmed in large epidemiological studies, the presence of orthostatic hypotension in the high-risk population with idiopathic RBD predicts future development of Parkinson's (Palma & Kaufmann, 2014).

Sexual dysfunction can precede Parkinson's in both men and women. Symptoms include reduced libido, difficulty with sexual arousal, erectile dysfunction and anorgasmia. For example, in a large retrospective study, men with erectile dysfunction were at increased risk for developing Parkinson's (Gao et al., 2007).

Prodromal Parkinson's

The concept of prodromal Parkinson's has arisen from these observations:

- The discovery of monoallelic genetic forms of Parkinson's and other susceptibility genes in presymptomatic individuals
- The Braak hypothesis of rostral progression (from brainstem to cerebral cortex) of LB pathology involving extranigral locations before dopaminergic neurons
- Clinical and epidemiologic studies of NMSs preceding motor symptoms, with functional brain and cardiac imaging demonstrating support for these early NMSs
- Polysomnography for sleep disorders, particularly RBD

There is now strong evidence that early NMSs (loss of smell, RBD, autonomic symptoms and mood symptoms) can precede any motor signs or symptoms or be present when the motor symptoms are insufficient to fulfil diagnostic criteria.

The use of NMSs in the diagnosis of Parkinson's is undergoing evaluation. RBD has the highest predictive value for developing a LB disorder. Loss of smell, constipation and mood disorders have lower specificity owing to their common occurrence in the general population, particularly among the elderly. However, the combination of different NMSs may provide stronger risk stratification. For example, in the Honolulu Aging Study, impaired olfaction, constipation, slow reaction time, excessive daytime sleepiness and impaired executive function were associated with risk of clinical Parkinson's or incidental LB or neuronal loss in the substantia nigra or locus coeruleus (in the autopsy cohort). A combination of two or more of these premotor features was associated with an up to 10-fold risk of developing Parkinson's (Ross et al., 2012). The PREDICT-PD Parkinson's study (Noyce et al., 2017) examined prospective

Parkinson's risk using an online questionnaire, keyboard-tapping test and geno-typing. This study looked at the development of the premotor Parkinson's markers of anosmia, RBD and finger-tapping speed as well as incident Parkinson's. Development of Parkinson's on follow-up was significantly associated with the NMS risk score at baseline.

NMSs can have an important role in the early and accurate diagnosis of Parkinson's. This may involve the multidisciplinary involvement of other specialists and review of their previous investigations—for example, sleep specialists, the ear-nose-throat clinic or gastroenterology.

Motor symptoms and signs

Individuals report a wide variety of motor symptoms: for example, abnormal gait, balance, or posture; upper or lower limb tremor; impaired dexterity with fine motor tasks; limb stiffness, pain or cramping; change in handwriting; and altered speech or facial expression. Parkinson's can often be immediately evident on observing the individual in the waiting room, as he or she stands from sitting and then walks to the consulting room. Similarly, in many, the diagnosis is quickly evident during the examination for the typical motor features of tremor, rigidity and gait disturbance. In others, however, despite prolonged and thorough examination, the diagnosis remains unclear. For example:

- Several common tremor disorders can mimic Parkinson's.
- Other gait disorders—such as frontal gait disorder, widespread cerebro-vascular disease and musculoskeletal disorders—can complicate the gait assessment.
- Non-extrapyramidal rigidity, such as paratonia, occurs in cognitive disorders and in the elderly.
- Several other neurological and rheumatologic disorders can affect the assessment of dexterity or mimic bradykinesia.

Tremor

Tremor should be observed when the person is walking and then when sitting. When sitting, ask the person to gently rest the hands on the lap to assess resting tremor. Asking the person to perform mental tasks, such as serial seven subtraction, will accentuate a true resting tremor (therefore making the Parkinson's tremor more obvious) or reduce or eliminate, by distraction, any postural or functional component. The arms should then be held extended outward to assess postural tremor. It is important to note whether the tremor is immediate on posture or delayed for a number of seconds, a phenomenon called "re-emergence." Subsequently, observe for tremor in various positions of pronation-supination of the forearm and flexion-extension of the wrist or elbow. Carefully note whether the tremor is regular or jerky; the degree of symmetry or asymmetry; whether tremor is exacerbated in any position or absent in others; and whether there is any abnormal posturing of the digits or limbs (dystonic posturing). Then test for kinetic tremor—for example, by goal-directed tasks such as finger-nose testing. But it is important to make a distinction between incoordination, where relevant, and kinetic tremor. Next, observe for head, jaw, voice or palatal tremor. Make note of any abnormal posturing of the jaw or neck—for example, a tendency toward lateral neck rotation (torticollis), neck extension (retrocollis) or neck flexion (anterocollis). Finally, it is useful to examine for any tremor when the person is writing, also noting any abnormal pen grip or hand posturing and the nature of the handwriting itself. For example, micrographia is common in Parkinson's.

The typical tremor in Parkinson's is an asymmetric resting tremor. The "pill rolling" tremor is a tremor of thumb and index finger in close proximity. Parkinson's tremor often increases during walking; it can affect both arms and legs. Parkinson's rest tremor often worsens with distraction or mental exercises. There can be postural upper limb tremor, but this tends to be distal rather than proximal and often occurs after a delay of a few seconds (reemergence) and with similar frequency (4-6 Hz) to the resting tremor. Jaw tremor is also a common feature.

Differentiating a Parkinson's tremor from other common types of tremor, particularly essential tremor (ET) and dystonic tremor, can be difficult. For example, rest tremor occurs in about 30% of ET, and ET is often asymmetric. However, ET rarely affects the legs; if there is rest tremor, it is associated with longer disease duration and more marked severity; in ET, the postural tremor is generally more prominent than rest tremor, immediate on posture (not reemergent), and proximal as well as distal. ET is more likely to be associated with head tremor; it is reduced on walking and may be associated with bradykinesia, but there is generally preserved amplitude of repetitive movements and no freezing (Cohen et al., 2003). Jaw tremor occurs in ET, but this tends to be postural (mouth opening) or kinetic (speaking) rather than at rest. Conversely, head tremor occurs in Parkinson's, but whereas head tremor in ET is postural, Parkinson's head tremor persists when the person is supine and has similar frequency to the limb resting tremor, or 4 to 6 Hz (Roze et al., 2006).

Dystonia results from abnormal muscle tone, often in antagonistic muscles, leading to tremor or abnormal posturing. The tremor can occur in association with dystonia affecting the limb itself or dystonia elsewhere in the body. It is generally asymmetric, irregular in rhythm and amplitude, and often task-specific—for example, while the person is writing or playing a musical instrument. Dystonic tremor is usually exacerbated in certain limb positions and improved in others, sometimes with complete positional resolution, or a "null point"; in positions of maximal severity, the tremor can spread to other body segments, and individuals often exhibit a sensory trick or *geste antagoniste*, where light touch to the affected body part can relieve symptoms (Deuschl, 2003).

Rigidity

The extrapyramidal rigidity in Parkinson's is characterised by either "lead pipe" rigidity, where the increased limb tone is maintained throughout passive movement, or "cogwheel" rigidity, where there is increased tone with superimposed tremor. The person is assessed in the standing position for axial and limb rigidity; tone is tested at the wrist, elbow, shoulder and spine. In the early stages, this can be subtle and also inhibited by the person's ability to relax. Activation manoeuvres on the opposite side (synkinesis—for example, hand opening and closing or arm raising or lowering) can accentuate the increased tone, thus improving sensitivity.

Careful consideration should also be given to neurocognitive comorbidities—for example, dementia or previous stroke—through access to medical notes or previous psychometric assessments (as at the cognitive clinic). For example, paratonia is common in the elderly, particularly those with cognitive impairment. In paratonia, the person is unable to relax. This makes the assessment of true tone difficult, either because of resistance to passive movement, called *gegenhalten*, or involuntary assistance of movements, called *mitgehen*. In these individuals the presence of other signs such as primitive reflexes, utilisation (a form of environmental dependence, as when the person puts on a pair of glasses handed to him or her), or motor perseveration may be a clue that the rigidity is paratonic rather than extrapyramidal. Similarly, spasticity is a form of increased tone encountered in stroke and other structural brain and spine disorders; this is a velocity-dependent increased tone with sudden give-way, so-called "clasp-knife rigidity." Paratonia also acts in a velocity-dependent manner but without give-way.

Bradykinesia

Bradykinesia in Parkinson's is a progressive reduction in amplitude and velocity of repetitive movements and can include the freezing of movements. Bradykinesia can also manifest as impaired speech (hypophonia or dysprosody); reduced facial expression and hence apparent blunted emotional response (hypomimia); and more gross motor difficulties, as in getting out of a chair. The term "true bradykinesia" is sometimes used to acknowledge the difficulty in distinguishing this condition from other causes of slow movements or impaired dexterity. Assessment can be difficult for many reasons: the individual may, for example, have pre-existing motor impairment from any other cause; cognitive impairment or dysphasia can make it difficult for person to understand how to perform the tapping test correctly; co-existing tremor or coordination difficulties; disorders of praxis; and other non-neurological causes, such as deforming arthropathy secondary to rheumatoid arthritis.

Gait disorder

Parkinson's is characterised by difficulty in initiating gait, hesitation on turning and on changing direction, slow gait velocity with reduced stride length and reduced arm swing; the tendency to turn *en bloc* and stooped posture. At later stages, festination occurs, with progressively shorter but faster steps to maintain foot position with the anterior momentum of the body. Also, gait instability with impaired postural reflexes is seen as Parkinson's advances.

However, there are a number of other gait disorders, including cerebellar or sensory ataxia, hemiplegic gait following cerebral infarction, spastic gait, frontal gait disorder, myopathic gait and neuropathic gait. Frontal gait disorder (also termed "gait apraxia") in particular poses diagnostic challenges. The frontal lobes play an important role in balance and walking through connections to the basal ganglia, cerebellum and brainstem (Thompson, 2012). Frontal gait disorders may also involve a slow gait, short stride length, postural unsteadiness, initiation difficulties, and freezing. Causes include extensive subcortical vascular disease (Binswanger disease); hydrocephalus and normal-pressure hydrocephalus; dementias with frontal lobe atrophy; and other frontal lobe structural or degenerative pathology. Exclusively lower body Parkinsonism is a clue that there may be vascular pseudoparkinsonism.

A multidisciplinary approach—with input from a movement disorders specialist and experienced physiotherapist, who may have also observed the person performing functional activities in a natural setting—will therefore be helpful in the diagnosis of Parkinson's.

Imaging in Parkinson's

Parkinson's is predominantly a clinical diagnosis based on the examiner's clinical experience and interpretation of the physical signs. If there is diagnostic doubt, the clinical features usually become clearer with time, as this is a progressive neurodegenerative disorder. It is therefore entirely reasonable to defer diagnosis until a subsequent review.

Structural brain scanning with magnetic resonance imaging (MRI) is not usually helpful in the diagnosis of idiopathic Parkinson's. However, MRI can be useful if an atypical Parkinson's syndrome is suspected. For example, conditions such as progressive supranuclear palsy and multiple system atrophy can have characteristic radiologic features. When, for example, there is suspicion of pseudoparkinsonism, a frontal gait disorder, or gait impaired by widespread cerebrovascular change, or normal-pressure hydrocephalus, MRI will provide support for these alternative diagnoses. Also, MRI may be needed in conjunction with functional brain imaging to make sure that the apparent changes are not secondary to an underlying structural brain abnormality such as cerebrovascular disease.

Functional neuroimaging can be used to assist diagnosis. For example, DaTSCAN is a radionucleotide scan using single-photon emission computed tomography (SPECT) to measure presynaptic dopamine transporter levels; it is therefore a marker of dopaminergic neuronal loss. DaTSCAN can have incomplete sensitivity and specificity; in particular, there is a potential for false-negative results (lower sensitivity) in early Parkinson's. The UK Parkinson's Excellence Network has examined the use of DaTSCAN in the diagnosis of Parkinson's or its differentiation from other disorders. Identified limitations include the method of DaTSCAN interpretation (visual or semiquantitative) and interobserver reliability; the lack of a diagnostic gold standard in the majority of clinical studies (made on final clinical diagnosis rather than pathologic confirmation); absence of blinding of DaTSCAN interpretation in some studies; and publication bias (Galbraith, 2016). However, the UK Parkinson's Excellence Network concludes that moderate evidence shows DaTSCAN to be capable of diagnosing presynaptic dopaminergic loss accurately and that it can therefore differentiate neurodegenerative extrapyramidal disorders from other causes such as essential tremor. However, it is acknowledged that DaTSCAN may have lower sensitivity in early Parkinson's.

One circumstance in which DaTSCAN is often useful is when there is unequivocal Parkinsonism but difficulty differentiating between purely drug-induced Parkinsonism (for example, secondary to neuroleptic medication, dopaminergic anti-emetics or anti-vertigo medication) versus an underlying neurodegenerative cause that has been exacerbated by these medications.

False-positive DaTSCAN results are not uncommon. Frustratingly, in circumstances where DaTSCAN would be most useful and the neurological signs are equivocal, DaTSCAN can show mild asymmetry or possible subtle abnormalities. It can become evident, with lack of clinical progression over time or evolution of clinical signs, that there is an alternative diagnosis and the apparent DaTSCAN abnormality was due to positioning in the scanner (such as faulty head alignment leading to apparent asymmetry); inaccuracy of visual scan interpretation; or apparent change of uptake in the basal ganglia secondary to another cause, most commonly lacunar infarction or microvascular change. Performing a coregistered MRI or computed tomography scan of the head is recommended. See Figure 5.2 for examples of DaTSCANs and MRIs.

Making an accurate diagnosis

An accurate diagnosis of Parkinson's is important because this is a progressive neurodegenerative disorder with numerous life-altering implications. A correct diagnosis is particularly important in discussing the prognosis and making recommendations for the best treatment. Potential future development of disease-modifying (neuroprotective) therapies would make early and accurate diagnosis mandatory.

There are a number of Parkinson's diagnostic criteria, such as the Queen Square Brain Bank Criteria and Movement Disorder Society (MDS) Clinical Diagnostic Criteria (Postuma et al., 2015). For example, MDS criteria require

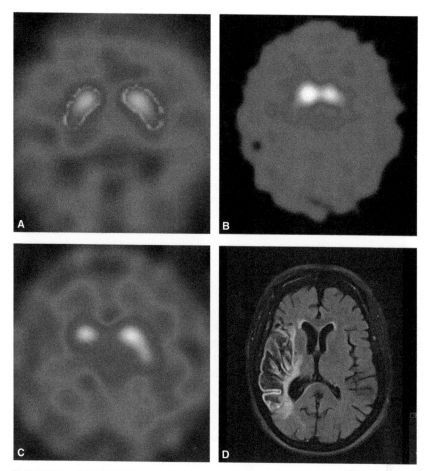

FIGURE 5.2 (A) DaTSCAN showing normal tracer uptake in caudate and putamen giving the typical "comma" shape in a person with dystonic neck and limb tremor; (B) Loss of putaminal tail giving "full stop" shape and also asymmetrical caudate uptake, in idiopathic PD; (C) Clearly demarcated loss of right putaminal uptake; (D) MRI scan on the same person shows right middle cerebral artery hemisphere stroke. This was a false positive DaTSCAN; the clinical examination features were spasticity on the left (from the stroke) and longstanding dystonic tremor in the right arm; but excellent left basal ganglia uptake excludes Parkinson's disease as the cause for the right-sided tremor.

1. Evidence of Parkinsonism: bradykinesia and also tremor or rigidity or both
2. Other supportive criteria, including response to dopaminergic therapy, levodopa-induced dyskinesia, olfactory loss or cardiac sympathetic denervation on metaiodobenzylguanidine scan
3. Absence of any absolute exclusion criteria; for example, cerebellar abnormalities, downward supranuclear gaze palsy, behavioural variant frontal dementia or primary progressive aphasia, purely lower limb Parkinsonism for 3 years, treatment with a dopamine receptor blocker, lack of levodopa response, corticosensory signs or limb dyspraxia or normal functional imaging

Additionally, there are a number of "red flags" for alternative diagnoses:

- Rapid progression to wheelchair use within 5 years
- Lack of significant progression over 5 years
- Inspiratory respiratory symptoms
- Early severe autonomic failure
- Early recurrent falls
- Disproportionate anterocollis
- Absence of common NMSs
- Unexplained pyramidal signs
- Bilateral highly symmetric signs

These absolute exclusion criteria and red flags allude to atypical Parkinson's disorders and other causes of secondary Parkinsonism.

It is noteworthy that a significant proportion of individuals with presumptive Parkinson's—diagnosed in specialist centres and who were recruited to clinical studies using functional imaging as a biomarker of neurodegeneration—were found to have normal functional imaging. This has led to the concept of scans without evidence of dopaminergic deficit (SWEDD), although this likely reflects diagnostic inaccuracy rather than a novel disease entity. For example, when Erro and others (2016) reviewed the literature on SWEDD cases, the ultimate correct diagnoses included adult-onset dystonia (determined by normal DaTSCAN and consistent electrophysiology or alternative genetic disease); other tremor disorders (such as ET), vascular or drug-induced pseudoparkinsonism, psychogenic causes, soft extrapyramidal signs in the elderly and issues with DAT interpretation.

This provides further support for a detailed history of symptoms (including NMSs); full medication and family history; and, importantly, a thorough and systematic clinical examination.

Receiving and giving the diagnosis

It is important to leave sufficient time to give and explain the implications of the diagnosis. Many individuals have already consulted their family doctors and sought a specialist opinion because of the suspicion that they have Parkinson's. Indeed, in individuals with any type of tremor, this is usually the diagnosis they are most familiar with and are thus keen to have confirmed or excluded. This is usually clear during the consultation. In others, the diagnosis will be totally unexpected. Therefore it is helpful to clarify the person's thoughts and expectations on the cause of the symptoms first, and this will guide delivery of the diagnosis. The process in arriving at the diagnosis should be explained carefully. It is important to show empathy, as this is a major life-altering diagnosis, and time should be given for the person to assimilate the information and then ask any questions. It should be emphasised that there are a number of effective medications and non-pharmacological interventions, including lifestyle modifications, that can be of help. Individuals should be given written information and a list of the national Parkinson's organisations. In the United Kingdom, the charity Parkinson's UK is a valuable source of information, and its website (www.parkinsons.org.uk), offers details regarding the implications of the condition, employment issues, driving regulations, available support structures, and financial help. Parkinson's UK also enables people to find their local Parkinson's support group. At the end of the consultation, it should be explained that the family doctor will receive a full report and that the newly diagnosed person will also receive a copy. Neverthless, it will be useful to provide a separate explanatory report for the individual in non-technical language. A follow-up plan should be given, along with contact details for the local Parkinson's disease nurse specialist (PDNS).

Medication

At diagnosis, motor symptoms may be insufficiently severe to affect quality of life (QoL) or require treatment, which can be deferred. The person may also prefer to research the different medication options personally and discuss them with others.

There is no known treatment that can slow or reverse the progressive neuronal loss that occurs in Parkinson's (Fox et al., 2018). However, there are several medications that improve symptoms and enhance QoL. Levodopa was the main treatment for many years and is still considered the most effective. Monoamine oxidase inhibitors type b (MAO-B) and dopamine agonists can also be used as monotherapy to treat early Parkinson's. However, dopamine agonists can have more side effects. A person starting levodopa may immediately have better symptom control and fewer side effects over the early years. However, immediate levodopa use has a stronger association with earlier development of motor fluctuations and dyskinesias. When dopamine agonists were directly compared with levodopa as the starting treatment for Parkinson's, motor fluctuations occurred later or were less severe (Table 5.1).

However, dopamine agonists can also cause more side effects. These include impulse control disorders such as difficulty resisting pleasurable impulses such as hypersexuality, pathologic gambling, compulsive computer gaming or internet use or impulsive shopping and eating.

The National Institute for Health and Care Excellence suggests offering a choice of dopamine agonists, levodopa or MAO-B inhibitors, for people in the early stages of Parkinson's whose motor symptoms do not affect their QoL (www.nice.org.uk) but to offer levodopa to people whose motor symptoms do affect their QoL. In practice, the person's age and comorbidities will affect this decision.

The National Institute for Health and Care Excellence also recommends giving individuals and their families or caregivers oral and written information

TABLE 5.1 Medication options for the initial treatment of Parkinson's

Drug class	Examples	Efficacy	Risk of dyskinesia	Risk of ICD	Confusion/ hallucinations
Levodopa + AADI	Co-beneldopa Co-careldopa	+++	++	+	+
Dopamine agonists	Ropinirole Rotigotine Pramipexole	++	+	++	++
MAO-B	Rasagiline Selegiline Safinamide	++	+/-	+	+

AADI = aromatic acid decarboxylase inhibitor, MAO-B = monoamine oxidase inhibitor type b, ICD = impulse control disorder

about certain risks and to record that these discussions have taken place. Topics to be discussed include (1) impulse control disorders with all-dopaminergic therapy (increased risk with dopamine agonists), (2) excessive sleepiness and sudden onset of sleep with dopamine agonists, and (3) psychotic symptoms (such hallucinations and delusions) with all Parkinson's medication (and again higher risk with dopamine agonists).

Parkinson's medications can often cause nausea. The risk is lessened by starting at a low dose and building up slowly. Usually, an antiemetic is not required. Following a warning from the Medicines and Healthcare products Regulatory Agency, domperidone should not be prescribed routinely on starting dopaminergic medication and particularly not for those over 60 years of age or those with serious underlying conditions such as congestive heart failure, severe hepatic impairment or significant electrolyte disturbance. A baseline electrocardiogram should be performed before domperidone is prescribed to make sure that the QT interval is normal. The potential benefits and risks should be discussed, and there should be vigilance for other medications that prolong the QT interval.

Psychological impact and adjustment

A new diagnosis of Parkinson's will have a major psychological impact on the individual and his or her family; this will require adjustment to the immediate and long-term consequences. This process continues through all the stages of Parkinson's and can be eased by support from friends and family, charitable organisations such as Parkinson's UK, professional counsellors and psychologists. Consideration of adjustment and psychological care, however, is a task for all members of the Parkinson's multidisciplinary team (MDT), who can be an important source of psychological support for people with Parkinson's. Each person's experience is unique, so clinicians should take time to understand what the diagnosis means for the individual. Factors such as personality, previous experience of distress, existing coping strategies, social support and attitudes or expectations of living with a disability all influence how an individual adjusts.

Psychological adjustment should be understood as a dynamic process over time and not as a set of "stages" that every person will work through; however, common themes can be identified. Ways to approach them are listed in Table 5.2 (Parkinson's Foundation).

Identification of non-motor symptoms

There should be ongoing vigilance for NMSs, and screening tools have been developed for this. For example, the NMS questionnaire is a specifically designed 30-item questionnaire for NMSs (Martinez-Martin et al., 2007). Individuals are also encouraged to identify their three most important symptoms for focused discussion during the consultation. The NMS questionnaire is available for download from the Parkinson's UK website. Compared with more extensive validated scales, full cognitive and behavioural assessments and detailed neurological examination, the NMS questionnaire has shown low sensitivity for some

TABLE 5.2 Common themes in psychological adjustment to life with Parkinson's

Psychological theme	Additional information
Denial or disbelief	This may be an early feature, particularly if symptoms are mild. Individuals are encouraged to be honest with themselves and others, obtain as much accurate information on Parkinson's as possible, and focus on things they can continue to achieve (including employment and relationships) rather than potential disabilities.
Discouragement and searching for an explanation	As they try to make sense of why Parkinson's has come into their lives (a question that is usually not fully answered), people can feel anger, blame, shame or sadness. Depression is common and can respond to psychological therapies or, if marked, antidepressant medication.
Adjustment to one's changed ability or role in employment and relationships	This can lead to frustration and emotional distress. Individuals should consider adjustments to their household or employment tasks and the need for additional help. Couples or family therapy can be helpful, and members of the Parkinson's MDT often build up therapeutic relationships with couples.
Realization of the full impact of Parkinson's	Communicating openly about priorities and having realistic expectations are key to successful adjustment.

items (for example, hyposmia and sleepiness). However, one study (Romenets et al., 2012) reports a mean sensitivity of about 70% for "clinically significant" symptoms and a high overall specificity about 90%. Such screening tools are useful; however, there is no substitute for a thorough exploration of symptoms and the assistance of other specialists—for example, psychologist, speech and language therapist, sleep physician, etc.

Driving

People with Parkinson's must inform their driving regulatory authority. In the United Kingdom, people newly diagnosed with Parkinson's must inform the Driver and Vehicle Licencing Agency. They are asked to perform a self-completed questionnaire, and their neurologist also completes a report. The latter covers the motor severity of their condition; presence or absence of motor fluctuations and whether these are unpredictable or sufficient to impair driving; presence of excessive daytime somnolence; and cognitive or behavioural symptoms such as compromised attention, impulsivity, or visuoperceptual symptoms. Guidelines for physicians are provided by the Driver and Vehicle Licencing Agency (www.gov.uk/dvla/fitnesstodrive) and emphasise the need to treat and continually monitor the condition with respect to driving. People newly diagnosed with Parkinson's should also inform their insurance companies so that they are appropriately covered.

At diagnosis, impairment of driving is rarely an issue, but the driving regulatory authority will stipulate a review at intervals of 1 to 3 years. In cases where a formal driving assessment is required, individuals can be referred to a regional driving assessment centre, either by direct self-referral or via a doctor (www.rdac.co.uk). This assessment is performed by a specially trained driving instructor and an occupational therapist (OT) and incorporates a physical assessment of ability to operate the controls. A full report is provided, including recommendations for adaptations to driver controls where necessary.

Employment

Employment provides an important role not only for financial security but also social interaction; it also promotes confidence and mental well-being. Most people are able to continue in their normal work for several years, while their condition remains well controlled on medication. This should be emphasised at diagnosis.

In the United Kingdom, the Equality Act 2010 (www.gov.uk) defines disability as a physical or mental impairment that has a substantial long-term negative effect on one's ability to pursue normal daily activities. Progressive conditions, such as Parkinson's, can be classified as disabilities. Therefore employers are legally obliged to make reasonable adjustments so that Parkinson's individuals can obtain employment or are not disadvantaged in performing their jobs. Such adjustments include changing the recruitment process when applying for work, making physical changes to the workplace (for example, to facilitate access or make ergonomic adaptations), permitting a phased return to work following illness, allowing flexible or part-time work and offering training opportunities and appropriate recreation and refreshment facilities. These adaptations can be arranged through discussions with the person's manager, occupational health department or human resources. Input from an occupational health specialist to perform a detailed assessment in the workplace, to assess need for adaptations, is recommended.

All working individuals should be informed that detailed information is available from Parkinsons UK (www.parkinsons.org.uk) highlighting their legal rights, the responsibilities of employers, and how to access support if there are difficulties.

Intervention by the multidisciplinary team

Parkinson's disease nurse specialist

The PDNS's role differs around the world, but broadly the PDNS acts as a care coordinator for the person with Parkinson's. Associated duties include

- Post-diagnostic counselling
- Regular assessment of motor and non-motor symptoms
- Checking if medication is being prescribed and taken correctly
- Enquiry about medication-related side effects

A PDNS prescriber or advanced nurse practitioner might make medication adjustments and prescribe a new medication, following consideration and discussion of benefits and risk of side effects, in order to optimise symptom control and maximise QoL. The PDNS will usually act as the main point of contact for the person with Parkinson's, providing telephone advice and support as needed, referral on to MDT members as appropriate and signposting to external support organisations.

Post-diagnostic counselling. The PDNS should make contact with a newly diagnosed individual promptly, either by telephone or face to face, to offer an introduction, check the person's understanding, and invite any immediate questions relating to the new diagnosis and medication. If this initial contact is by telephone, it should be followed by a face-to-face consultation where the PDNS can assess the individual's level of understanding relating to the diagnosis, correct any misunderstandings, and answer questions. It is important to promote a feeling of optimism and try to make sure that the person leaves the consultation feeling more positive about the future with Parkinson's. During this consultation, an assessment can be made of the level of acceptance of the diagnosis. If distress caused by the diagnosis is excessive or interferes with the individual's relationships or work performance, the person may have an adjustment disorder. Usually this can be managed by correcting misunderstandings about the condition, reassuring the person about sources of help and support, and encouraging him or her to draw on the existing social networks. Relaxation therapy and cognitive behavioural therapy (CBT) can also be helpful. In some services, occupational therapists (OTs) provide this kind of support. In some cases, referral to a clinical psychologist is needed. Individuals differ in the amount of information they want in relation to prognosis, how symptoms will progress over time, the effect of Parkinson's on life expectancy, and the likelihood of significant disability. Building up good rapport, so that the individual feels comfortable raising these questions if desired, is very important. Discussions in this regard should be led by the individual.

Symptom review

Those commenced on medication may notice an improvement in movement, dexterity, and the ability to carry out day-to-day activities; they may feel more like their old selves, find that their thinking is clearer or sharper, notice an improvement in tremor, or feel steadier on their feet. Many notice a significant improvement, but others (especially if diagnosed very early, with few deficits) do not. If there is are significant deficits at diagnosis without discernible benefit from medication, this should be reported back to the diagnosing clinician.

Medication concordance

It is important to check that any planned medication has in fact been prescribed and is being taken correctly. It is worth spending time to make sure that the individual has a good understanding of the medication regimen. Checking to see whether medication led to an improvement in symptoms is helpful, as a good response is in keeping with a diagnosis of Parkinson's.

Medication side effects

If present, side effects are often reported voluntarily. Non-etheless, the PDNS should ask specifically about the side effects listed in Table 5.3.

Taking the time, at this point, to discuss impulsive and compulsive behaviours in detail is key to reducing the risk of significant problems in this regard in the future. With the individual's permission, it is helpful to include the caregiver in these discussions. The caregiver can help monitor for behavioural change. The individual and caregiver should be advised that the emergence of impulsive behaviours is likely to be medication-related and should be reported to the Parkinson's specialist or PDNS.

Driving

The PDNS should check if the individual drives and should reinforce driving advice, as mentioned earlier.

TABLE 5.3 Common adverse effects of Parkinson's medications
Nausea
Excessive daytime sleepiness
Dizziness or light-headedness on standing
Confusion
Hallucinations
Behavioural change
Increased spending
Increased sexual appetite
Gambling
Compulsive eating
Obsessive interest in hobbies

Establishing rapport

This initial consultation with a newly diagnosed individual is the start of what will hopefully be a long and fruitful therapeutic relationship. It is important to begin to build a trusting relationship, to be honest about what Parkinson's means, but also promote optimism for the person's future with Parkinson's. Individuals often want to know what they can do to help themselves. Advice regarding exercise is very important, along with tips for healthy eating and good hydration. Advice on remaining both physically and mentally active and socially engaged can be helpful.

Education

Signposting to good-quality information, especially that available from Parkinson's charities (Parkinson's UK, the Parkinson's Foundation, the European Parkinson's Disease Association) and local support groups is also very important. The education of a newly diagnosed individual enables self-management in the future, and it is the responsibility of all members of the MDT to deliver education at every consultation. An education programme can further support the goal of self-management. Such group education programmes are an efficient use of heath professionals' time and, by bringing newly diagnosed individuals together, facilitate the development of peer support networks. The PDNS should encourage newly diagnosed individuals to attend the programme. If no programme exists locally, the PDNS will be just the person to set it up. (See Chapter 3 for what to include.)

Referral to the multidisciplinary team

The PDNS should offer early referral to the MDT. The potential benefits of this include expert advice on keeping active; a personal exercise prescription; and early detection of problems with posture, gait, mood, cognition, speech, and activities of daily living. The Parkinson's MDT can help the individual to get the very best from life with Parkinson's.

Physiotherapy

Exercise and physical activity

Different types of exercises are recommended in Parkinson's, including

- Aerobic exercise
- Resistance training for strength
- Balance exercises for posture and the prevention of falls

A meta-analysis by Uhrbrand and colleagues (2015) of controlled studies of intensive exercise therapy in Parkinson's has shown there is strong evidence that resistance training improves muscle strength; moderate evidence that endurance training improves cardiovascular fitness; and an indication that all exercise therapies may benefit balance, gait and motor function (Unified Parkinson Disease Rating Scale). Other systematic reviews have shown that aerobic exercise is immediately beneficial for balance, gait and motor function, although evidence of more prolonged benefit will require randomised controlled trials (Shu et al., 2014).

It has been proposed that early intensive exercise may have a protective benefit, but this will require further research and longer-term follow-up. The MDS task force has highlighted methodologic deficiencies in these studies (Fox et al., 2018). Importantly, a study of an exercise regimen in Parkinson's to target risk factors for falls showed no overall reduction in falls in the intervention group. In the lower severity group, however, there were significantly fewer falls, whereas in the higher severity group there was a trend to have more falls. This supports benefit from these physical exercises at the diagnosis phase of Parkinson's (Canning et al., 2015) but caution at later stages of physical disability.

Physical activity is also likely to have benefits in other domains including attention, cognition, sleep, fatigue and mental well-being. Falling in Parkinson's is further discussed in Chapter 10 and exercise in Chapter 11.

In early Parkinson's, vigourous exercise is recommended, such as running, cycling or gym classes, including circuit training; this should be sufficient for the participant to feel hot and sweaty and to cause a rise in the heart and respiratory rates. A recommended minimum is 2.5 hours per week.

Assessment and intervention

The physiotherapist can provide specialist assessment of physical needs, a tailored regimen to achieve the required level of fitness, assistance in motivation and advice on continuing self-exercising.

At initial assessment, an important question to ask the individual is "what is your biggest problem?" Understanding an individual's perspective is crucial for shared goal setting. The initial assessment should also ascertain baseline measurements of gait, balance, transfers, and physical function.

Even in the early stages of Parkinson's, changes in posture may be noted. These can be due to a combination of factors, including rigidity and disruption of the brain's automatic processes, which remind the individual of the upright midline posture. The individual's shoulders may become slightly stooped and the chin protracted without the individual's awareness. The tragus-to-wall (Heuft-Dorenbosch et al., 2004) measure can be used as a baseline to give the individual an awareness of the extent of the problem. Exercises and stretches can often improve posture, and seeing the improvement, measured in centimeters from the wall, can encourage and motivate the individual to continue with an exercise programme. Signposting to information and exercise opportunities is important; the Parkinson's Foundation fact sheet on posture includes exercises and tips for maintaining and improving posture. There may also be local (or online) exercise groups, such as Pilates, that the individual can be encouraged to join.

Once goals have been agreed on, intervention by the therapist may include one-on-one exercise programmes or groups such as high-intensity interval training, tai chi or dance. Education is an important aspect of intervention for both the individual with Parkinson's and the caregiver, as it can facilitate autonomy and adjustment. This may be offered by the MDT, or there may be an opportunity to attend an in-person or online programme run by Parkinson's UK locally.

Occupational therapy

Initial assessment

Initial assessment by an OT aims to gain a full and comprehensive picture of the individual's medical history, current symptoms, psychological health, and social and work situations.

The Canadian Occupational Performance Measure is a suitable tool for use in the Parkinson's service. It is a well-evidenced structured interview that covers, self-care, domestic activities, leisure and productivity. In addition to this, to ensure that more specific issues relating to Parkinson's are covered, assessment should include

- Sleep history
- Upper limb function, including use of cutlery and handwriting
- Mood (depression and anxiety)
- Cognition
- Sexual dysfunction (if not covered by the PDNS)

Upper limb assessment may include a nine-hole peg test to measure speed and accuracy, grip strength measurement, and a handwriting assessment to identify micrographia.

Comprehensive assessment of cognition and mood should be completed. The prevalence of psychiatric symptoms exceeds 60% even in Hoehn-Yahr stage 1 (early stage) Parkinson's (Barone et al., 2009). Suitable screening tools for depression in Parkinson's include the Beck Depression Inventory, Hospital Anxiety and Depression Scale, and Geriatric Depression Scale (Schrag et al., 2007).

There are a number of assessments to choose from for cognitive screening. The Montreal Cognitive Assessment has been used widely but there are issues currently with authority and training to use it. The Mini-Mental State Examination is quick to complete but does not adequately assess visuospatial skills and executive function. Addenbrooke's Cognitive Examination, version 3, is a suitable tool but takes longer than the Montreal Cognitive Assessment to complete.

Education

Some explanation, in simple terms, of the function of the basal ganglia can help the person with Parkinson's better understand the symptoms. For example, it might be useful for such a person to think of the basal ganglia as an autopilot. When the autopilot is broken, the person must pay more attention to the task at hand. This might explain why people with Parkinson's struggle to multitask. Moreover, paying attention all the time is tiring, so they may experience fatigue. It is helpful for individuals with Parkinson's and their caregivers to understand that cognitive processing is slowed, so it may take a little longer to respond to questions and complete tasks. Attention, concentration, and the ability to learn new things might also be affected. Planning, organisation and sequencing are required for any movement or activity. When skills such as problem solving and multitasking are required, activities can become difficult.

Cognitive strategies

Cognitive strategies can be taught at this stage, encouraging individuals to use the STOP, THINK, PLAN, DO strategy when they find that they are struggling to manage any activity (Table 5.4). This could involve tying shoelaces or trying to get out of a chair. Problems typically occur when a person is multitasking and not focusing on the task at hand or when anxiety supervenes.

Inability to manage everyday activities normally might lead to anxiety, which worsens function further. Palpitations linked to anxiety can be frightening. Relaxation techniques and CBT may be useful.

The OT assesses mood and discusses the practical aspects of managing the condition. It is important to make sure that the condition and symptoms are fully explained in order to reduce anxiety. Any identified low mood needs to be addressed, discussing possible triggers for both anxiety and depression.

TABLE 5.4 "Stop, think, plan, do" cognitive strategy

STOP	As soon as the activity is proving difficult, stop and take a breath. Continuing to try will only cause more anxiety.
THINK	Work out the end aim; for example tying a shoelace or going to the bathroom.
PLAN	Plan how to complete the activity, identify stages of the activity and identify strategies for transfers.
DO	Complete the activity with full focused attention.

The OT can initiate conversations to assist with this adjustment but, if necessary, the neuropsychologist and OT can work together to look at specific symptoms.

Self-management training

Even at this early stage of the condition, the concept of self-management can be introduced. This is about giving individuals the autonomy to manage their own condition throughout its course. The aim is to promote a positive attitude toward daily activities that enhances function. Self-management skills reduce anxiety and engender confidence in seeking support. By providing education and advice early, the MDT can help individuals to take responsibility for their condition and be prepared for changes in symptoms.

Speech and language therapy

Issues with speech are common in Parkinson's, including low speech volume (hypophonia), lack of speech intonation (dysprosody), and articulation difficulty (dysarthria), which can affect intelligibility and consequently communication. Referral to a specialist speech and language therapist is recommended, and interventions such as Lee Silverman Voice Therapy (LSVT) can be very beneficial. LSVT is an intensive speech therapy regimen with four 1-hour SLT sessions per week for 4 consecutive weeks. The treatment focuses on sensory feedback, readjusting the individuals' perception of how loud other people find their speech, and reinforcing that louder speech is more audible for communication partners. On the completion of therapy, participants are encouraged to continue daily short 10- to 15-minute sessions of voice projection practice using the LSVT protocol. An evidence-based review of randomised controlled trials of LSVT has shown improvement in the vocal sound pressure level and also benefit in other outcomes including speech rate, prosody, voice quality, intelligibility, vocal cord movements, swallowing, and facial expression (Mahler et al., 2015).

Top tips for the diagnostic stage

1. The following NMSs may precede motor symptoms:
   a. REM sleep behaviour disorder
   b. Anosmia
   c. Autonomic symptoms (constipation, erectile dysfunction)
   d. Depression

2. NMS enquiry may lead to an earlier and more accurate diagnosis of Parkinson's.

3. MDS criteria for a diagnosis require
   a. Bradykinesia and either rest tremor or rigidity (or both)
   b. Supportive features such as anosmia, good response to dopaminergic therapy, levodopa-induced dyskinesia
   c. Absence of absolute exclusion criteria such cerebellar signs, downward gaze palsy, purely lower limb Parkinsonism for 3 years, normal functional imaging

4. A cognitive task makes a true Parkinson's tremor more obvious but lessens functional tremor.

5. Leg tremor is less common in essential tremor than in Parkinson's.

6. Comorbidities such as stroke or arthritis may impair movement and confound the assessment of bradykinesia.

7. On functional imaging, a false-negative DaTSCAN may occur early in the condition; false-positive DaTSCANs may be due to technical issues or comorbidity, particularly lacunar infarction.

8. If symptoms are minimal and not affecting function, drug therapy can be deferred.

9. If there is functional impairment, initial drug therapy should be levodopa.

10. Early referral for multidisciplinary assessment can help to promote self-management skills, establish good exercise habits, and identify mood, cognitive, and functional issues.

11. All newly diagnosed individuals should be referred to the PDNS, who acts as a point of contact and provides post-diagnostic counselling.

12. All members of the MDT should be alert to the possibility of an adjustment disorder. Individuals should be encouraged to make use of their social networks for support. Signposting to peer support groups, CBT and relaxation therapy may help.

13. All Parkinson's services should have a self-management and education programme that includes recommendations on having a will and power of attorney.

Abbreviations: CBT, cognitive behavioural therapy; MDS, Movement Disorder Society; MDT, multidisciplinary team; NMS, non-motor symptom; PDNS, Parkinson's disease nurse specialist; REM, rapid eye movement

References

Adams-Carr, K. L., Bestwick, J. P., Shribman, S., Lees, A., Schrag, A., & Noyce, A. J. (2016). Constipation preceding Parkinson's disease: a systematic review and meta-analysis. *Journal of Neurology, Neurosurgery, and Psychiatry, 87*(7), 710–716.

Barone, P., Antonini, A., Colosimo, C., Marconi, R., Morgante, L., Avarello, T. P., et al. (2009). The PRIAMO study: a multicentre assessment of nonmotor symptoms and their impact on quality of life in Parkinson's disease. *Movement Disorders, 24*(11), 1641–1649.

Braak, H., Bohl, J. R., Muller, C. M., Rub, U., de Vos, R. A., & Del Tredici, K. (2006). Stanley Fahn Lecture 2005: the staging procedure for the inclusion body pathology associated with sporadic Parkinson's disease reconsidered. *Movement Disorders, 21*(12), 2042–2051.

Canning, C. G., Sherrington, C., Lord, S. R., Close, J. C., Heritier, S., Heller, G. Z., et al. (2015). Exercise for falls prevention in Parkinson's disease: a randomised controlled trial. *Neurology, 84*(3), 304–312.

Chen, H., Shrestha, S., Huang, X., Jain, S., Guo, X., Tranah, G. J., et al. (2017). Olfaction and incident Parkinson disease in US white and black older adults. *Neurology, 89*(14), 1441–1447.

Cohen, O., Pullman, S., Jurewicz, E., Watner, D., & Louis, E. D. (2003). Rest tremor in patients with essential tremor: prevalence, clinical correlates, and electrophysiologic characteristics. *Archives of Neurology, 60*(3), 405–410.

Deuschl, G. (2003). Dystonic tremor. *Revue neurologique (Paris), 159*(10 Pt 1), 900–905.

Erro, R., Schneider, S. A., Stamelou, M., Quinn, N. P., & Bhatia, K. P. (2016). What do patients with scans without evidence of dopaminergic deficit (SWEDD) have? New evidence and continuing controversies. *Journal of Neurology, Neurosurgery, and Psychiatry, 87*(3), 319–323.

Fox, S. H., Katzenschlager, R., Lim, S. Y., Barton, B., de Bie, R. M. A., Seppi, K., et al. (2018). International Parkinson and movement disorder society evidence-based medicine review: update on treatments for the motor symptoms of Parkinson's disease. *Movement Disorders, 33*(8), 1248–1266.

Galbraith, K. (2016). *Diagnostic accuracy of DaTSCAN in Parkinson's and clinically uncertain parkinsonism.* Available at https://www.parkinsons.org.uk/sites/default/files/2017-07/RD2734 DaTCAT accuracy.pdf.

Gao, X., Chen, H., Schwarzschild, M. A., Glasser, D. B., Logroscino, G., Rimm, E. B., et al. (2007). Erectile function and risk of Parkinson's disease. *Amarican Journal of Epidemiology, 166*(12), 1446–1450.

Heuft-Dorenbosch, L., Vosse, D., Landewe, R., Spoorenberg, A., Dougados, M., Mielants, H., et al. (2004). Measurement of spinal mobility in ankylosing spondylitis: comparison of occiput-to-wall and tragus-to-wall distance. *Journal of Rheumatology, 31*(9), 1779–1784.

Iranzo, A., Santamaria, J., Valldeoriola, F., Serradell, M., Salamero, M., Gaig, C., et al. (2017). Dopamine transporter imaging deficit predicts early transition to synucleinopathy in idiopathic rapid eye movement sleep behaviour disorder. *Annals of Neurology, 82*(3), 419–428.

Ishihara, L., & Brayne, C. (2006). A systematic review of depression and mental illness preceding Parkinson's disease. *Acta Neurologica Scandinavica, 113*(4), 211–220.

Jennings, D., Siderowf, A., Stern, M., Seibyl, J., Eberly, S., Oakes, D., et al. (2014). Imaging prodromal Parkinson disease: the Parkinson Associated Risk Syndrome Study. *Neurology, 83*(19), 1739–1746.

Mahler, L. A., Ramig, L. O., & Fox, C. (2015). Evidence-based treatment of voice and speech disorders in Parkinson disease. *Current Opinion in Otolaryngology & Head and Neck Surgery, 23*(3), 209–215.

Martinez-Martin, P., Schapira, A. H., Stocchi, F., Sethi, K., Odin, P., MacPhee, G., et al. (2007). Prevalence of nonmotor symptoms in Parkinson's disease in an international setting: study using nonmotor symptoms questionnaire in 545 patients. *Movement Disorders, 22*(11), 1623–1629.

Noyce, A. J., R'Bibo, L., Peress, L., Bestwick, J. P., Adams-Carr, K. L., Mencacci, N. E., et al. (2017). PREDICT-PD: an online approach to prospectively identify risk indicators of Parkinson's disease. *Movement Disorders, 32*(2), 219–226.

Olson, E. J., Boeve, B. F., & Silber, M. H. (2000). Rapid eye movement sleep behaviour disorder: demographic, clinical and laboratory findings in 93 cases. *Brain*, *123*(Pt 2), 331–339.

Palma, J. A., & Kaufmann, H. (2014). Autonomic disorders predicting Parkinson's disease. *Parkinsonism and Related Disorders*, *20*(Suppl 1), S94–S98.

Parkinson's Foundation. *Posture and Parkinson's*. Retrieved November 20, 2020, from https://www.parkinson.org/sites/default/files/attachments/Posture_and_Parkinsons.pdf.

Parkinson's Foundation. *Stages of Adjustment to Parkinson's*. Retrieved November 19, 2020, from https://www.parkinson.org/sites/default/files/Stages of Adjustment to Parkinson%27s.pdf.

Postuma, R. B., Berg, D., Stern, M., Poewe, W., Olanow, C. W., Oertel, W., et al. (2015). MDS clinical diagnostic criteria for Parkinson's disease. *Movement Disorders*, *30*(12), 1591–1601.

Romenets, S. R., Wolfson, C., Galatas, C., Pelletier, A., Altman, R., Wadup, L., et al. (2012). Validation of the non-motor symptoms questionnaire (NMS-Quest). *Parkinsonism and Related Disorders*, *18*(1), 54–58.

Ross, G. W., Abbott, R. D., Petrovitch, H., Tanner, C. M., & White, L. R. (2012). Pre-motor features of Parkinson's disease: the Honolulu-Asia Aging Study experience. *Parkinsonism and Related Disorders*, *18*(Suppl 1), S199–S202.

Ross, G. W., Petrovitch, H., Abbott, R. D., Tanner, C. M., Popper, J., Masaki, K., et al. (2008). Association of olfactory dysfunction with risk for future Parkinson's disease. *Annals of Neurology*, *63*(2), 167–173.

Roze, E., Coelho-Braga, M. C., Gayraud, D., Legrand, A. P., Trocello, J. M., Fenelon, G., et al. (2006). Head tremor in Parkinson's disease. *Movement Disorders*, *21*(8), 1245–1248.

Schrag, A., Barone, P., Brown, R. G., Leentjens, A. F., McDonald, W. M., Starkstein, S., et al. (2007). Depression rating scales in Parkinson's disease: critique and recommendations. *Movement Disorders*, *22*(8), 1077–1092.

Shu, H. F., Yang, T., Yu, S. X., Huang, H. D., Jiang, L. L., Gu, J. W., et al. (2014). Aerobic exercise for Parkinson's disease: a systematic review and meta-analysis of randomised controlled trials. *PLoS ONE*, *9*(7), e100503.

Sommer, U., Hummel, T., Cormann, K., Mueller, A., Frasnelli, J., Kropp, J., et al. (2004). Detection of presymptomatic Parkinson's disease: combining smell tests, transcranial sonography, and SPECT. *Movement Disorders*, *19*(10), 1196–1202.

Thompson, P. D. (2012). Frontal lobe ataxia. *Handbook of Clinical Neurology*, *103*, 619–622.

Uhrbrand, A., Stenager, E., Pedersen, M. S., & Dalgas, U. (2015). Parkinson's disease and intensive exercise therapy: a systematic review and meta-analysis of randomised controlled trials. *Journal of Neurological Science*, *353*(1–2), 9–19.

Chapter 6

Multidisciplinary Work in the Maintenance Stage

Fiona Lindop, Lisa Brown, Andrew Paget, Jess Marsh, Clare Johnson, Caroline Bartliff and Rob Skelly

Chapter outline

Introduction

The maintenance stage of Parkinson's begins when the diagnosis is established and accepted. It is a period of relative stability; but as time passes, a variety of both motor and non-motor symptoms (NMSs), may be encountered (see Fig. 6.1). It is often the NMSs that are the most burdensome.

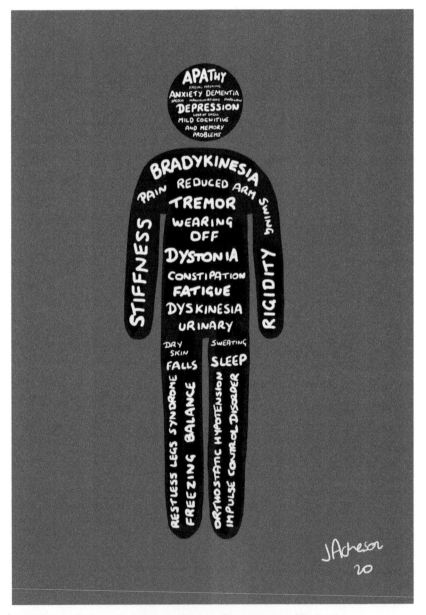

FIGURE 6.1   Parkinson's symptoms. *Figure used by permission of Dr. J. Acheson.*

The impact of Parkinson's on the individual depends not just on Parkinson's-related impairments but on comorbidities as well as environmental and social factors. The condition may affect activities of daily living (ADLs), performance at work, and work-life balance. Individuals will benefit from assessment by a multidisciplinary team (MDT), whose focus is the promotion of independence, management of symptoms and maintenance of health and well-being. Such an assessment may identify targets for intervention and education, which can be key to successful self-management. It may take time for an individual to adjust to this diagnosis, and further adjustments may be needed as the condition progresses. Physiotherapists, occupational therapists (OTs), Parkinson's disease nurse specialists (PDNSs), speech and language therapists (SLTs), psychologists and physicians all have a part to play in supporting the individual with Parkinson's, enabling him or her to participate fully in work and social activities and achieve the best possible quality of life (QoL). This chapter provides an overview of the problems encountered in the maintenance stage and describes an integrated MDT approach to their management.

Motor symptoms in the maintenance stage

The motor signs of Parkinson's are rest tremor, bradykinesia (poverty of movement) and rigidity (muscle stiffness). A combination of these signs may cause a variety of problems as the condition progresses. Reduced dexterity, for example, can lead to difficulty managing cutlery, illegible handwriting or struggling with buttons on clothing. Tasks that require repetition of a movement, such as brushing one's teeth or beating eggs, may be particularly difficult. Individuals may be independent in all ADLs but report "slowing down," taking longer to get washed and dressed. Often, they report weakness (but usually there is no objective muscle weakness) and may notice changes in gait, including, for some, the onset of freezing of gait (FOG). Posture may become more flexed and turning over in bed at night may be difficult. The MDT can offer interventions to address these problems.

Symptoms that are due to stiffness and bradykinesia often improve with dopaminergic treatments (that stimulate the dopamine system) such as levodopa (L-dopa). As time passes, owing to the continued loss of striatal dopamine, motor symptoms may worsen and an increase in medication may be necessary. Therapy interventions should be considered alongside changes to medication. Indeed, intensive multidisciplinary rehabilitation may enable the reduction of dopaminergic medications (Ferrazzoli et al., 2018). When worsening function prompts consideration of a medication increase, it is important to consider whether "wearing off" (a worsening of symptoms that occurs before the next medication dose is due) is present, as this will influence drug strategy: for example, more frequent L-dopa dosing or the use of long-acting treatments such as dopamine agonists and monoamine oxidase inhibitors. The drug management of "wearing off" is covered in Chapter 7. Before increasing a person's medication, it is essential to inquire about side effects and to be mindful that the higher the L-dopa dose, the greater the risk of subsequent motor side effects such as motor fluctuations and dyskinesia. In general, we try not to exceed 600 mg/d of L-dopa, but it is sometimes necessary to use more than this.

Interventions from therapists can help to limit drug increases by suggesting alternative solutions to problems and by improving fitness and general conditioning. For example, practicing difficult transfers may improve performance on these tasks. An integrated multidisciplinary approach to problems can enable the individual to achieve the best outcome.

Tremor

The characteristics of tremor are described in Chapter 5. Tremor can be a significant symptom and may have a negative impact on the individual's QoL. It is often resistant to dopaminergic therapy, and an escalation of medication can lead to unwanted side effects (e.g., dyskinesia) without improving the tremor. Embarrassment about tremor can increase anxiety and limit social interactions and work-related activities.

The MDT can offer strategies, such as manipulating a small object in the hand (coin, keys), or applying pressure through the affected limb: this can temporarily halt the tremor. Weighted cutlery for mealtimes and a weighted pen for handwriting can be beneficial. The OT can help the individual understand what situations are likely to increase the tremor and how to reduce potentially stressful situations. Advance planning and adjustments should be considered. For example, an individual can be advised to try breathing exercises before delivering a work presentation, to use the tremor-affected hand during the presentation, and to speak slowly throughout. Therapists can teach upper limb exercises, including large-amplitude movements to improve strength and dexterity and to reduce tremor. Five quick finger flicks, with fully extended stretches from shoulders to fingertips, can encourage better movement and a more relaxed limb. Flexing the hand by squeezing a ball is not advised, as it can encourage a flexor pattern to evolve.

If tremor remains a significant problem despite medication changes and therapy input, referral for neurosurgical intervention should be considered. Thalamic deep brain stimulation can be very effective, and focussed ultrasound treatments are also being used.

Freezing of gait

Gait changes include reduced or absent arm swing, variable step length, freezing and difficulty with turning. These changes may be more pronounced when the person is dual tasking, such as walking and talking or walking and carrying. Freezing of gait (FOG) can be defined as "a brief, episodic absence or marked reduction of forward progression of the feet despite the intention to walk" (Bloem et al., 2004); the individual will often feel that his or her feet have been "glued to the floor." FOG can be unpredictable, lasting from a few seconds to several minutes. It can lead to heightened anxiety, loss of confidence, and reduced activities outside the home, such as shopping or going to a restaurant. It is important to ascertain when and where FOG occurs and to establish whether FOG is "on freezing" or "off freezing." "On freezing" occurs when medication is optimal, whereas "off freezing" can occur when medication is wearing off; it may respond to a change in medication. "On freezing" is less responsive to medication changes; therefore non-pharmacological interventions may be indicated.

FOG is often preceded by festination, whereby the individual involuntarily takes short, increasingly fast steps that can lead to walking on tiptoes. This is accompanied by flexion at the trunk, hips, and knees. FOG can reduce independence, mobility, and QoL and increase the risk of falling (Okuma et al., 2018). It can occur in many circumstances, such as:

- Walking in a straight line
- Approaching a destination, such as a chair
- Turning
- Walking through a doorway
- Initiating a first step
- Attempting to recommence walking after stopping

There is now preliminary evidence for distinct phenotypes within FOG: asymmetric motor, anxious and sensory-attention types (Ehgoetz Martens et al., 2018). The "cross-talk model" provides a helpful framework for understanding these profiles (Lewis & Barker, 2009). This suggests that the processing of information from cognitive, motor, and limbic pathways occurs in a parallel and integrated way across the circuits of the basal ganglia, modulated by striatal dopamine. Where striatal dopamine is already depleted, inputs from each of these circuits compete for the available dopamine and, in certain situations, the striatum's processing capacity can become overloaded, resulting in faulty output from the relevant motor nuclei and producing gait changes and potentially FOG (Lewis & Barker, 2009). Reflecting the multiple pathways involved, FOG benefits from a multidisciplinary perspective.

Assessment and intervention by the multidisciplinary team

The assessment of FOG can be difficult owing to the episodic nature of the problem; common triggers experienced at home may not be replicated in a clinical setting. Tools to measure of severity include the Movement Disorders Society - Unified Parkinson's Disease Rating Scale (MDS-UPDRS) (Goetz et al., 2008) or the New Freezing of Gait Questionnaire (Nieuwboer et al., 2009). A comprehensive assessment would include cognitive testing and measures of affect (emotion and mood) in addition to spatiotemporal gait parameters (step and stride length, cadence, speed) as well as a detailed clinical history. Typically, intervention comprises the optimisation of medication (Schaafsma et al., 2003) and use of cues (visual or auditory). Detailed multidisciplinary assessment allows for more robust and targeted interventions, such as cognitive training (Walton et al., 2018), techniques for the management of anxiety (Paget, 2019), and physical training (Canning et al., 2015), which have evidenced longer-lasting effects (Delgado-Alvarado et al., 2020). The complex and overlapping nature of FOG lends itself well to collaborative work that supports individually tailored interventions—for example, by involving neuropsychologists who can provide support when anxiety (e.g., fear of falling) or cognitive difficulties are interfering with physical training interventions. A combination of various approaches is likely to have a greater impact on the management of FOG.

FOG increases the risk of falling. It is important for the therapists to identify when and where FOG occurs so as to be able to offer the appropriate cue or strategy. Teaching individuals to recognise when festination begins may enable them to avoid progressing to FOG. Adopting "marching" steps (an attentional cue) or employing a wider arc can reduce FOG on turning. Visual cues, such as by using a laser pen, may also help. Further examples of cueing strategy are shown in Table 6.1.

Non-motor symptoms

NMSs can be more troublesome than motor symptoms; individuals may experience several NMSs simultaneously. It is helpful to screen for NMSs. The NMS questionnaire (NMSQuest), a self-completion tool with 30 items, is suitable for annual screening (Chaudhuri et al., 2006) and can be downloaded from the Parkinson's UK website. Table 6.2 lists the main NMSs typically associated with Parkinson's. This section covers the MDT's management of specific NMSs.

Behavioural and cognitive symptoms

Psychiatric symptoms, particularly low mood and anxiety, are common in Parkinson's and are attributed to both psychological factors (such as adjustment to the condition) and biochemical factors (neurodegenerative endogenous mono-amine depletion).

Depression

Studies have consistently shown depression to be a major determinant of adverse QoL in Parkinson's. Diagnostic criteria used in relation to the general population (e.g., the *Diagnostic and Statistical Manual of Mental Disorders*, 5th ed. [DSM-V]) can be applied to Parkinson's or adapted for such use. DSM-V criteria for depression are either low mood or reduced interest or pleasure in most activities together with a combination of other symptoms. These include weight change, insomnia or hypersomnia, slowing of thought or physical

TABLE 6.1 Suggested mobility cueing strategies

Problem	Cues/ strategies type	Examples
Open walkway freezing	Auditory	Metronome or music (four beats in bar music works best).
Gait initiation failure	Attentional	Imagining taking a big step then taking a big step.
	Proprioceptive	Weight transference (rocking), from foot to foot before attempting first step *or* taking small step backward before attempting first step.
	Visual	Laser pen/laser shoes/laser walking aid.
	Auditory	Another person saying "big steps" loudly and firmly.
Doorway freezing	Visual	Place a bright, sticky note at the individual's eye level on the wall of room beyond the doorway. The individual can then focus on the sticky note while approaching and going through doorway.
Destination freezing	Attentional	Individuals concentrate on big steps as they approach their destination, including marching steps for any turning required.
	Visual	Place markers (sticky tape) on the floor at the destination. As the individual approaches, he or she steps on the markers until the destination is reached.
Freezing of gait during turning	Attentional	The individual recites a poem or beats a rhythm in his or her head and steps in time to this. Or the individual practises walking around a stationary person and then, without the person there, walks around an imaginary person, maintaining a wider arc for turning.
	Visual	Use a walking aid with integral laser *or*, for an area where frequent turning is required such as bathroom or kitchen, place sticky notes on an imaginary clock face on the floor in the area where the turn is required, placing markers at 12, 6, 3, and 9 o'clock (extra markers may be required between these points). The individual then steps on the sticky notes while making the turn. The sticky notes can be replaced with sticky tape when the correct positioning has been ascertained.

TABLE 6.2 Non-motor symptoms in Parkinson's

Emotion, behaviour and thinking symptoms	Depression Anxiety Apathy Psychosis Hallucinations Mild cognitive impairment and dementia
Sleep-related symptoms	Rapid-eye-movement sleep behaviour disorder (i.e., the acting out of dreams) Excessive daytime somnolence (sleepiness) Insomnia
Autonomic dysfunction	Constipation Urinary symptoms (e.g., urgency, frequency) Sexual dysfunction Swallowing problems and drooling Delayed gastric emptying leading to nausea and erratic absorption of medication Postural hypotension Hyperhidrosis (excessive sweating) Heat/cold intolerance
Abnormal sensation	Pain Anosmia
Miscellaneous	Fatigue Seborrhaeic dermatitis

movement, fatigue, feelings of worthlessness or inappropriate guilt, impaired concentration or indecisiveness and thoughts of death or suicide. Depression in the context of Parkinson's is best understood as a continuum; a person may experience low mood and feelings associated with depression but not meet criteria for a clinical diagnosis.

Cognitive behavioural therapy (CBT) as well as mindfulness and relaxation—which can be accessed at Improving Access to Psychological Therapies (IAPT) and private providers—may have a role in the management of depression in Parkinson's. In CBT, individuals are taught to recognise and challenge negative thoughts and behavioural responses. CBT for depressive symptoms in Parkinson's has shown benefit in controlled clinical trials (Dobkin et al., 2019). CBT delivered by telephone is also effective (Dobkin et al., 2020), as are group therapy and third-wave CBT (Zarotti et al., 2020).

The effect of psychiatric and dopaminergic medications for depressed mood in Parkinson's has been assessed by a Movement Disorder Society (MDS) evidence-based review (Seppi et al., 2019). For example, the tricyclic antidepressants (TCAs) nortriptyline and desipramine and the selective serotonin-norepinephrine reuptake inhibitor (SNRI) venlafaxine have shown benefit in well-designed studies. Surprisingly, evidence for many other commonly used antidepressants is insufficient for the Parkinson's population, although they may be efficacious. There are other considerations—such as the anticholinergic side effects of TCAs, particularly in the elderly, and the potential for SNRI medications to worsen tremor and, more rarely, Parkinsonism (Bharucha & Sethi, 2004).

Anxiety

General anxiety disorder is defined as excessive anxiety or apprehension associated with physiological symptoms including restlessness, fatigue, concentration difficulty, irritability, muscular tension and sleep disturbance. Clearly there is considerable overlap between the psychological and physical symptoms of depression and anxiety as well as with the symptoms of Parkinson's itself. Careful assessment is required, and formal psychology review may be indicated. Anxiety symptoms may worsen as Parkinson's medication wears off and may respond to adjustment in dopaminergic treatment.

CBT, mindfulness, and relaxation provide clinically useful frameworks to help anxiety management in Parkinson's (Zarotti et al., 2020). Strategies from Acceptance and Commitment Therapy (ACT), a third-wave CBT, have also been shown to increase emotional well-being for people with Parkinson's (Ghielen et al., 2017).

OT intervention for anxiety may include relaxation and breathing techniques such as square breathing (breathing in for a count of 4, pausing for 4, breathing out for 4 and pausing for 4). The tense-relax relaxation technique, progressively tensing and relaxing muscles throughout the body, can also enable individuals to recognise a relaxed state and aid sleep. A CBT approach can help the individual to challenge negative thinking by detailing specific situations and identifying their exact thoughts about it. There are four stages to this approach:

1. Identifying the physical symptoms (e.g., increased tremor)
2. Identifying the exact thought
3. Challenging the thought
4. Practising change of thought

Apathy

Apathy has been defined as a reduction in motivation and goal-directed behaviour. Around 40% of people with Parkinson's experience apathy (den Brok et al., 2015), which is associated with increased distress for caregivers (Leroi et al., 2012). In individuals with apathy, it is important to consider depression and dementia; but apathy can occur in the absence of these conditions. Treatment of underlying depression may lead to an improvement in apathy. Both serotonergic and dopaminergic deficits are linked to apathy (Schrag & Politis, 2016). Rivastigmine may be helpful (Seppi et al., 2019). The model proposed by Levy and Dubois (2006) can be helpful to the MDT in conceptualising the role of apathy in an individual's behaviour and his or her likely engagement in rehabilitation. This highlights three key subtypes of apathy: autoactivation (lack of activity or initiation of thought), emotional affective apathy (emotional indifference and blunting) and cognitive apathy (inability to expand on plans, to organise or pursue a plan). Parkinson's seems to be characterised by cognitive apathy and autoactivation apathy (Radakovic et al., 2018). The dimensional apathy scale (Radakovic et al., 2018), validated for use in Parkinson's, can be a helpful tool to clarify an individual's behaviour and provide appropriate psychoeducation to the individual and his or her loved ones.

As part of MDT intervention, the OT can offer advice regarding external motivation, including using a diary and planning activities into the day or week as well as supporting the caregiver to motivate the individual. Thinking about and exploring the rewards gained from completing an activity can support motivation. A person is more likely to complete an activity that offers a better reward, such as a pleasure-related or financial one.

Cognitive problems

Cognition may be impaired in more than a third of individuals at or soon after diagnosis (Foltynie et al., 2004). Mild cognitive impairment in Parkinson's (PD-MCI) occurs when:

- Gradual cognitive decline is observed by the individual, caregiver, or clinician
- There are objective deficits on formal cognitive testing
- These deficits are insufficient to affect the person's functional independence (Litvan et al., 2012)

Assessment tools include the Montreal Cognitive Assessment (MOCA) and Addenbrooke's Cognitive Evaluation III (ACE-III). Some 25% of people with Parkinson's have PD-MCI, and these are at greater risk of developing Parkinson's dementia (Aarsland et al., 2010). However, cognition can be understood as a spectrum and continuum of function in comparison to an individual's earlier level of function. An individual's ability to plan and organise complex tasks may be impaired, so therapists should assess this aspect of cognition and provide compensatory cognitive rehabilitation. Discussion about cognition is helpful to make sense of the subtle yet significant changes an individual may be experiencing. If cognitive function is affecting ADLs or the ability to work, the OT can explore these difficulties, advise on adaptation, and offer strategies. Management includes helping the individual to understand that executive skills are integral to carrying out everyday tasks such as getting dressed, and that these tasks require planning, organisation and sequencing as well as problem solving and multitasking skills. Stress and fatigue can affect cognitive skills, and education regarding this is essential.

Neuropsychological assessment is required if someone is reporting difficulties with cognition, but screening and assessments have not been sensitive enough to detect problems. A more thorough search would be especially necessary for a person in a high-functioning occupation. Cognitive decline sufficient to affect functional independence (dementia) is covered in Chapter 9.

Sleep

Rapid-eye-movement sleep behaviour disorder

RBD is characterised by the acting out of dreams, which may be violent, and there may be vigorous limb jerking or shouting during sleep. There is a risk of self-injury or injury to the bed partner. It occurs in 15% to 24% of individuals with Parkinson's and is linked to hallucinations, autonomic dysfunction, and more rapid cognitive decline (Kim et al., 2018). Clonazepam appears to be effective at reducing bothersome RBD, but it can increase the risk of falls. Melatonin may also be helpful, but robust evidence is lacking. The option of separate beds or bedrooms for the person with Parkinson's and the carer should be discussed.

Excessive daytime somnolence

Excessive daytime somnolence (EDS) is a risk factor for the development of Parkinson's and occurs in 20% to 60% of individuals with this condition. The prevalence of EDS increases over time and is more common in men. EDS can impair ADLs, QoL, social activity, and work effectiveness; it also increases the burden of the carer. EDS, particularly the sudden onset of sleep, may make driving unsafe. EDS can also lead to insomnia. EDS can be assessed using the Epworth Sleepiness Scale. EDS may be exacerbated by dopaminergic medication, particularly dopamine agonists. Other medications causing drowsiness include antipsychotic medications such as quetiapine and clozapine and drugs used to treat depression, RBD (clonazepam), and anxiety. Depression itself can cause drowsiness. It is important to identify and treat potential causes—for example, by reducing the dosage of a dopamine agonist. The National Institute for Health and Care Excellence (NICE) (2017) recommends that modafinil can be considered for the treatment of EDS. We suggest a trial of caffeine (coffee) but warn of urinary symptoms. Continuous positive airway pressure (CPAP) treatment is effective for those with obstructive sleep apoea. Bright-light therapy can be useful and is likely to be safe (Videnovic et al., 2017).

Insomnia

Insomnia may involve difficulty getting to sleep, maintaining sleep, or early-morning waking. Poor sleep during the night may affect wakefulness and performance at work during the day. Indeed, sleep quality has a significant effect on QoL. The prevalence of insomnia in Parkinson's was 37% in the PRIAMO (a multicentre study of Parkinson's and non-motor symptoms) study of Parkinson's

TABLE 6.3 Factors contributing to insomnia

Motor symptoms	Akinesia may cause the individual to wake to turn over.
	Early-morning foot and leg dystonia may wake an individual up.
	Tremor may start on waking during the night and impede a return to sleep.
Anxiety and depression	These may lead to insomnia.
	Depression probably has the greatest effect on sleep.
Other non-motor symptoms	Pain or nocturia may interfere with sleep.
Medications	There is a positive association between daily L-dopa dose and insomnia.
	Dopamine agonists, well known to cause daytime somnolence, may also cause insomnia.
	Other medications that might be alerting or activating include cholinesterase inhibitors (e.g., rivastigmine) and some antidepressants, including sertraline, fluoxetine and venlafaxine.
	Selegiline has amphetamine-like metabolites and may therefore reduce sleep, particularly if it is taken late in the day.
Comorbid sleep disorders	Restless legs syndrome, periodic leg movements of sleep, and sleep-disordered breathing (e.g., obstructive sleep apnoea) may interrupt sleep and reduce sleep hours and quality.
	When these conditions are suspected, referral to a sleep clinic can help confirm the diagnosis.

and NMSs (Barone et al., 2009). Disordered sleep maintenance appears to be the most common problem. Table 6.3 shows factors that may contribute to insomnia (Wallace et al., 2020).

In the treatment of insomnia, the factors in Table 6.3 should be considered and treated first. Members of the MDT should be able to offer advice on sleep hygiene (Table 6.4). CBT for insomnia (CBTi), is available online at www.sleepstation.org.uk/nhs-options/ or www.veterantraining.va.gov/insomnia and should be offered. There is evidence that physical exercise may be beneficial for sleep (Amara et al., 2020), as may tai chi and bright-light therapy. The latter (at 10,000 lux) for 1 hour twice during the day simulates sunlight and improves sleep quality in people with Parkinson's (Videnovic et al., 2017). Sedative medication is occasionally needed but should be used with caution in the elderly, as it may increase the risk of falls. Controlled-release melatonin at 2 mg may be helpful, and we sometimes prescribe zopiclone.

TABLE 6.4 Sleep hygiene: advice and strategies

General advice

Avoid worrying about sleeping.	Encourage a relaxed approach to managing sleep problems.
Make sure that the environment is comfortable.	The bedroom should be dark and not too warm or too cold. Make sure that the bed is comfortable.
Establish a sleep routine.	Go to bed and get up at the same time each day. (Circadian rhythm is habitual and responds better to routine.)
Avoid caffeine.	Avoid caffeine-containing tea or coffee later in the day.
Keep physically active.	Engage in moderate exercise, as it will improve sleep.
Avoid vigorous exercise before bedtime.	Avoid exercise for 2 hours before bedtime.

Struggling to get to sleep

Keep a sleep diary.	Helps identify patterns of sleep problems
Write issues or problems down.	This will prevent your thoughts from interrupting your sleep.
Create a "wind down" routine.	Avoid stimulant activities (e.g., working or using a computer). Engage in relaxing activities (e.g., bathing or using relaxation techniques).
Use distraction	Reading before going to sleep can be relaxing, but put your down book at least an hour before going to sleep. that Use a radio with a sleep function automatically switches off after a set time.

Waking during the night and being unable to get back to sleep

Don't have a clock at the bedside.	Looking at the time on waking can cause the circadian rhythm to wake you up at the same time every night.
If you are awake, do not remain in bed longer than 20 minutes.	Try to get back to sleep using relaxation therapy; if you are unable to do so after 20 minutes, move to a spare bed or quiet room to relax.
Avoid activities during night that would usually be done during the day.	This can cause the circadian rhythm to become habitual, waking you up to complete stimulating activities.
Take a nap every day.	Daytime sleep of up to 1 hour taken between 11 am & 3 pm reduces fatigue. If taken later, may affect sleep at night. Individuals sometimes wake during night due to being overtired.

Assessment and intervention from the OT can improve sleep quality, and a 24-hour sleep-pattern diary can point to the reasons for the impairment. The Parkinson's Disease Sleep Scale (PDSS) identifies symptoms contributing to disturbed sleep and provides an objective method for targeted therapeutic approaches for management of nocturnal symptoms (Chaudhuri et al., 2002). In particular, therapists can teach bed mobility strategies—for example, breaking the movement into its component parts.

Anxiety may prevent an individual from getting to sleep or returning to sleep if awakened. Fatigue may also affect sleep. The management of anxiety and fatigue may therefore help to improve sleep quality. It is advisable to back up verbal advice on sleep hygiene (see Table 6.4) with a printed information sheet.

Autonomic dysfunction

Constipation

Constipation should be considered in the presence of hard stools, straining, passage of two or fewer stools per week, or the sensation of incomplete emptying. It occurs frequently, affecting up to 50% of people with Parkinson's; its prevalence tends to increase with disease progression. There are two main mechanisms for constipation in Parkinson's: slow colonic transit and defecatory dysfunction. Normal bowel opening involves the coordinated contraction of abdominal and diaphragmatic muscles and relaxation of the puborectalis muscles and the anal sphincter. In Parkinson's, failure of the puborectalis to relax and contraction of the anal sphincter during attempts to open the bowels may lead to a sensation of outflow obstruction. Failure of the pelvic floor (puborectalis) to relax can be considered a form of dystonia and has been shown to improve with Parkinson's medications (Mukherjee et al., 2016).

Several other factors may contribute to constipation, including poor fluid intake, reduced activity levels, reduced food intake and effects of medications such as opioid analgesics and anticholinergics. Constipation can result in discomfort, affect ADLs, and cause psychological as well as social distress, consequently affecting QoL. It can delay gastric emptying, leading to impaired absorption of Parkinson's medication and poor control of Parkinson's symptoms. It is important to consider constipation as a potential factor when there is a sudden deterioration in Parkinson's symptoms.

Simple lifestyle modifications include increasing daily physical activity, adopting the optimal position for bowel opening (feet on small block to raise the knees toward the chest) and increasing the intake of fluid and fibre. All MDT members should be able to deliver simple dietary advice—for example, suggesting the consumption of at least five portions of fruit and vegetables per day. Natural remedies such as prune juice or syrup of figs can be helpful. If the stool is hard and pellet-like, then increased fluid intake should be advised; if it is soft but difficult to pass, a stimulant laxative such as senna along with an increased fibre intake can be helpful. For hard and large stools, increased fluid and fibre plus an osmotic laxative is advisable. For Parkinson's-related constipation, there is evidence for the safety and effectiveness of the following:

- Macrogol (Zangaglia et al., 2007)
- Fibre in conjunction with a probiotic (Barichella et al., 2016)
- Lubiprostone (Ondo et al., 2012)

Prucalopride may be effective, but trial evidence in Parkinson's is lacking. If defecatory dysfunction is suspected, dispersible L-dopa or apomorphine taken 30 minutes beforehand may help with bowel opening (Stocchi & Torti, 2014). Botulinum toxin can also be considered.

Urinary symptoms

Lower urinary tract symptoms (LUTS), are common in Parkinson's and are linked to reduced QoL and institutionalisation. In early Parkinson's, Hoehn-Yahr stage 1, the prevalence of LUTS is 43%, and it increases thereafter (Barone et al., 2009). Urinary incontinence is not common in the maintenance stage, appearing on average 12 years after a Parkinson's diagnosis. LUTS in people with Parkinson's could be due to Parkinson's or to comorbidity, such as stress incontinence in women and prostatic enlargement in men. Severe urinary symptoms should lead the clinician to consider multisystem atrophy as an alternative diagnosis.

The bladder stores urine until the person finds it convenient to pass the urine. Storage symptoms include urgency, frequency, nocturia (getting up at night to pass urine) and incontinence. Voiding symptoms include hesitancy, poor stream, straining, a sensation of incomplete emptying and terminal dribbling. Urodynamic studies show detrusor hyperactivity in more than half of newly diagnosed people with Parkinson's (McDonald et al., 2017). The neurological basis of LUTS in Parkinson's is failure of the basal ganglia to suppress micturition, but pathology in numerous other brain regions may contribute. The autonomic nervous system may also be affected. Nocturia is the most common urinary symptom reported in people with Parkinson's. When nocturia is present, the clinician should determine whether there is nocturnal polyuria, the passage of more than one-third of the daily urine between midnight and 8 am. Nocturnal polyuria may be a clue to a fluid-overload state with increased clearance of fluid at night, as, for example, in heart failure. In this case, a diuretic, timed to clear the excess fluid well before bedtime can help.

Assessment

Although the NMSQuest is an adequate screening tool for urinary symptoms in Parkinson's, a more detailed inquiry is needed when such symptoms are present. Although not validated in Parkinson's specifically, the International Prostate Symptom Score may be useful (Pavy-Le Traon et al., 2018). It is important to find out how bothersome the symptoms are, as a conservative management strategy can be adopted for symptoms that are not bothersome. A 3-day frequency-volume chart should be considered if the individual appears well motivated and has good cognition. For men with obstructive symptoms, renal function (urea and electrolytes) should be assessed and a prostate-specific antigen (PSA) test offered. An abdominal examination can show a distended bladder or suggest constipation. A digital rectal examination may give information about the size and nature of the prostate or may highlight constipation. A postvoid bladder scan should be available in the clinic. It can identify incomplete bladder emptying, which may contribute to urinary frequency and may indicate voiding difficulties.

Intervention

Lifestyle measures that may improve symptoms of detrusor hyperactivity include sufficient fluid intake (as concentrated urine may be more irritant to the bladder), treating constipation, and avoidance of drinks containing caffeine. Bladder training incorporates urge suppression, distraction, pelvic floor exercises and a personalised voiding schedule. Such bladder training can lead to subjective improvement in LUTS and reduce the number of voids per 24 hours (McDonald et al., 2020).

Dopaminergic medications may help LUTS in Parkinson's. Anticholinergic medication can be effective in treating detrusor instability in the general population, but side effects such as dry mouth, blurred vision, constipation, and confusion limit its appeal for people with Parkinson's, who already have a cholinergic deficit and a high risk of dementia. Selective M3 muscarinic receptor antagonists (e.g., solifenacin) and anticholinergics that have poor central nervous system penetration (e.g., trospium), have fewer side effects than oxybutynin, but we recommend against their use in people with cognitive impairment. The beta-3 adrenoceptor agonist mirabegron is a suitable alternative, reducing bladder contractility without anticholinergic side effects. Studies proving its efficacy in Parkinson's are awaited, but our experience of using this drug has been good. Desmopressin, an anti-diuretic hormone, reduces urine production by the kidneys and has been used under specialist supervision to treat troublesome nocturia. Clearly it should not be used in those with heart failure. It appears relatively safe and effective in the general population and could be considered for troublesome nocturia in Parkinson's, but concerns persist about hyponatraemia and use in the elderly.

In men with comorbid benign prostatic hyperplasia that causes voiding symptoms (and sometimes secondary detrusor instability), alpha blockers such as doxazosin or tamsulosin can reduce smooth muscle tone in the bladder neck, urethra, and prostate and improve urine flow. Alpha blockers may cause postural hypotension, so they should be used with caution. For prostatic enlargement, finasteride or other 5-α reductase inhibitors can be used to reduce prostate size. If medication is unsuccessful, surgical prostatectomy might be considered.

Drugs that reduce bladder contractility, such as anticholinergics, may cause acute retention of urine in those with high postvoid residual volumes. Double voiding can be tried, and intermittent self-catheterisation may be used. Referral to a urologist should be considered if troublesome voiding symptoms continue.

Intravesical botulinum toxin injection can be effective for detrusor hyperactivity, but the effect wears off after some months. Sometimes botulinum toxin treatment is complicated by urinary retention, in which case the individual will have to self-catheterise until the toxin has worn off. Transcutaneous tibial nerve stimulation (TTNS) is a form of neuromodulation that has been used safely and successfully to treat overactive bladder symptoms in people with multiple sclerosis. A trial of home-based TTNS in Parkinson's is under way (McClurg et al., 2020).

Sexual dysfunction

Sexual dysfunction in Parkinson's is linked to the depletion of central dopamine and to peripheral autonomic neuropathy. Both men and women with Parkinson's report sexual dissatisfaction more commonly than controls—the major determinants being age, severity of Parkinson's, and depression (Meco et al., 2008). Sexuality is a significant determinant of QoL for people with chronic conditions. Bronner et al. (2004) have reported that 41.9% of men and 28.2% of women ceased sexual activity after being diagnosed with Parkinson's. In Parkinson's, a healthy sex life is associated with overall life satisfaction (Moore et al., 2002).

Sex and intimacy are key issues that should be discussed and addressed as part of a Parkinson's consultation. When Parkinson's medications are prescribed, the risk of hypersexuality should be highlighted. The mention of hypersexuality offers an opportunity to discuss sex and intimacy more broadly.

For both the individual and his or her partner, their physical relationship may alter. Sex may become less or more important to them. Parkinson's can affect individuals' self-esteem, making them feel less attractive or desirable. Partners may struggle with their changing role and be so busy "caring for" that they forget to "care about" their loved one. All these factors can affect intimacy. It is especially important to provide opportunities to talk about and solve problems.

Factors affecting sex and intimacy

Problems affecting intimacy in Parkinson's may become more prominent as the condition progresses. These include:

- Loss of fluidity of movement and difficulties in sustaining movement
- Increased tremor or dyskinesia during arousal
- Vaginal dryness
- Erectile problems
- Issues with reaching climax
- Excessive sweating or drooling
- Fear of urination
- Difficulty focusing attention
- Reduced libido
- Reduced sexual self-image

Intimacy can also be affected by other factors, including growing older, mood, stress and anxiety, disparity in sexual appetite and no longer sharing a bed or bedroom because of sleep disturbances.

Communication is key to a good relationship, and helping couples to see things from each other's perspective is a good starting point in addressing intimacy issues. Where there is a disparity in sexual appetite, a frank and open discussion can be helpful and may facilitate ongoing open discussion. Signposting and referral to relationship counselling or support may also be indicated.

Practical tips to improve intimacy include planning for sex when medication is optimal (not necessarily at bedtime), finding a position that reduces the burden of repetitive movement for the individual with Parkinson's, using silk or satin sheets to aid movement, employing lubricants to aid penetration or massage oils to aid movement. Referral to a sex therapist may also be indicated.

Erectile dysfunction

Erectile dysfunction (ED), or the inability to achieve or maintain an erection sufficient for satisfactory sexual performance, is common among older males and increases with age. The prevalence of ED in the general population exceeds 50% in those above age 70 years (Kessler et al., 2019). The prevalence of ED among those with Parkinson's may be higher still. Factors contributing to ED include stress, fatigue, anxiety, and the excessive use of alcohol. Advice includes losing weight (if overweight), stopping smoking, maintaining a healthy diet, exercising regularly and using various strategies to manage stress and anxiety.

ED may be associated with Parkinson's or with the use of medications such as thiazide diuretics and beta blockers. Long-standing high blood pressure, prostate problems, and diabetes can also contribute to erectile problems. Finally, antidepressants can affect ability to reach climax.

Selective medications such as type-5 cyclic guanosine monophosphate phosphodiesterase inhibitors used to treat erectile problems can be effective in Parkinson's. Raffaele et al. (2002) reported that men with Parkinson's and depression taking sildenafil achieved an erection sufficient for intercourse on 85% of attempts. Apomorphine injection may be helpful as an alternative to sildenafil (O'Sullivan, 2002).

These drugs should be used with caution if there is a history of cardiovascular disease and should not be prescribed if nitrates are being taken, in cases of retinitis pigmentosa (a rare eye condition causing blindness), or in men with a history of priapism (abnormally sustained and painful erection). It is important to be cautious if the individual has postural hypotension.

The most common adverse effects of sildenafil are headache, flushing, and indigestion. Temporary visual problems (e.g., color-vision disturbances) may occur with higher doses. Adverse effects occur mostly at a low level and are short lived.

Impulse control disorder and sexual function

Increased sexual drive or lack of sexual impulse control is thought to occur in 2% to 8.8% of people with Parkinson's who are on dopaminergic medication, especially but not exclusively dopamine agonists (Bronner & Vodusek, 2011).

A greater sexual drive can be helpful in a relationship if it improves both partners' satisfaction and QoL but it can also cause problems. Lack of control of sexual impulses can lead to significant issues, including:

- A preoccupation with sexual thoughts
- Greater sexual demands on an unwilling partner
- Promiscuity and unsafe sexual encounters
- Habitual use of internet pornography and telephone or internet sex lines
- Contact with sex workers

These problems can cause considerable tension within the family and lead to relationship breakdown. Early reporting and intervention are vital to reduce potential harm. Every consultation should include questions and discussion regarding the risks of impulse control disorder.

When such issues are reported by the individual or family, it is important that they understand that the behaviour is a medication-related side effect and likely to be beyond the individual's control. The individual often feels a sense of shame, and there may be judgment on the part of the family. Therefore a clear understanding of the causes can reduce potentially harmful attitudes of blame and shame.

When such problems arise, a prompt review and adjustment of medication is indicated. Gradually reducing and stopping dopamine agonists and adjusting other medications should be considered, alongside psychological help and support. If hypersexual behaviour persists after the removal of dopamine agonist medication, referral to clinical neuropsychology or CBT can be considered (Okai et al., 2013). Quetiapine is also an option (Rees et al., 2007).

Advice for the multidisciplinary team

It can be difficult to address problems relating to sexual function and intimacy within a routine consultation owing to time constraints and the lack of clinician confidence. A good option for the MDT is to identify one team member who can specialise in this area and thus be able to discuss sexual health issues, carry out assessments, and offer appropriate treatment advice, signposting, and onward referral.

Fatigue

Fatigue is a sense of tiredness or exhaustion brought on by repeated activity; it naturally impairs performance. In healthy individuals, fatigue improves following rest and does not affect everyday activity; but in Parkinson's, fatigue is brought on by minimal exertion, is chronic, improves little with rest and has a huge impact on daily function (Kluger & Friedman, 2014). Fatigue may precede the motor symptoms of Parkinson's and is present in about one-third of individuals in the early stages and more than 80% of those in late stages (Barone et al., 2009). The biology of fatigue is not well understood, but there are physical and psychological components. Sleep disturbance, medications and low mood might be implicated. Although there is some overlap between the symptoms of fatigue and depression, fatigue commonly occurs in those who are not depressed. L-dopa might have a beneficial effect on fatigue (Schifitto et al., 2008). In terms of drug treatment, a small trial of methylphenidate has shown some benefits (Mendonca et al., 2007), but this drug is not widely used. In a Movement Disorder Society evidence-based review, rasagiline was considered efficacious and possibly useful, but modafinil and testosterone were not efficacious (Seppi et al., 2019). Many members of the MDT may contribute to the management of fatigue. The physician should consider the possibility of comorbidities, including anemia, chronic infections, thyroid disorders, renal failure, cardiac failure, vitamin D deficiency, depression and adverse effects of medication.

The OT should consider the daily routine, sleep hygiene, depression management, and need for social support. This will include identifying the individual's current level of participation in the home and community and possibly introducing a graded programme to facilitate increasing activities and participation. Sleep hygiene can help to establish a routine, and daytime sleep can reduce the buildup of fatigue during the day. Engaging in daily mental and physical activities is important, and individuals should be encouraged to go outdoors daily for a walk or run. The physiotherapist can implement a graded exercise programme.

Psychological care and the multidisciplinary team's stepped-care model

Psychological care

Psychological care focuses on emotional, cognitive, and behavioural changes that may be experienced by the individual. The neurochemical changes that occur in people with Parkinson's have been directly associated with changes in behaviour, thinking, and emotional experience. It is shortsighted, however, to only look at the emotional experience of people with Parkinson's from a biological model. In living with Parkinson's, people experience challenges in fulfilling the meaningful roles in their lives. Managing the impact of the condition requires a concept of the understandable and expected emotional reactions that people experience. These include shock, anger, and sadness. Difficulty with executive function may make it harder for an individual to put into action the strategies suggested to manage emotional distress. Individual differences in personality, previous experience of distress and varying coping resources mean that people with similar symptoms may have different psychological experiences. An individual's thoughts, feelings, and appraisal of how to cope require a customised approach.

Understanding the psychological adjustment process is key for the MDT. This is essential to working in a psychologically minded way and is part of the psychological care that each member has a responsibility to provide.

As well as considering the adjustment process, the term *psychological distress* or simply *distress* can help the clinician to communicate about the individual's emotional experience without resorting to making a diagnosis such as anxiety or depression (although this may be appropriate in some cases). Beyond diagnosis, however, we need an understanding of what an individual's experience means to him or her personally to be able to provide the needed support and psychological care.

The progressive nature of Parkinson's can mean that individuals experience repeated cycles of an adjustment process as they come to understand and experience the changes in their condition. Uncertainty about progression may add to an individual's distress.

A shared biopsychosocial understanding for the MDT and the person with Parkinson's is a key tool in making sense of the individual's situation and may also act as an intervention (Wilson et al., 2009).

Table 6.5 lists examples of biological, psychological, and social factors and how they may interact with one another.

TABLE 6.5 Examples of biological, psychological, and social factors	
Biological factors	Dopaminergic pathways have a role in mediating several non-motor symptoms affecting cognition, sleep and pain. Dopaminergic medication can have a beneficial effect on mood and apathy as well as motor symptoms. Anxiety can be associated with "wearing off" effect of medication (Chaudhuri & Schapira, 2009). Impulsive or compulsive behaviours and hallucinations can be side effects of medication.
Psychological factors	Psychological adjustment, condition acceptance, and mood have been shown to be associated with quality of life (Rosinczuk & Koltuniuk, 2017). Difficulties with psychological adjustment were found to be associated with rates of anxiety and depression for people with Parkinson's (Garlovsky, Overton, & Simpson, 2016). An association between anxiety and difficulties with cognition has also been shown for people with Parkinson's (Dissanayaka et al., 2017). It is important to be aware of the interaction of emotional and cognitive processes in seeking to understand a person's changes in behaviour.
Social factors	The impact on family and social relationships requires consideration. How the individual and their social network understand their condition could impact the confidence to manage day-to-day life alongside the condition. Support for the individual's social network (family, friends, carers) is essential.

Care from the multidisciplinary team: the stepped-care model

Psychological care is "everyone's business." in the MDT and at the heart of a holistic and person-centred approach to neurorehabilitation. Members of the MDT may feel more confident in providing psychological care if there is a clear referral pathway for additional support—for example, a clinical psychologist within the team.

A stepped-care model of psychological well-being provides structure. The individual should have access to the appropriate service matched to his or her needs. Figure 6.2 is an example of a stepped-care model for a Parkinson's service with access to clinical neuropsychology.

Psychological interventions

There are several approaches to providing psychological support, including education through support groups, social support from family and Parkinson's

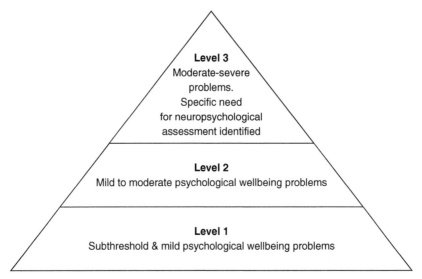

Level 3
Moderate-severe problems.
Specific need for neuropsychological assessment identified

Level 2
Mild to moderate psychological wellbeing problems

Level 1
Subthreshold & mild psychological wellbeing problems

FIGURE 6.2   The stepped-care model Level 1: An individual is experiencing general difficulties with mood, cognition, or understanding of his or her condition. MDT members should inquire about mood and cognition. NMSQuest is a useful screening tool. If issues are identified, more detailed assessment using tools such as the MoCA and the Hospital Anxiety and Depression Scale may be required. Intervention may be offered by the MDT or through charitable sector. **Level 2**: Difficulties may be having impact on individual's engagement with rehabilitation or be a greater source of distress. Assessment should be by team member with expertise in assessment and treatment of psychological and cognitive difficulties, often the OT, but it may be another MDT member such as the PDNS or doctor. Use of more detailed assessment tools such as the Addenbrooks Cognitive Examination (ACE-III) may be appropriate. Where available, the clinical neuropsychologist provides a supporting or advisory role. **Level 3**: An individual experiencing moderate to severe emotional, cognitive, and behavioural issues. Clinical neuropsychologist assessment and intervention or referral to mental health services may be indicated.

charities as well as input from occupational therapy or social services to address anxiety related to financial stressors or physical difficulties at home or work. Lifestyle interventions are recommended, including regular exercise and eating a healthy diet. Relaxation therapies such as meditation, massage, acupuncture, or tai chi may also be beneficial. Zarotti et al. (2020) provide a review of psychological interventions for people with Parkinson's.

Formal psychological assessment and intervention can be provided by a clinical psychologist or neuropsychologist. Any mental health professional involved in the individual's care should be integrated into the MDT to ensure cohesive psychological care.

The multidisciplinary team's intervention and roles

This section addresses the roles of the various members of the MDT in the maintenance stage of Parkinson's. The different disciplines have specific skills, which are explored. All disciplines work closely together in an integrated way to support the individual with Parkinson's. An awareness of issues beyond traditional specialty boundaries enables each clinician to provide holistic care. The physiotherapist may issue an exercise prescription, but all MDT members should be aware of the importance of physical activity and should encourage the individual in this regard. Examples of integrated work have been described earlier, including joint-discipline assessment in the management of FOG, reinforcing dietary advice to address constipation, and fatigue management. Key principles of integrated multidisciplinary rehabilitation are also described in Chapter 3.

The consultant

NICE (2017) recommends that individuals with Parkinson's be medically reviewed every 6 to 12 months. The purpose of the review is to check that symptoms are well controlled, monitor for side effects of medications, and review the diagnosis. Not everyone with Parkinson's has a good response to L-dopa, but failure to improve with dopaminergic medication should raise concern: is the diagnosis correct? Atypical Parkinsonian conditions may present similarly to Parkinson's but often have a poor response to L-dopa (see Chapter 13). As a minimum, we recommend asking about urinary symptoms, erectile dysfunction, falls and behavioural change. The physical examination should include checking eye movements to look for evidence of progressive supranuclear palsy. Failure of voluntary downgaze with preservation of the vestibular ocular reflex is typical, but an early sign may be slowing of vertical saccades. Large declines in blood pressure on standing ($>30/15$), which can occur in Parkinson's, might suggest multisystem atrophy. If dementia develops within a year of the onset of motor symptoms, the individual may well have dementia with Lewy bodies rather than Parkinson's.

Medical reviews can be undertaken by the Parkinson's disease nurse specialist (PDNS) or the neurologist/geriatrician. If the PDNS feels the diagnosis to be in doubt, he or she should refer back to the neurologist/geriatrician.

Parkinson's disease nurse specialist

The PDNS's review should focus on enabling the individual to live a full and active life. Review of motor symptoms—including examination of tremor, upper limb tone, and bradykinesia—is important, as well as noting any changes in gait and balance. Advice on non-drug strategies to help with mild stiffness and slow movement should be considered before medications are escalated. Such strategies would include exercise and advice from the physiotherapist and OT for problems related to upper limb function, gait or balance. If gait difficulties are affecting day-to-day function or if wearing-off phenomena are beginning to develop, a small increase in medication may be indicated.

A thorough assessment of NMSs should be undertaken. The NMSQuest can be completed by the individual prior to the consultation and can help to identify specific symptoms of concern. Cognition, mood, sleep, bladder, and bowel issues as well as sex and intimacy should all be considered as part of the PDNS's review.

It is important to have an accurate and complete list of medications; some Parkinson's MDTs include a pharmacist to ensure best practice with respect to medication management. The efficacy of an individual's medication in maintaining QoL should be established. A good rule of thumb is to prescribe just enough medication to enable the person live a full and active life yet not too much to avoid the risk of developing side effects.

Potential side effects of medications

Potential side effects of medications should be explored and discussed (see Table 6.6). Individuals should be given printed information or a copy letter that includes benefits and potential side effects of medication.

Telephone advice

During the maintenance stage an annual face-to-face review with the PDNS may suffice, but provision of a responsive PDNS telephone advice service is essential for answering any interim questions or concerns, promptly reviewing any issues that may arise, adjusting medication, or arranging for a review from another member of the MDT.

Physiotherapist

The physiotherapist should take an accurate history and carry out a detailed assessment, ensuring that the main problems from the individual's perspective are understood. Shared goals, time scales, and an intervention programme can

TABLE 6.6 Common side effects of Parkinson's medication and suggested interventions

Adverse Effect	Suggested Interventions
Nausea	Nausea is often short-lived, so people with Parkinson's should be reassured and encouraged to continue with dopaminergic medication.
	Taking dopaminergic medication with food can reduce nausea.
	Anti-emetics can be offered. Domperidone is an option, but there are serious safety concerns (Simeonova et al., 2018); this drug should not be used in those with cardiac disease or a prolonged QTc (an electrocardiographic abnormality). Despite its anticholinergic activity, we often prescribe cyclizine. Ondansetron is sometimes used but may prolong the QTc and worsen constipation.
	Prochlorperazine and metoclopramide are contraindicated in Parkinson's.
Somnolence	If this is severe or sudden in onset, the individual should be advised not to drive.
	Dose reduction should be considered, particularly for dopamine agonists.
Postural dizziness or light-headedness	Postural blood pressure (BP) should be checked. The individual should lie or sit for 10 to 15 minutes before BP is measured lying or sitting. BP is then measured after standing for 1 and 3 minutes.
	If postural hypotension is identified, the individual should initially be advised to keep well hydrated and offered an information sheet on lifestyle measures (Parkinson's UK, 2020) (see Chapter 10).
Hallucinations	These should be discussed and assessed no matter how transient, especially if medications have been newly commenced or escalated. It may be helpful to introduce questions about hallucinations by asking about vision in general. Normalising the experience may help to elicit an open response. For example, "Lots of people with Parkinson's experience hallucinations. Has that ever happened to you?"
Confusion	This can be induced by medication, especially if it is sudden in onset and outside the context of dementia.
	Consideration should be given to other potential causes (infection, dehydration, constipation).
Impulsive and compulsive behaviours	These should be considered at each consultation, with direct questioning of the individual and, if possible, a family member or caregiver. These include changes in behaviour, especially impulsive spending, compulsive gambling, hobbying, cleaning, excessive eating, or any increase in sexual appetite. If gambling is an issue, the individual should be signposted to support services such as BeGambleAware for information regarding environmental protections such as voluntary limits on stakes and credit card payments.

(Continued)

Driving

Individuals who drive should have regular cognitive assessments. It is usually a family member who identifies any difficulties with driving, although some individuals recognise changes and stop driving for safety reasons. The Rookwood driving assessment is a cognitive scale validated for use in stroke and, though imperfect, is the best predictor of on-road driving assessment outcome currently available for Parkinson's (Lloyd et al., 2020). The Parkinson's driving questionnaire, available on the Parkinson's UK website, is a useful tool. If a practical assessment is required, referral to a driving assessment centre should be made. All individuals who drive should be asked about sleep. If they have excessive daytime sleepiness as assessed by the Epworth Sleepiness Scale, they should be advised not to drive.

The speech and language therapist

Speech problems

Despite the NICE guidelines stating that referral to a speech and language therapist (SLT) should be considered early, the Parkinson's UK National Audit (2019) identified that the majority of SLT referrals occurred in the maintenance stage. Offering earlier advice enables the person with Parkinson's to establish new speech habits or strategies that can offset further complications as the condition progresses. Various speech, voice, and communication changes occur over the course of the condition, and these are prevalent in 75% to 90% of people with Parkinson's (Schalling et al., 2017, Theodoros & Ramig, 2011).

The SLT addresses hypokinetic dysarthria, which includes fast, rushed speech, changes to voice quality (harsh/breathy/rough), reduced vocal loudness, limited dynamic pitch range, poor breath support and neurogenic dysfluency (Duffy, 2019). Language difficulties are also common, primarily characterised by the individual forgetting the idea that is being conveyed or experiencing word retrieval difficulties. Conversation involves multiple cognitive processes, as illustrated in Fig. 6.4. Describing these processes in layman's language can help caregivers understand the difficulties the person with Parkinson's experiences when their "autopilot" is not working effectively and helps explain why adjustments are necessary to improve communication. The idea may be forgotten, meaning that any subsequent language will not be formulated. Next, the individual may not be able to recall a specific word, thus disrupting the flow of conversation. This can be managed with listener awareness and strategies. Breakdowns can occur anywhere in this sequence.

SLTs have a number of effective therapy approaches ranging from breath support treatments including expiratory muscle strength training (Sapienza et al., 2011), semioccluded vocal tract therapy (Meerschman et al., 2019), intensive voice training programs such as Speak Out (Boutsen et al., 2018), and Lee

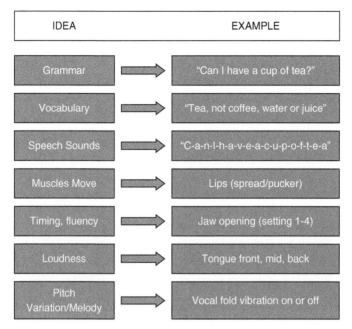

IDEA	EXAMPLE
Grammar	"Can I have a cup of tea?"
Vocabulary	"Tea, not coffee, water or juice"
Speech Sounds	"C-a-n-I-h-a-v-e-a-c-u-p-o-f-t-e-a"
Muscles Move	Lips (spread/pucker)
Timing, fluency	Jaw opening (setting 1-4)
Loudness	Tongue front, mid, back
Pitch Variation/Melody	Vocal fold vibration on or off

FIGURE 6.4 The demands of language processing.

Silverman Voice Therapy (LSVT), (Ramig et al., 2018). The aim of these programs is to increase vocal loudness, enhance pitch range, and improve speech intelligibility. LSVT is the best-evidenced of these treatments and is considered the gold standard.

When an individual presents with a soft voice, it is essential to provide audiovisual feedback so that he or she can hear, see, and feel what it is like speak louder. In Parkinson's, the voice has been noted to be around 2 to 4 dB quieter (Fox & Ramig, 1997). This is a subtle and gradual shift that the individual may acknowledge but not fully appreciate. In a single session, the SLT can demonstrate that the individual's voice can be strengthened with increased internal physical drive. However, individuals must develop strong self-monitoring skills to align the way they hear themselves with how others perceive them. These concepts are fundamental to effective voice treatment in Parkinson's. Technology also provides an opportunity for audiovisual-kinesthetic feedback, including apps such as a decibel meter (e.g., Decibel X). Over time, individuals should progress from visual feedback to internalising the feeling, so that they can easily generate and feel comfortable with a louder conversational voice.

Communication subskills can be effectively practised in an individual consultation; however, group work, particularly for the maintenance of therapeutic targets, can be beneficial. Parkinson's group therapy can focus on carryover, social connection, and identity; it can have psychosocial benefits, as evidenced by a number of studies. One example is the singing group format combining singing, voice projection and body movements using a multisensory approach to enhance speech intelligibility (Vella-Burrows & Hancox, 2012).

Swallowing (Dysphagia)

Dysphagia occurs in over 80% of people with Parkinson's (Suttrup & Warnecke, 2016). Although swallowing difficulties can occur at any stage, pharyngeal and esophageal changes frequently precede clinical symptoms (Sung et al., 2010). Dysphagia management entails a range of strategies including education and advice, texture modification, environmental adjustments, postural moves (chin tuck, head turn) and specific exercises. Promising emerging therapies include Chin Tuck with Resistance (Yoon et al., 2014) and Expiratory Muscle Strength Training, which, over a 4-week period, improved swallowing (Sapienza et al., 2011). There is also strong evidence for the Shaker exercise (Logemann et al., 2009) and Masako technique (pharyngeal strengthening exercise). Pressure training devices such as the IQoro and Iowa Oral Performance Instrument (IOPI), are also generating interest among SLTs but require further research to show efficacy.

Dietitian

The dietitian has a role in assessing the individual for optimal weight and nutrition. People on Mediterranean diets are at lower risk of developing Parkinson's (Alcalay et al., 2012). A Mediterranean diet appears to be safe, but the benefits for people who already have Parkinson's are unclear. Paknahad (2020) reported improvements in cognition. Ketogenic diets may also improve cognition in the short term (Phillips et al., 2018), but long-term effects have not been studied. Advice regarding constipation may be important at this stage of Parkinson's. Where swallowing problems have been identified, liaison between SLT, dietitian, and the person with Parkinson's will pay dividends.

Personal perspective: Tim's story

When I was first diagnosed with Parkinson's disease in 2014, I was 57 years old, fit, active, and on the leadership team of a large Christian church. Over the last 6 years, as I have struggled with various symptoms and the side effects of medication, the regular visits to the Derby Parkinson's MDT have proven invaluable.

The speech therapist has helped me cope with the reduction of power in my voice—a critical tool in my very public job. The dietitian has encouraged me to eat more healthily and given me advice to cope with the growing problem of constipation. An OT has seen me regularly, and we have chatted about numerous issues including sleep patterns, mood swings, exercise, rest routines, work patterns and even libido levels! My wife has also been to see the OT to discuss what it's like caring for someone with Parkinson's. I'm due to see a clinical psychologist to talk about strategies to cope with the impulsive behaviours caused by some of the medications. The specialist physiotherapist has enabled me to keep moving well by giving me exercises specific to certain muscles and limbs and has also measured my movements on a regular basis to watch out for any deterioration. Finally, the nurses have cheerfully weighed me and taken my blood pressure without making me feel that I'm an invalid or inadequate.

All this—and more—occurred in a relaxed atmosphere of genuine care and concern alongside professionalism of the highest level.

Living with Parkinson's is not easy. The Derby Parkinson's MDT has made it more than manageable so far. I don't know what the future holds, but to have the team available when I need it is a great comfort and support.

Tim Gunn

Top tips in the maintenance stage

1. All members of the MDT should encourage physical activity and exercise.
2. Identify whether FOG is "on" or "off" and where it occurs most frequently. An MDT approach to the management of FOG is recommended.
3. Cues can be useful for dealing with FOG. These may be attentional, proprioceptive, visual, or auditory.
4. The self-completed NMSQuest is a useful tool in screening for non-motor symptoms.
5. CBT is effective for treating depression in Parkinson's. It can be delivered remotely.
6. Exercise and bright-light therapy are both effective for dealing with insomnia in Parkinson's.
7. Constipation can lead to delayed gastric emptying. Consider constipation as a cause of the dose failures.
8. A postvoid bladder scan can help to identify those with incomplete voiding. In such cases try "double voiding" and avoid anticholinergic medications.
9. Identify one member of the MDT to deal with sexual health issues.
10. The MDT should develop one-page information sheets with lifestyle advice for common problems such as medication side effects, constipation, postural hypotension, bladder symptoms, and insomnia. Parkinson's UK, the Parkinson's Excellence Network and the Parkinson's Foundation also have useful resources.
11. Understanding the psychological adjustment process is key for the MDT.
12. Consider biological, psychological, and social factors when symptoms are being assessed.
13. It is important to always have an accurate record of each individual's medications. Every such list should be checked carefully by the doctor or nurse at each visit. Including a pharmacist in the team should be considered.
14. Before taking posture blood pressure measurements, allow time for the individual to achieve a normal resting blood pressure, ideally while lying down.
15. Make a recording of the individual's voice and play it back; the shift in awareness can be rapid.

Abbreviations: CBT, cognitive behavioural therapy; FOG, freezing of gait; MDT, multidisciplinary team; NMSQuest, non-motor symptom questionnaire

Levy, R., & Dubois, B. (2006). Apathy and the functional anatomy of the prefrontal cortex-basal ganglia circuits. *Cerebral Cortex*, *16*(7), 916–928.

Lewis, S. J., & Barker, R. A. (2009). A pathophysiological model of freezing of gait in Parkinson's disease. *Parkinsonism and Related Disorders*, *15*(5), 333–338.

Litvan, I., Goldman, J. G., Troster, A. I., Schmand, B. A., Weintraub, D., Petersen, R. C., et al. (2012). Diagnostic criteria for mild cognitive impairment in Parkinson's disease: Movement Disorder Society Task Force guidelines. *Movement Disorders*, *27*(3), 349–356.

Lloyd, K., Gaunt, D., Haunton, V., Skelly, R., Mann, H., Ben-Shlomo, Y., et al. (2020). Driving in Parkinson's disease: a retrospective study of driving and mobility assessments. *Age and Ageing*, *49*(6), 1097–1101.

Logemann, J. A., Rademaker, A., Pauloski, B. R., Kelly, A., Stangl-McBreen, C., Antinoja, J., et al. (2009). A randomised study comparing the Shaker exercise with traditional therapy: a preliminary study. *Dysphagia*, *24*(4), 403–411.

McClurg, D., Panicker, J., Walker, R. W., Cunnington, A., Deane, K. H. O., Harari, D., et al. (2020). Stimulation of the tibial nerve: a protocol for a multicentred randomised controlled trial for urinary problems associated with Parkinson's disease-STARTUP. *BMJ Open 10*(2) e034887.

McDonald, C., Rees, J., Winge, K., Newton, J. L. & Burn, D. J. (2020). Bladder training for urinary tract symptoms in Parkinson disease: A randomized controlled trial. *Neurology 94*(13) e1427-e1433

Meco, G., Rubino, A., Caravona, N., & Valente, M. (2008). Sexual dysfunction in Parkinson's disease. *Parkinsonism and Related Disorders*, *14*(6), 451–456.

Meerschman, I., Van Lierde, K., Ketels, J., Coppieters, C., Claeys, S., & D'Haeseleer, E. (2019). Effect of three semi-occluded vocal tract therapy programmes on the phonation of patients with dysphonia: lip trill, water-resistance therapy and straw phonation. *International Journal of Language and Communication Disorders*, *54*(1), 50–61.

Mendonca, D. A., Menezes, K., & Jog, M. S. (2007). Methylphenidate improves fatigue scores in Parkinson disease: a randomised controlled trial. *Movement Disorders*, *22*(14), 2070–2076.

Miller-Koop, M., Rosenfeldt, A. B., & Alberts, J. L. (2019). Mobility improves after high intensity aerobic exercise in individuals with Parkinson's disease. *Journal of Neurological Science*, *399*(15), 187–193.

Mirelman, A., Rochester, L., Maidan, I., Del Din, S., Alcock, L., Nieuwhof, F., et al. (2016). Addition of a non-immersive virtual reality component to treadmill training to reduce fall risk in older adults (V-TIME): a randomised controlled trial. *Lancet*, *388*(10050), 1170–1182.

Moore, O., Gurevich, T., Korczyn, A. D., Anca, M., Shabtai, H., & Giladi, N. (2002). Quality of sexual life in Parkinson's disease. *Parkinsonism and Related Disorders*, *8*(4), 243–246.

Mukherjee, A., Biswas, A., & Das, S. K. (2016). Gut dysfunction in Parkinson's disease. *World Journal of Gastroenterology*, *22*(25), 5742–5752.

National Institute for Health and Care Excellence (NICE), (2017). Parkinson's disease in adults: NICE guideline [NG71]. Retrieved June 7, 2020, from https://www.nice.org.uk/guidance/ng71/resources/parkinsons-disease-in-adults-pdf-1837629189061.

Ni, M., Hazzard, J. B., Signorile, J. F., & Luca, C. (2018). Exercise guidelines for gait function in Parkinson's disease: a systematic review and meta-analysis. *Neurorehabilitation and Neural Repair*, *32*(10), 872–886.

Nieuwboer, A., Rochester, L., Herman, T., Vandenberghe, W., Emil, G. E., Thomaes, T., et al. (2009). Reliability of the new freezing of gait questionnaire: agreement between patients with Parkinson's disease and their carers. *Gait and Posture*, *30*(4), 459–463.

O'Sullivan, J. D. (2002). Apomorphine as an alternative to sildenafil in Parkinson's disease. *Journal of Neurology, Neurosurgery, and Psychiatry*, *72*(5), 681.

O'Sullivan, J. D. (2020). Too much of a good thing: hedonistic homoeostatic dysregulation and other behavioural consequences of excessive dopamine replacement therapy in Parkinson's disease. *Journal of Neurology, Neurosurgery, and Psychiatry*, *91*(6), 566–567.

Okai, D., Askey-Jones, S., Samuel, M., O'Sullivan, S. S., Chaudhuri, K. R., Martin, A., et al. (2013). Trial of CBT for impulse control behaviours affecting Parkinson patients and their caregivers. *Neurology*, *80*(9), 792–799.

Okuma, Y., Silva de Lima, A. L., Fukae, J., Bloem, B. R., & Snijders, A. H. (2018). A prospective study of falls in relation to freezing of gait and response fluctuations in Parkinson's disease. *Parkinsonism and Related Disorders*, *46*, 30–35.

Ondo, W. G., Kenney, C., Sullivan, K., Davidson, A., Hunter, C., Jahan, I., et al. (2012). Placebo-controlled trial of lubiprostone for constipation associated with Parkinson disease. *Neurology*, *78*(21), 1650–1654.

Paget, A. T. (2019). *Cognitive therapy for anxiety-related freezing of gait in Parkinson's disease: a retrospective clinical case study*. London, UK: Parkinson's Excellence Network Mental Health Conference.

Paknahad, Z., Sheklabadi, E., Derakhshan, Y., Bagherniya, M., & Chitsaz, A. (2020). The effect of the Mediterranean diet on cognitive function in patients with Parkinson's disease: A randomised clinical controlled trial. *Complement Ther Med*, *50*, 102366.

Parkinson's UK (2019). UK Parkinson's Audit - Summary Report https://www.parkinsons.org.uk/sites/default/files/2020-01/CS3524%20Parkinson%27s%20UK%20Audit-Summary%20Report%202019%20%281%29.pdf.

Parkinson's UK. (2020). Low Blood Pressure and Parkinson's [online]. Retrieved November 19, 2020, from https://www.parkinsons.org.uk/sites/default/files/2018-09/FS50%20Low%20blood%20pressure_WEB.pdf.

Pavy-Le Traon, A., Cotterill, N., Amarenco, G., Duerr, S., Kaufmann, H., Lahrmann, H., et al. (2018). Clinical Rating Scales for Urinary Symptoms in Parkinson Disease: Critique and Recommendations. *Mov Disord Clin Pract 5*(5) 479–491.

Peterka, M., Odorfer, T., Schwab, M., Volkmann, J., & Zeller, D. (2020). LSVT-BIG therapy in Parkinson's disease: physiological evidence for proprioceptive recalibration. *Boston Medical Centre Neurology*, *20*(1), 276.

Phillips, M. C. L., Murtagh, D. K. J., Gilbertson, L. J., Asztely, F. J. S., & Lynch, C. D. P. (2018). Low-fat versus ketogenic diet in Parkinson's disease: a pilot randomised controlled trial. *Movement Disorders*, *33*(8), 1306–1314.

Radakovic, R., Davenport, R., Starr, J. M., & Abrahams, S. (2018). Apathy dimensions in Parkinson's disease. *International Journal of Geriatric Psychiatry*, *33*(1), 151–158.

Raffaele, R., Vecchio, I., Giammusso, B., Morgia, G., Brunetto, M. B., & Rampello, L. (2002). Efficacy and safety of fixed-dose oral sildenafil in the treatment of sexual dysfunction in depressed patients with idiopathic Parkinson's disease. *European Urology*, *41*(4), 382–386.

Ramig, L., Halpern, A., Spielman, J., Fox, C., & Freeman, K. (2018). Speech treatment in Parkinson's disease: randomised controlled trial (RCT). *Movement Disorders*, *33*(11), 1777–1791.

Rees, P. M., Fowler, C. J., & Maas, C. P. (2007). Sexual function in men and women with neurological disorders. *Lancet*, *369*(9560), 512–525.

Rosinczuk, J., & Koltuniuk, A. (2017). The influence of depression, level of functioning in everyday life, and illness acceptance on quality of life in patients with Parkinson's disease: a preliminary study. *Neuropsychiatric Disease and Treatment*, *13*, 881–887.10.2147/NDT.S132757.

Sapienza, C., Troche, M., Pitts, T., & Davenport, P. (2011). Respiratory strength training: concept and intervention outcomes. *Seminars in Speech and Language*, *32*(1), 21–30.

Schaafsma, J. D., Balash, Y., Gurevich, T., Bartels, A. L., Hausdorff, J. M., & Giladi, N. (2003). Characterisation of freezing of gait subtypes and the response of each to levodopa in Parkinson's disease. *European Journal of Neurology*, *10*(4), 391–398.

Schalling, E., Johansson, K., & Hartelius, L. (2017). Speech and communication changes reported by people with Parkinson's disease. *Folia Phoniatrica et Logopaedia*, *69*(3), 131–141.

Schifitto, G., Friedman, J. H., Oakes, D., Shulman, L., Comella, C. L., Marek, K., et al. (2008). Fatigue in levodopa-naive subjects with Parkinson disease. *Neurology*, *71*(7), 481–485.

Schrag, A., & Politis, M. (2016). Serotonergic loss underlying apathy in Parkinson's disease. *Brain*, *139*(Pt 9), 2338–2339.

Seppi, K., Ray Chaudhuri, K., Coelho, M., Fox, S. H., Katzenschlager, R., Perez Lloret, S., et al. (2019). Update on treatments for nonmotor symptoms of Parkinson's disease-an evidence-based medicine review. *Movement Disorders*, *34*(2), 180–198.

Simeonova, M., de Vries, F., Pouwels, S., Driessen, J. H. M., Leufkens, H. G. M., Cadarette, S. M., et al. (2018). Increased risk of all-cause mortality associated with domperidone use in Parkinson's patients: a population-based cohort study in the UK. *British Journal of Clinical Pharmacology*, *84*(11), 2551–2561.

Stocchi, F., & Torti, M. (2014). Gastrointestinal dysfunctions in Parkinson's disease. In K. R. Chaudhuri, E. Tolosa, A. H. V. Schapira, & W. Poewe (Eds.), *Non-motor symptoms of Parkinson's disease* Oxford, United Kingdom: Oxford University Press.

Sung, H. Y., Kim, J. S., Lee, K. S., Kim, Y. I., Song, I. U., Chung, S. W., et al. (2010). The prevalence and patterns of pharyngoesophageal dysmotility in patients with early stage Parkinson's disease. *Movement Disorders*, *25*(14), 2361–2368.

Suttrup, I., & Warnecke, T. (2016). Dysphagia in Parkinson's disease. *Dysphagia*, *31*(1), 24–32.

Theodoros, D., & Ramig, L. (2011). *Communication and swallowing in Parkinson's disease,* San Diego, CA: Plural Publishing.

Vella-Burrows, P., & Hancox, G. (2012). *Singing and People with Parkinson's*: No. 4 (Singing, Wellbeing and Health). Canterbury Christ Church University.

Videnovic, A., Klerman, E. B., Wang, W., Marconi, A., Kuhta, T., & Zee, P. C. (2017). Timed light therapy for sleep and daytime sleepiness associated with Parkinson disease: a Randomised Clinical Trial. *Journal of the American Medical Association Neurology*, *74*(4), 411–418.

Wallace, D. M., Wohlgemuth, W. K., Trotti, L. M., Amara, A. W., Malaty, I. A., Factor, S. A., et al. (2020). Practical evaluation and management of insomnia in Parkinson's disease: a review. *Movement Disorders, Clinical Practice*, *7*(3), 250–266.

Walton, C. C., Mowszowski, L., Gilat, M., Hall, J. M., O'Callaghan, C., Muller, A. J., Georgiades, M., et al. (2018). Cognitive training for freezing of gait in Parkinson's disease: a randomised controlled trial. *Nature Portfolio Journal Parkinson's Disease*, *4*, 15. https://doi.org/10.1038/s41531-018-0052-6.

Wilson, B. A., Gracey, F., Evans, J. J., & Bateman, A. (2009). *Neuropsychological rehabilitation: theory, models: therapy and outcome*. Cambridge, United Kingdom: Cambridge University Press.

Yoon, W. L., Khoo, J. K., & Rickard Liow, S. J. (2014). Chin tuck against resistance (CTAR): new method for enhancing suprahyoid muscle activity using a Shaker-type exercise. *Dysphagia*, *29*(2), 243–248.

Zangaglia, R., Martignoni, E., Glorioso, M., Ossola, M., Riboldazzi, G., Calandrella, D., et al. (2007). Macrogol for the treatment of constipation in Parkinson's disease. A randomised placebo-controlled study. *Movement Disorders*, *22*(9), 1239–1244.

Zarotti, N., Eccles, F. J. R., Foley, J. A., Paget, A., Gunn, S., Leroi, I., et al. (2020). Psychological interventions for people with Parkinson's disease in the early 2020s: where do we stand? *Psychology and Psychotherapy: Theory, Research and Practice*. 2021 Sep 30;94(3):760-797.

Chapter 7

The Complex Stage of Parkinson's

Clare Johnson, Lisa Brown, Maxine Kavanagh, Caroline Bartliff,
Fiona Lindop, Jess Marsh, Suzanne Filon and Rob Skelly

Chapter outline

Motor symptoms in the complex stage

Wearing-off symptoms

When levodopa treatment is started, it is usually given three times a day. A good response to treatment is expected, which, if it occurs, supports the clinical diagnosis. Improvements in tremor may be less than hoped for, but people with Parkinson's often find that their other motor symptoms (stiffness, slow movement) and functional state (ability to wash, dress, write, walk) improve significantly. The serum half-life of levodopa is only about 90 minutes, but typically the improvements in motor function last throughout the day. This suggests that dopamine nerves have some way of storing the dopamine for later use. Over the following few months or years, the benefits of levodopa treatment seem to last less long. People with Parkinson's report that a levodopa dose does not last long enough, as the beneficial effects appear to wear off before the next dose is due. Eventually the clinical effects of a dose of levodopa start to mirror the serum half-life (see Fig. 7.1). Individuals in this situation become very dependent on their medication.

Often the simplest and preferred remedy is to add another dose in the day and thus reduce the interval between doses. Alternatively, increasing the dose may help. Using a higher dose of levodopa means that the peak serum level of levodopa will be higher but also that the levodopa will last longer, as levels stay above the threshold required for clinical benefit for longer. Increasing the dose may also be the preferred option when a general decline in response to levodopa throughout the day is reported.

Other options (Table 7.2) include adding drugs such as long-acting dopamine agonists (DAs such as ropinirole XL, pramipexole modified release, rotigotine patch), type b monoamine oxidase inhibitors (selegiline, rasagiline, safinamide) or catechol-O-methyl transferase inhibitors (entacapone, opicapone, tolcapone). The choice will depend on the risk of side effects, which varies from person to person. For example, an elderly person with cognitive impairment might be at high risk of confusion, hallucinations and somnolence from a DA; therefore reducing the dose interval of levodopa might be preferred. The orange staining of secretions from the use of entacapone may not be an issue for most people, but those with troublesome drooling or urinary incontinence may find their clothing ruined.

Using an extended-release levodopa preparation (e.g., Madopar CR) might seem a logical approach, but clinical trials have shown no reduction in "off" time compared with standard levodopa (MacMahon et al., 1990). Melevodopa-carbidopa (Rytary, IPX-066, not available in the United Kingdom at the time of publication) is a newer modified-release formulation that may be more effective at reducing "off" time than levodopa-carbidopa-entacapone (LCE), but LCE dosing was not optimised in the study reporting this finding (Stocchi et al., 2014). Istradefylline, an adenosine A2A receptor agonist available in Japan and the United States but not yet in the United Kingdom, is effective for wearing-off symptoms.

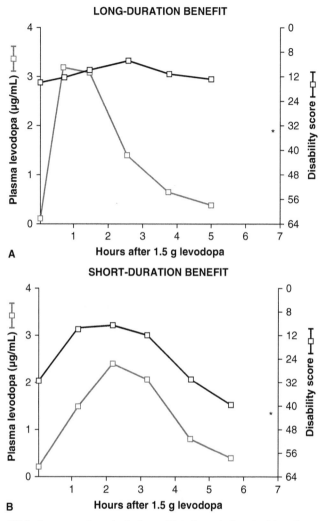

FIGURE 7.1   Clinical response to a single dose of levodopa. A. Sustained benefit associated with no wearing off B. Short-duration benefit associated with wearing-off symptoms Image from Muenter, M. D., & Tyce, G. M. (1971). L-dopa therapy of Parkinson's disease: plasma L-dopa concentration, therapeutic response, and side effects. *Mayo Clinic Proceedings, 46*, 231–239.

Early-morning dystonia

Dystonia is an abnormal contraction of a muscle or group of muscles. It can be uncomfortable and results in abnormal posture. The most common dystonia seen in Parkinson's is early-morning foot or leg dystonia, which responds well to dopamine. The use of extended-release levodopa (e.g., Sinemet CR) at night can be effective. Long-acting dopamine agonists are also effective. Some people

TABLE 7.2 Drug management of motor complications of levodopa therapy

Motor complications	Drug management options
Wearing off	Reduce time interval between levodopa doses Increase levodopa dose Add a MOAIB Add a long-acting dopamine agonist (e.g., Ropinirole XL) Add a COMT inhibitor (e.g., entacapone) Modified release levodopa: melevodopa/carbidopa
Early morning dystonia	Controlled-release levodopa at night (e.g. Sinemet CR) Long-acting dopamine agonists or rotigotine patch Dispersible co-beneldopa on waking Apomorphine subcutaneous injection in the morning Apomorphine sublingual
Dose failures: "No on"	Check concordance Medication to be taken on an empty stomach Change levodopa extended-release to standard levodopa Rescue medication: - Dispersible co-beneldopa - Apomorphine (e.g., Apo-Go Pen) Protein redistribution diet
Peak-dose dyskinesia	Reduce levodopa dose Change levodopa extended-release to the standard preparation (e.g., change Sinemet CR to Sinemet Plus) Stop COMT inhibitor Add amantadine Clozapine (monitoring required)
On-off fluctuations	Dose fractionation: give more frequent doses but lower doses Add COMT inhibitor, MOAIB, or long-acting dopamine agonist but also lower the levodopa dose Avoid levodopa extended release (e.g., Sinemet CR) Liquid levodopa (see text) Consider advanced treatment including: - DBS - LCIG - Apomorphine infusion
Biphasic dyskinesia	Reduce the number of doses of levodopa in the day Try using a long-acting dopamine agonist

Abbreviations: COMT, catechol-O-methyl transferase; DBS, deep brain stimulation; LCIG, levodopa-carbidopa intestinal gel; MOAIB, monoamine oxidase inhibitor type b.

with Parkinson's prefer to take levodopa medication during the night rather than having to wake up with painful dystonia.

Dose failures, "no on"

Sometimes a dose of levodopa does not seem to work at all. This can be due to delayed gastric emptying, dietary protein competing for absorption, or use of a controlled-release medication. It is also worth checking that the medication has actually been taken, as the prevalence of cognitive decline increases as Parkinson's progresses. Poor medication concordance is linked to worse motor symptoms (Grosset et al., 2009). Strategies to reduce the risk of dose failures include compliance aids, switching from extended-release to standard-release levodopa, treating constipation, and taking medication on an empty stomach. Occasionally protein redistribution diets are required, in which case supervision from a dietitian would be called for. Fast-acting rescue medication may be required for dose failures (see Table 7.2).

Peak-dose dyskinesia

Chorea is the most common dyskinesia (abnormal movement) caused by levodopa. This is an excessive, unwanted, dancelike, writhing or fidgety movement. The side more affected by Parkinson's symptoms is also more affected by dyskinesia. The neck and upper limbs are more affected than the lower limbs. Most commonly, levodopa-induced chorea occurs at peak serum levodopa concentrations, which occur about 30 minutes after dosing. Peak-dose dystonias and chorea can occur concurrently. Risk factors for the development of peak-dose dyskinesia include young age, condition severity, levodopa dose, and duration of levodopa therapy. In one study, the risk of dyskinesia after 5 years of levodopa treatment was 50% in those aged 40 to 59 years, 26% in those aged 60 to 69 years, and 16% in those aged above 70 years (Kumar et al., 2005). Non-physiological pulsatile stimulation of dopamine receptors and changes in receptor sensitivity may be involved in the development of dyskinesia.

Many people with Parkinson's tolerate dyskinesia very well. Although dyskinesia may affect some 60% of people after 10 years of treatment, it is often not troublesome. If troublesome, the dyskinesia might easily be controlled with medication adjustment (Van Gerpen et al., 2006). Drug management options are shown in Table 7.2. Some individuals find that glasses with blue lenses can reduce dyskinesia, but objective evidence of benefit is lacking.

On-off fluctuations

As Parkinson's progresses, an individual's ability to move may vary from normal movement when medication is working well (an "on" state) to severe stiffness and poverty of movement (an "off" state). Along with struggling to move, in an off state an individual might experience a sudden change in mood (anxiety, depression, or a panic attack) as well as autonomic changes (e.g., sweating). These sudden "offs" can be unpredictable. Sometimes an individual will change from troublesome dyskinesia to sudden "off" with little useful "on" time in between. These are on-off fluctuations, which can be difficult to manage. People with Parkinson's usually prefer dyskinesia to bradykinesia; this should be borne in mind when adjustments in medication are being made (see Table 7.2). Aiming for continuous dopamine stimulation is a logical strategy. Smaller but more frequent doses of levodopa can be tried. To achieve small changes in dose, some specialists recommend making up a solution of levodopa using four pills of co-careldopa 25/250 in 1 L of water with vitamin C added. This solution contains 1mg/mL of levodopa. The solution must be refrigerated, stirred thoroughly before use, and freshly prepared each day. It has a fast onset of action and improves on-off fluctuations (Pappert et al., 1996). However, many people find the preparation steps to be onerous and discontinue its use.

Biphasic dyskinesia

Sometimes individuals report the worsening of walking or other motor symptoms shortly after taking levodopa and again as the medication wears off. Leg dystonias causing walking difficulty are typical. They are hard to explain and difficult to treat. Use of a long-acting dopamine agonist rather than levodopa may be helpful.

Advanced treatments

If motor fluctuations and dyskinesias remain difficult to manage despite the strategies outlined in Table 7.2, advanced treatment options should be considered, such as:

- Subcutaneous apomorphine infusion
- Deep brain stimulation (DBS)
- Levodopa-carbidopa intestinal gel (Duodopa)

Subcutaneous apomorphine

Apomorphine has similar efficacy to levodopa for the treatment of Parkinson's motor symptoms. It can be used by intermittent subcutaneous injection for "off" periods and early-morning akinesia or as a continuous subcutaneous infusion via a pump in advanced disease. Subcutaneous apomorphine infusion therapy can lead to a remarkable decrease of time spent in the "off" state without any increase in dyskinesia (Carbone et al., 2019).

Selection criteria

An apomorphine pump should be considered in individuals who have one or more of the following:

- Significant and unpredictable "off" periods that are no longer controlled with optimised oral therapy
- Significant dyskinesia limiting further oral medication adjustments
- A need for frequent apomorphine rescue

The person with Parkinson's or a caregiver must be trained and available to commence and discontinue the infusion morning and evening. Apomorphine can be considered with caution in those with neuropsychiatric features (hallucinations, paranoia, impulse control disorder). There is some evidence that it is well tolerated with no worsening of neuropsychiatric features and may even have a positive effect on visual hallucinations (Borgemeester et al., 2016). Apomorphine therapy seems to be associated with a lower incidence of emergent impulse control disorders than oral dopamine agonists (Barbosa, et al., 2017). Those with excessive daytime somnolence or troublesome postural hypotension may not tolerate apomorphine, in which case alternative advanced treatments should be considered.

Procedure for starting treatment (test dose, how to determine dose for infusion)

Apomorphine therapy should be initiated following an apomorphine response test in order to establish the dose at which the individual responds without prohibitive side effects. An effective apomorphine response test should include the following:

- Pretreatment with domperidone 10 mg three times daily for 5 days (an electrocardiogram [ECG] to check for prolonged QTc should be completed). Domperidone is not usually needed long-term and can be discontinued gradually once the individual is on a stable regime.
- Individuals should attend for the response test in an "off" state. This can be achieved by withholding dopaminergic medications until after the test is complete. This should be individualised (i.e., for a planned 10 a.m. response test, it may be advisable to allow an early-morning dose and advise no medication after 7 a.m. so as to enable to the individual to get to the clinic).
- Pre-assessment should be undertaken, including the Unified Parkinson's Disease Rating Scale (UPDRS) motor score, timed walk and blood pressure lying and standing.
- Administration of a 1-mg test dose to ensure no adverse reaction.
- A gradual increase in injection by 1 to 2 mg at 45- to 60-minute intervals until the desired motor response is achieved without adverse effect.

- Monitoring of time to onset of effect, duration of effect, and any adverse effects at each dose increase should be undertaken, including recording of postural blood pressures.
- The optimal dose for most individuals usually ranges from 2 to 6 mg. Once a good motor response has been achieved, the UPDRS and timed walk can be remeasured and percentage improvement calculated.
- Pump treatment can be commenced in an individual who is already using frequent apomorphine injections by starting an hourly infusion at the rate of 2 to 3 mg per hour and gradually titrating upward depending on the response. The usual pump rate for continuous infusion is 3 to 7 mg per hour. The maximal daily dose is 100 mg.
- If the apomorphine pump is being initiated in an individual who has not had apomorphine previously, the response test can be carried out by giving an initial 1mg bolus and commencing the infusion at 1 to 2 mg per hour with gradual upward titration of the infusion rate.
- Injection or pump training should be carried out during the response test and is fundamental to therapy compliance and the prevention of adverse events.
- Ongoing community support is also helpful and can often be arranged through company nurse advisors.

Complications and monitoring

The most common complications of apomorphine therapy are related to the injection site; they include bruising, inflammation, and the formation of subcutaneous nodules. Rarely, abscess or necrosis can occur. The risk can be reduced by good injection technique, thorough hygiene, and effective site rotation. Localised massage and the use of ultrasound therapy (see discussion of physiotherapy, further on) can be helpful. Sedative effects are also common; if severe, they can lead to the discontinuation of therapy. Apomorphine should be used carefully in those with preexisting orthostatic hypotension because its ability to lower blood pressure may worsen symptoms. Autoimmune hemolytic anemia is a rare complication of apomorphine infusion therapy and should be monitored with full blood counts. If anemia is detected, a hematologist should be consulted and tests for hemolysis, such as a Coombs test, should be undertaken. How frequently these tests should be performed during chronic treatment with apomorphine is somewhat controversial (Carbone et al., 2019). We check the full blood count before treatment commences and every 6 to 12 months or if the individual reports breathlessness or fatigue. Eosinophilia may occur.

Possible drug interactions should be considered, particularly the concomitant administration of ondansetron, which can induce hypotension and syncope. Care should be taken to minimise the use of other drugs that might induce prolongation of the QTc interval. This is especially important in individuals with preexisting cardiac disease (Renoux et al., 2016).

Deep brain stimulation

DBS is considered for people with advanced Parkinson's whose symptoms are not adequately controlled by best medical therapy (National Institute for Health and Care Excellence [NICE], 2017). It is also commonly used to treat dystonia and essential tremor. DBS entails stereotactic implantation of permanent electrodes into the brain. Most commonly the electrodes are sited in the subthalamic nucleus (STN), but they may also sometimes be sited in the globus pallidus interna or thalamus. DBS aims to correct the imbalance created by diminished function of the substantia nigra. Dopamine depletion in the basal ganglia leads to abnormally high inhibitory output from the STN. High-frequency DBS overrides these signal patterns, creating a functional lesion. Thus these signals are replaced with a still abnormal but less pathologic signal.

The selection of candidates for deep brain stimulation

The key to good outcomes is selecting the right candidates. This procedure improves only those symptoms that are responsive to levodopa (motor symptoms). The best someone can be with DBS is the same as the best they can be with levodopa. Although surgery will hopefully improve the levodopa-responsive symptoms and "backtrack" these for a few years, the Parkinson's motor symptoms usually continue to progress at the same rate as they did before DBS. DBS does not delay or prevent the occurrence of dementia (Krishnan et al., 2019). DBS is not curative but may improve QoL for a few years. The PD Surg trial reported improved QoL 12 months after DBS to the STN (Williams et al., 2010).

The NHS Commissioning Board (2013) developed a policy for DBS in movement disorders, advising that all best medical therapy options should have been considered or tried by a movement disorder neurologist before considering a non-oral therapy (DBS, Duodopa, and apomorphine). According to the criteria shown in Table 7.3, DBS is routinely commissioned for people with this condition.

Sometimes it can be difficult for clinicians to get a clear picture of the Parkinson's symptoms. In such instances objective measures of movement and tremor may help. Wearable devices with appropriate software (e.g., Personal Kinetigraph or PKG) are sometimes used to confirm suitability for DBS or other advanced treatments.

The NHS Commissioning Board recommends that STN DBS should not be performed in individuals with marked postural instability, "on" freezing, or "on" falls. As depression can be a potential side effect of DBS, those with a history of severe depression should be assessed by a psychiatrist in advance of DBS. People over the age of 70 are poor candidates, as good outcomes are less likely in this age group. If an individual has an impulse control disorder due to a high dose of dopamine agonist, this should be addressed prior to surgery.

Many hours are spent in determining whether the individual is a suitable candidate and ensuring that he or she has the relevant information to make an

---

TABLE 7.3 National Health Service criteria for deep brain stimulation in Parkinson's

- A diagnosis of Parkinson's, assessed by the UK Parkinson's Disease Society Brain Bank criteria.
- The individual is fit to undergo DBS surgery under general anaesthesia with no contraindications for surgery as assessed by an anaesthetist.
- A life expectancy of 5 or more years as assessed by medical history and liaison with other professionals.
- Symptoms of severe motor complications that compromise function and QoL, including symptoms that are responsive to DBS.
  - On/off fluctuations
  - Levodopa-induced dyskinesias - (with 30% of a 24-hour period in either a disabling "off" state or with disabling dyskinesia)
  - Functionally impairing medication resistance, tremor
- A minimal 40% improvement in the UPDRS motor scale subscores in response to levodopa following a practically defined period off medication. If the indication is a functionally impairing tremor, assessment should show that it significantly impairs ADLs and affects QoL.
- No evidence of a clinically significant cognitive impairment. This is assessed by a psychologist at most centres.

Abbreviations: ADLs, activities of daily living; DBS, deep brain stimulation; QoL, quality of life: UPDRS, Unified Parkinson's Disease Rating Scale

---

informed decision regarding the surgery. Unrealistic expectations as to the potential benefits of DBS may later contribute to reduced satisfaction and a poor clinical outcome following surgery (Geraedts et al., 2019). The individual is finally discussed at a multidisciplinary meeting to assess suitability.

The procedure

DBS surgery usually requires the individual to wake up midsurgery so that symptoms can be assessed when the trial lead is placed. The two head wounds tend have a small, permanent bump due to the plastic caps covering the surgical site. Wires under the skin connect to the battery, which is usually situated in the upper left chest but varies depending on the implant centre. Battery replacements are required every few years, depending on the voltage used. Rechargeable systems have been developed that can stay in place for a minimum of 15 years, but the individual must be trusted to recharge such a system at least once weekly.

Immediately postsurgery

Individuals often feel an "impact effect," also known as a "honeymoon period," when their symptoms improve because of the amount of stimulation delivered in theatre. This can last for several weeks. However, the length of time is not indicative of how much improvement will be gained. The individual goes home after a few days with the DBS switched off.

Follow-up in the clinic

Several weeks later, the individual attends the DBS centre for "mapping," when each contact is assessed to ascertain which one gives the best result and at what voltage symptoms improve or side effects appear. The voltage will be increased incrementally by a handheld programmer given to the individual and caregiver with instructions on its use. The DBS specialist will set the parameters so that the individual can increase or decrease only a certain amount, as advised. Some people will have smaller parameters depending on any impulsiveness and side effects identified on mapping. The therapeutic voltage level must be reached before a benefit will be noticed. At this point, medications can start to be reduced. It can take up to a year to optimise the medication and DBS voltage. Some people require more support than others, so post-DBS care is tailored individually.

The goal is improvement in QoL. Some people are able to reduce their medications more than others. The advantage of decreasing medications is that any side effects will be diminished and there will be more options to add medications back in as the condition progresses.

Individuals may develop apathy in the first few months, which tends to settle, and medication reduction is thought to contribute to this. It would be very rare for anyone to completely stop all Parkinson's medications: most tend to feel better on some levodopa.

Complications

The spread of stimulation can cause sensory disturbance, muscle contractions, dizziness, diplopia, walking problems and dyskinesia. This can be improved by altering the shape of the electrical field so the person should be advised to contact the DBS specialist team. Psychiatric side effects of DBS can also occur, including depression, anxiety, psychosis and impulsive disorders. Affected individuals should alert the DBS team so that treatments and settings can be adjusted accordingly. Over time, when levodopa-responsive symptoms start to improve post-DBS, the individual may start to notice other symptoms. It is likely that these will have been present for a while but were overshadowed by a more problematic symptom.

Speech is affected by DBS in 50% of people, either immediately after the DBS or a few years later. Dysarthria may be due to the spread of electricity beyond the target area of stimulation: sometimes this can be improved by changing the DBS field. Some people have two different programs (e.g., one for talking and one for mobility). SLT input is beneficial for advising on strategies and taking baseline recordings to monitor for progression.

Having DBS may affect relationship dynamics. The improvement in symptoms may affect both partners as their roles change. Caregivers can find it difficult to step back from their caring role to allow the individual to become more independent, and they may feel that they are no longer needed.

Weight gain is common post-DBS. This is multifactorial but partially due to reduced dyskinesia. Balestrino et al., (2017) reported that over half of their subjects were overweight at 1 year post-DBS compared to the baseline of 19%. This may affect functional ability.

Walking speed usually improves after surgery, but other important aspects of gait may not. Balance may become worse and falls may increase after STN-DBS (Duncan, Van Dillen, Garbutt, Earhart, & Perlmutter, 2018).

Individuals benefit from a multidisciplinary approach before and after surgery. Individuals often require help to increase their confidence in being independent with ADLs. Multidisciplinary rehabilitation is important in helping to improve specific functional impairments associated with DBS (Tassorelli et al., 2009).

Levodopa-carbidopa intestinal gel

Treatment with LCIG (Duodopa, Duopa) aims to reduce motor fluctuations by providing continuous dopamine stimulation. The gel is more stable than levodopa-carbidopa dissolved in water and the volume is much smaller. LCIG is delivered directly to the jejunum (the site of absorption) via a percutaneous jejunostomy tube. Stable serum levodopa levels can be achieved. LCIG can achieve significant reductions in "off" time, and improvements in ADLs and QoL have been reported (Olanow et al., 2014).

Candidate selection

People suitable for LCIG therapy are those with an established diagnosis of Parkinson's, a good response to levodopa, motor fluctuations unresponsive to best medical treatment, and at least 3 hours of "off" time per day. Mild dementia is not a contraindication, but dementia may increase the risk of the device tubing being pulled out. Such an individual or his or her caregiver must recognise and respond to device alarms (Burack et al., 2018). Expectations must be realistic. In the United Kingdom, only specialist neuroscience hubs can select people for LCIG therapy, but it is important for other clinicians to refer appropriately. The PDNS may have an important role in supporting people through the preprocedure assessment, dose titration, and follow up.

Percutaneous jejunostomy

The jejunal tube is usually sited by an endoscopist. Often a trial of treatment via a nasojejunostomy tube is undertaken. This helps to establish the effectiveness of LCIG before percutaneous jejunostomy is attempted. A hospital stay of a few days can be expected. Usually the infusion is run over 16 hours during waking hours. The starting dose of LCIG can be estimated from calculating the equivalent daily dose of levodopa. The dose is then titrated.

Complications

Complication related to the jejunostomy tube are very common, with 95% of those treated in the only double-blind randomised controlled trial held thus far reporting side effects (Olanow et al., 2014). Kinking, blockage, and dislodgement occur commonly. Prophylactic administration of vitamin B12, pyridoxine and folic acid might reduce the risk of polyneuropathy. Tube infections, if they occur, are most likely in the first 2 to 4 weeks.

Choosing among advanced treatments

Choosing from among the different advanced treatments largely depends on the individual's age, comorbid conditions, NMSs, and social support (Table 7.4). For further practical guidance, see Worth (2013).

TABLE 7.4 Comparison of advanced treatments for Parkinson's

	Apomorphine infusion	Deep brain stimulation	Levodopa-carbidopa intestinal gel
Suitable for those aged >70 years	Yes	No	Yes
Suitable in mild dementia	No	No	Yes
Suitable in depression	Yes	No (may be suitable after detailed psychiatric evaluation)	Yes
Suitable in those with history of intolerance to dopamine agonists	Usually not	Yes	Yes
Invasiveness	+	++	++
Location for start of treatment	District general hospital	Neuroscience centre	Neuroscience centre
Side effects	Subcutaneous nodules Hallucinations Psychosis Hypotension Haemolytic anaemia Impulse control disorder	Speech problems Stroke (when electrode inserted) Lead infection Weight gain	Tube kinking, blockage or displacement (common) Polyneuropathy Peritonitis Stoma site infection Stoma site hematoma Weight loss Levodopa side effects
Blood monitoring	Full blood count	-	Vitamins B6 and B12
Cost	+++	++	++++

Non-motor symptoms in the complex stage

All the NMSs described in Parkinson's may occur in this stage. In particular, dementia and psychosis can be considered markers of complexity, as their presence complicates management of other symptoms. This section covers psychosis and selected other NMSs that are particularly troublesome in advanced Parkinson's. Dementia is covered in Chapter 9.

Fatigue

Fatigue is a sense of tiredness or exhaustion brought on by repeated activity and leading to impaired performance. In healthy individuals, fatigue improves following rest and does not affect everyday activity, but in Parkinson's fatigue is brought on by minimal exertion, is chronic, improves little with rest and has a huge impact on daily function (Kluger & Friedman, 2014). Fatigue may precede the motor symptoms of Parkinson's. It is present in around 33% of individuals in the early stages and more that 80% of those in late stages (Barone et al., 2009). The biology of fatigue is not well understood, but there are physical and psychological components. Sleep disturbance, medications, and low mood might be implicated. Although there is some overlap between the symptoms of fatigue and depression, fatigue occurs commonly in those who are not depressed. Although Parkinson's medications commonly cause daytime somnolence, most have little effect on fatigue. Levodopa might have a beneficial effect on fatigue (Schifitto et al., 2008). In terms of drug treatment, a small trial of methylphenidate has shown some benefit (Mendonca et al., 2007), but this drug is not widely used. Rasagiline was considered efficacious and possibly useful in a recent review (Seppi et al., 2019). Modafinil and testosterone are not helpful. Many members of the MDT may contribute to the management of fatigue. The physician must consider the possibility of such comorbidities as anemia, chronic infection, thyroid disorders, renal failure, cardiac failure, vitamin D deficiency, depression and adverse effects of medication. The OT should consider the daily routine, sleep hygiene, depression management and need for social support. The physiotherapist should consider a graded exercise programme.

Pain

Pain is a common symptom affecting around 60% of individuals with Parkinson's (Broen at al., 2012). Chronic pain is more common in Parkinson's than in age-matched individuals with other chronic diseases and is linked with depression and reduced QoL. It may be difficult to determine whether the pain is due to Parkinson's or common comorbidities such as osteoarthritis, osteoporotic vertebral fractures, or painful neuropathies. Pain is likely to be Parkinson's-related if it started after the Parkinson's appeared, is worse on the side more affected by the Parkinson's, and improves with levodopa or other dopaminergic (dopamine-like) medications (Perez-Lloret et al., 2014). Pain sensitivity is increased in individuals with Parkinson's who are off medication (Sung at al., 2018); therefore optimising the Parkinson's medication is often helpful.

It is important to remember that his or her pain may not be voluntarily reported by the individual; thus should be included as a key issue in assessments and reviews. The NMS questionnaire has a screening question for chronic pain and, if this highlights an issue, a clinical evaluation should follow. Use of a more detailed pain assessment tool such as King's Parkinson's disease pain questionnaire should be considered at this stage (Martinez-Martin et al., 2018). It is important to identify, if possible, the root cause of the pain being experienced and to be aware that more than one area or type of pain may be involved. Five types of pain are commonly associated with Parkinson's (Ford, 2010):

- *Musculoskeletal pain* can be intensified in Parkinson's owing to rigidity and reduced mobility. It can improve with exercise and increased activity, and may also be relieved by levodopa. Simple analgesia or an intra-articular steroid injection may help. Orthopedic or rheumatological review should be considered.
- *Radicular/neuropathic pain* is pain in a nerve root causing motor and/or sensory signs. Further investigation should be considered, including the ascertainment of vitamin B12 level, glycosylated hemoglobin, alcohol history. Testing might include serum protein electrophoresis, autoantibody screen, imaging, neurophysiologic assessment. Gabapentin or amitriptyline can be helpful.
- *Dystonia* can affect limbs, trunk, neck, face, and jaw; it often occurs in "off" periods. An adjustment in dopaminergic medication may help. In the case of limb dystonia, holding the affected part in the neutral position and applying a stretch and hold for 2 minutes can bring temporary relief.
- *Central pain* is felt as a burning or stabbing pain, often in the abdomen, chest, mouth, or legs. Medication adjustment may be helpful.
- *Akasthesia* is a subjective restlessness that can lead to the inability to sit still, lie in bed, drive a car, eat at a table, or attend social gatherings (thus risking social isolation). It may improve with medication adjustment.

Pain thresholds and therefore the subjective experience of pain differs among individuals, so assessment and measurement can be difficult. The visual analogue scale is a useful tool to identify the severity of subjective pain, but it is also important to consider whether the pain is acute or chronic, how often and when it occurs, as well as whether it is an ache or a sharp pain. Identifying what makes it worse as well as what can improve it (e.g., rest, medication) can also help to direct intervention. A body chart can be of assistance in documenting affected body parts.

Depending on the information gained during the assessment, intervention may include advice regarding the application of heat or ice, exercise, hydrotherapy, and consideration of a medication review.

Drooling

Drooling can occur in up to 50% of people with Parkinson's, although in the early stages the impact may be small. Saliva flow tends to be normal or even decreased compared to that in people without Parkinson's. Drooling in Parkinson's is thought to be caused by a combination of factors, including orofacial rigidity, unintentional mouth opening, lingual bradykinesia, stooped posture and antecollis (dropped head). Cognitive and attentional factors may also contribute (Miller et al., 2019). For those affected, it represents a challenging and distressing symptom that can lead to poor oral hygiene, bad breath, eating and speaking difficulty, and an increased rate of respiratory tract infection from silent aspiration of saliva. From a psychosocial perspective, drooling leads to embarrassment, increasing emotional distress, reduced participation in social events and poorer QoL. Caregivers are also affected, for example, by increased clothes washing, restricted social life, and effects on intimacy.

The NICE Parkinson's Guideline (National Institute for Health and Care Excellence [NICE], 2017) advocates behavioural methods of intervention in the first instance, followed by consideration of pharmacological or surgical options if and when the former are ineffective. Behavioural methods include

- Attention to posture, with regular prompts to correct it (from self or caregiver).
- Raising the eye level of reading material or the computer screen.
- If the individual is sleeping in a chair, it is important to ensure that the head is properly supported in midline and that the back support is tilted back slightly.
- Using cues such as remembering to swallow as much saliva as possible before attempting to rise from the chair or to swallow before talking.
- Using a swallow prompt app as a training device to remind the person to increase the frequency of the resting swallow.
- Use of a pastille or chewing gum can alert the brain that there is something in the mouth that needs to be swallowed.
- Lip-seal exercises.

Anticholinergic medication can be used, but most systemic agents are not selective for M3 receptors and therefore carry undesirable adverse effects such as confusion, hallucinations, constipation, urinary retention and drowsiness in people with Parkinson's. Hyoscine patches can be effective but tend to be poorly tolerated. Sublingual administration of atropine eye drops and sublingual ipratropium bromide (e.g., the Atrovent inhaler) can be effective. Individuals with

Parkinson's should be made aware that these preparations are not licenced for the treatment of drooling. There is an obvious risk that atropine eye drops will be put in the eyes rather than used sublingually as intended by the prescriber. For that reason we advise against their use. Oral glycopyrrolate is efficacious (Arbouw et al., 2010) and is first line in the United Kingdom. Glycopyrrolate crosses the blood-brain barrier poorly and thus poses a low risk of side effects. If this is ineffective, not tolerated, or contraindicated, referral to a specialist service for botulinum toxin injections to submandibular or parotid glands or both can be an effective option (Miller et al., 2019). All treatments that reduce saliva production may have unwanted effects, including an increased risk of dental caries and dysphagia.

Psychosis

Criteria for a diagnosis of psychosis in Parkinson's include the presence of at least one of the following: illusions, false sense of presence, hallucinations and/or delusions. These symptoms should occur after the diagnosis of Parkinson's, be recurrent or continuous for at least a month, and not be triggered by a general medical condition such as infection (Ravina et al., 2007). Visual hallucinations are common, occurring in about one-third of people with Parkinson's. Visual hallucinations in Parkinson's are typically of people or animals moving about. Hallucinations in other modalities (auditory, tactile, olfactory) may also occur. First symptoms may be visual misinterpretations. Sensations of presence (feeling the presence of another person) or of passage (movement in the peripheral visual field) are also common. Often insight is preserved when hallucinations first appear, but over subsequent years individuals struggle to determine what is real and what is hallucinatory—they lose insight. Visual hallucinations are associated with increased caregiver burden and nursing home placement. Normalising the experience by stating that hallucinations are very common and can be treated may help individuals open up about their hallucinations.

Occasionally delusional interpretations of the hallucinations occur and the individual believes that he or she is being attacked or robbed, for example. Delusions occur in about 5% to 15% of people with Parkinson's and are common in those with dementia. Paranoid delusions may occur. Delusions of the partner being unfaithful may lead to pathologic jealousy (Othello syndrome), in which case a risk assessment should be undertaken and mental health referral considered. Delusional misidentification syndromes such as Capgras syndrome are not uncommon, particularly in those with dementia. In Capgras syndrome, the individual mistakes familiar people for impostors or doubles. They recognise the face but lack the usual emotional connection associated with the face.

The cause of psychosis in Parkinson's is unclear, but dopaminergic medications, damage to cholinergic neurons, sleep disturbance, cognitive decline and visual impairment all play a part.

Management depends to an extent on how well the symptoms are tolerated but might include the following:

- Exclusion of general medical causes of acute deterioration.
- In a medication review, possibly
  — Reduce the number of medications.
  — Reverse any recent medication change that could have precipitated psychosis.
  — Stop anticholinergic medications.
  — In stages, withdraw amantadine and selegiline, then other MAOIBs and dopamine agonists, then COMT inhibitors, and finally reduce the levodopa dose.
- Optimising vision. Correct refractive errors, treat cataracts, ensure rooms are well lit.
- Offering advice on sleep hygiene.
- Consider rivastigmine, which can effectively reduce hallucinations in those with Parkinson's and dementia. It has been used to treat psychosis in individuals without dementia, but evidence for this approach is lacking.
- Quetiapine may be helpful. Check QTc is normal before prescribing. It can be started at 12.5 mg twice daily and increased to 25 mg twice daily if needed. Further dose increments may be needed, but dosing is lower than in other psychotic conditions. Quetiapine may cause drowsiness and postural hypotension. Use of antipsychotic medications increases mortality risk; therefore a careful consideration of risks and benefits is indicated. Continued need for the medication should be reviewed regularly.
- Clozapine is highly effective in treating Parkinson's psychosis, but there is a risk of agranulocytosis; therefore those taking clozapine must be registered with a blood monitoring service.
- Pimavanserin, which is licenced in the United States (Seppi et al., 2019).
- Ondansetron was helpful for Parkinson's psychosis and found to be well tolerated in an open-label study (Zoldan at al., 1995).

Abnormal temperature control and sweating

Disorders of body temperature regulation can occur in Parkinson's. Hyperthermia is more common than hypothermia. General medical conditions such as infection and dehydration can contribute to high body temperature; these should be considered first. Anticholinergic medication may also contribute. Dopamine receptors in the hypothalamus are involved in the regulation of body temperature: stimulation of these receptors lowers body temperature and blockade of the receptors raises body temperature. This helps explain the rare but serious neuroleptic malignant syndrome and Parkinson's hyperpyrexia syndrome (see Chapter 12). High body temperature may also be a feature of serotonin syndrome, a rare complication of MOAIs used with antidepressants.

Disorders of sweating occur in around 50% of those with Parkinson's. Drenching sweats (hyperhidrosis) are more often reported, but reduced sweating in the palms may be more common. Sweating episodes may cause social embarrassment. If sweating symptoms fluctuate in relation to motor "off" periods, strategies to reduce motor fluctuations may also improve sweating symptoms. Often there is no correlation between sweating and motor control (Mostile & Jankovic, 2014).

It may help to adjust the person's clothing as well as the room temperature. Antiperspirants containing aluminium chloride hexahydrate should be tried. Anticholinergic medication such as glycopyrronium may be effective. Iontophoresis can be very effective. This electrical treatment is sometimes offered by dermatology departments, and machines for home use can be purchased. Usually two or three 20- to 30-minute treatments each week are needed for the first month. If the treatments are successful, top-up treatments may be needed on a weekly or monthly basis (British Association of Dermatologists, 2019). Injection of botulinum toxin A can be effective, but repeat injections are needed.

Intervention and support from the multidisciplinary team

Parkinson's disease nurse specialist

Review by the PDNS during the complex stage should focus on a thorough assessment of both motor symptoms and NMSs as well as any other complications; the nurse should assess how these difficulties are affecting the person's day-to-day function. It can be very helpful to spend some time talking through a typical day with the individual to develop a picture of the interplay between medication doses (particularly levodopa) and symptoms to determine how they fluctuate and affect day-to-day function. Creating a time line (see Figure 7.2) or using an "on/off" chart can help in carrying out this assessment and may suggest helpful medication adjustments (timing/dose-interval adjustments, dose increases, new medication options). It is vital that a risk/benefit analysis be carried out with the individual so as to identify potential problems that may arise from medication escalation, particularly the potential for worsening neuropsychiatric features. Even though motor symptoms can be troublesome, the risk of further

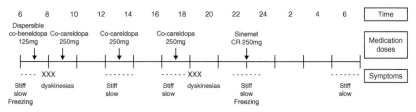

FIGURE 7.2   Time line showing time of each medication dose and timing and duration of symptoms. Key: - - - - "off" symptoms such as stiffness, slowness and freezing. XXX dyskinesia.

escalation may outweigh any benefit. If gaining a good understanding of fluctuations is proving to be very difficult, objective measures (e.g., the PKG) can be considered. Thought should be given to the person's suitability for advanced therapies; if appropriate, this should be discussed with the individual and appropriate referrals made.

When neuropsychiatric features predominate, the consultation should focus on how best to manage and support both the individual and caregiver in coping with hallucinations, psychosis, dementia (see Chapter 9) and impulsive/compulsive behaviours.

In this stage, the individual is likely to have complex health needs that can increase the risk of hospital admission and consideration of a care facility (nursing home). The PDNS is an important source of advice, support, and practical help in such instances. Caregivers will experience multidimensional changes within their expanding roles and increased responsibilities. They should be supported and involved through any process of change (Hand, 2017). A feeling of "loss of former self" and elements of grief can be experienced by caregivers who carry a higher Parkinson's burden and face greater psychosocial needs in the later stages of the condition (Fox et al., 2017). The PDNS can help by encouraging the caregivers to remember the positives of each day, to focus on what they are learning, and to acknowledge their good work.

For a person with Parkinson's, having a caregiver is linked with a better QoL. The caregiver reports additional information about symptoms and also encourages medication adherence and social engagement (Prizer et al., 2020). The PDNS should therefore encourage caregiver involvement. More symptoms in the person with Parkinson's, particularly immobility and NMSs, lead to a greater burden and more mental health symptoms for the caregiver. On the other hand, greater social support for the caregiver is associated with resilience and better mental health (Tyler et al., 2020). MDTs should offer educational interventions for caregivers. Such education should cover the scheduling of pleasant activities, communication strategies, and stress management (Simons at al., 2006). Fellowship with other caregivers through support groups may be helpful, and cognitive behavioural therapy (CBT) can be effective for caregivers with symptoms of psychological strain (Secker & Brown, 2005).

Psychological well-being

The biopsychosocial formulation (Evans et al., 2006)—which is described in more detail Chapter 6, on the maintenance stage—is a model that can be helpful in shaping a neurorehabilitation approach for persons with Parkinson's and the professionals who work with them. This approach helps to consider the interaction of several important factors (see Figure 7.3).

Understanding the interaction between an individual's mild cognitive impairment and emotional distress, for example, is very important. A holistic view

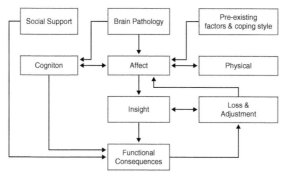

FIGURE 7.3   The biopsychosocial model of neurorehabilitation (Evans, 2006). Figure 7.3 de-
picts a biopsychosocial model of the consequences of Parkinson's based on the model for brain
injury described by Evans (2006). It can be used to map assessment results across the team; develop a shared formulation; and help to clarify events as they are viewed by the individual, family,
and professional. Arrows represent relationships and interactions between these areas; these may
change on an individual basis and may be bidirectional in some cases. ILS, independent living
skills. *Reproduced with permission from Wilson, B. A., Gracey, F., Evans, J., & Bateman, A. (eds.)*
(2009). Neuropsychological rehabilitation: theory, models, therapy & outcome. Cambridge, UK:
Cambridge University Press.

can help to ensure that the most suitable coping strategy to improve psychological well-being is recommended. An individual's cognitive resources and insight
will influence what intervention strategy is best. For example, one individual
may be able to learn and use self-directed strategies whereas another would
benefit from changes to the environment. Such changes might include supported engagement from formal or informal carers in relaxation, mindfulness, or
cognitive stimulation activities. Understanding the individual's core values and
making sure that the goals of rehabilitation are met can help to prioritise the
person's identity and sense of self despite having to live with a complex set of
experiences and symptoms.

Confronted with an individual's experience of delusions and hallucinations,
the health professional should consider what these are communicating about
the individual and not simply see them as organic consequences of Parkinson's.
Personally meaningful and interconnected themes can be found in the delusional experiences of a person with Parkinson's (Todd at al., 2010). Being scared,
trapped, not feeling safe, and losing control may be potential themes; they can
also represent the more general effects that Parkinson's can have on an individual's life. Offering a psychological formulation for delusional experiences
can help the person to understand the delusions. The MDT should provide interventions that help to diminish the distress that the person experiences (anxiety,
low mood) and consider ways in which an individual can be supported to feel
safe or more emotionally contained. Working with the family network is also
important.

Assessment and intervention from clinical psychologists, neuropsychologists, cognitive behavioural therapists or other mental health professionals can

be complementary to the Parkinson's MDT. Joint sessions with multiple MDT members can be effective, and Parkinson's outpatient or neurorehabilitation services should establish strong relationships with their local mental health services to help bridge the gap between neurological and mental health care. This can help to establish clear and agreed on referral and care pathways. An example of joint work among these organisations is a "training swap," with the Parkinson's team providing mental health team workers with training on Parkinson's and the mental health team providing training on psychosis and unusual experiences.

Physiotherapy

Falls

Risk of falling increases as the condition progresses. Establishing details of the fall may help target interventions. Questions to individuals should include how many times they have fallen, when and where they fell, what they were doing at the time, which direction they fell in, and how they got up again. Establishing what the individual thinks caused the fall is important, as it can indicate their insight and any behavioural factors. Because of the combination of impaired postural responses and reaching outside the base of support, most falls occur when individuals are reaching up above the head, below the knees, or transferring (standing from sitting). Freezing of gait (FOG) also increases the risk for falls, and many individuals fall when turning. Therapy-led gait and balance intervention and training in cues and strategies may help to reduce falls (see Chapter 10).

Posture

Several factors can lead to a deterioration in posture. These include soft tissue changes, degenerative skeletal changes, reduced range of motion, rigidity, dystonia and proprioceptive impairment. An increasingly flexed posture can lead to complications with balance and mobility, and the individual may develop back and neck pain. The tragus-to-wall measurement (Heuft-Dorenbosch et al., 2004) to measure posture can allow the individual to understand the extent of their problem and set an achievable goal. An example of such a goal might be a 2-cm improvement within 2 months. This can help motivate a person to engage in therapy programs such as exercises targeting head, neck, and trunk flexibility and core strength. It is important to include assessment and intervention for posture as early as possible, as it can be difficult to achieve improvement in long-standing problems. Posture reminders (apps or vibrating sensors) have been developed with little evidence for efficacy. Hydrotherapy can be beneficial (Volpe et al., 2017). Provision of an appropriate walking aid (walking poles, a three- or four-wheel walker) can improve posture while mobilising. Camptocormia, Pisa syndrome and antecollis (Table 7.5) can be especially difficult to treat, and evidence for the effectiveness of interventions is scant, with no proven long-term effects (Barone at al, 2016). Specific

TABLE 7.5 Postural deformities in Parkinson's

Posture Type	Description	Intervention
Camptocormia	Marked flexion (minimum 45 degrees) thoracolumbar flexion when walking or standing but resolves when lying down (Doherty et al., 2011). Affects between 3% and 17.6% of people with Parkinson's, more commonly older individuals or those with more severe Parkinson's, and around 7 to 8 years after diagnosis (Doherty et al., 2011). Can make it difficult for persons to see where they are going when mobilising, and the degree of flexion can increase the longer they stand or walk.	On testing muscle strength, trunk and hip extension are often normal. Maintaining flexibility and muscle strength are essential to arresting further deterioration; physiotherapy programs should reflect this. Walking poles or forearm walkers can be useful.
Pisa syndrome	Marked lateral flexion in the trunk (no consensus on degree but Doherty proposes at least 10 degrees), leaning to one side, which resolves upon lying down (Doherty et al., 2011). May initially become apparent when the individual is sitting in a chair and tilts to one side.	It is essential to maintain flexibility and muscle strength to arrest further deterioration. Exercising in front of full-length mirror can provide feedback to help attain or come closer to midline.
Antecollis	Marked flexion of the neck, which cannot be fully extended against gravity (Doherty et al., 2011). It also occurs in multiple system atrophy. Seen in some 5% to 8% of people with Parkinson's (Ashour & Jankovic, 2006). Can be accompanied by a lateral tilt to one side and pain in the neck. Can cause difficulties in mobilising (such people are unable to see where they are going) and with eating and swallowing. Can affect communication, as the individual may be unable to see other people's facial expressions and, likewise, their own facial expressions may be hidden from view.	Requires an individually tailored exercise programme to target head and shoulder flexibility. Custom-made or soft collars (bean or foam) can improve resting posture and relieve pain. Some individuals may benefit from injections of botulinum toxin (Botox).

walking aids may prove useful, and some individuals may benefit from a custom vest or suit.

Problems with Transfers

People with Parkinson's can find it increasingly difficult to rise from a chair, turn over in bed, or get in and out of bed. Chair rising can be affected by leg muscle weakness as well as loss of automaticity of a complex movement. Difficulty with bed mobility may be due to the wearing off of medication during the night, but it can also be due to the dysfunction of the automatic processing of a complex movement. The ability to turn over is intact but is no longer automatically executed. This can lead to the individual having to sit up every time he or she wants to turn over, which may occur several times during the night, interrupting his or her sleep and that of the partner. Breaking down the movement into stages (transfer strategy) can help. The physiotherapist or OT can teach strategies for both bed and chair mobility (Table 7.6); it is also important to teach the individual how to get up from the floor in the event of a fall. In addition, advising the use of a silk or satin strip over the middle third of the bed can enable an easier turn (see Chapter 6, Fig. 6.3). However, such individuals should be advised not to wear satin or silk nightwear if using this technique, as this might cause them to slip out of bed. The OT can assess whether equipment such as a bed lever would be beneficial; this would depend on the type of bed and the individual's cognitive ability.

TABLE 7.6 Transfer strategies

Transfer Strategy	Step 1	Step 2	Step 3	Step 4
Standing from a chair	Bottom forward	Place feet correctly	Place hands in position	With momentum—chin forward over knees— push up
Turning over in bed	Bend knees keeping feet on the bed	Turn head in direction of turn	Keeping knees bent, reach opposite arm across to side of bed (knees will follow)	Adjust bottom to find comfortable position
Getting out of bed	Bend knees keeping feet on the bed	Turn head towards direction of turn	Keeping knees bent, reach opposite arm across to side of bed (knees will follow)	Push up onto elbow at the same time as dropping feet over edge of bed and sit up

Apomorphine nodules

For those on apomorphine pumps, therapeutic ultrasound can reduce the tenderness of nodules that form around the needle sites. Guidelines are available and must be interpreted within the context of a full assessment by a trained clinician (Poltawski et al., 2008). The optimal frequency of ultrasound treatment is uncertain, but treatment twice a week for 2 to 4 weeks has been suggested (Poltawski et al., 2009; Todd & James, 2008). It is important not to apply ultrasound near the sited needle or on inflamed nodules.

Occupational therapy

In the complex stage, people with Parkinson's are likely to experience difficulties with ADLs. These may arise because of immobility, impaired upper limb motor function or cognitive decline. Having someone prompt during washing and dressing may be all that is needed to maintain function and complete the activity, but prompts may be an indicator of cognitive decline. Cognitive strategies that were previously taught to the individual may now have to be taught to caregivers. Cognitive decline is often accompanied by postural instability and FOG.

Environmental assessment

The OT can help by advising on the optimal layout of furniture, lighting, and decor. The environment should be kept as clear of clutter as possible. Lighting should be bright enough to allow the individual to spot obstacles along the route and to reduce the risk of visual misinterpretation. The OT should advise that decor can cause overstimulation of the visual field, thus affecting the individual's ability to focus on his or her physical function. For those susceptible to hallucinations, solid-color unpatterned carpets and walls may be less hallucinogenic. A home visit can enable the OT to observe the individual navigating from room to room. Modifying a route to reduce the number of turns and, for example, organising the kitchen so that all items are easily accessible may reduce the risk for falls. Reducing clutter and using visual cues in the environment can reduce FOG.

Aids and appliances

When aids to assist self-care or domestic activities are being provided, the fact that the individual has less ability to learn new things must be taken into consideration. If using the equipment entails learning a new way of completing an activity, this can cause confusion. If the equipment allows completion of the activity in the same way as before, individuals will find it more helpful.

Sleep

Sleep patterns can change. Vivid dreams can be disturbing, sometimes more so for the sleep partner. During rapid-eye-motion sleep behaviour disorder, the individual may act out dreams, which can include talking, shouting, lashing out or falling out of bed. Dreams usually involve being threatened or chased, so the verbal reactions of the individual will be defensive rather than offensive. If the caregiver is being disturbed by such dreams, it would be advisable for him or her to sleep in another room for some duration of the night. The dreamer can be awakened if there are signs of distress or concerns about safety. It is important also to consider a 24-hour sleep regimen, as increased fatigue at night may exacerbate vivid dreams.

Fatigue

Fatigue is common in Parkinson's and has a big impact on daily function. It also affects motivation, which is already low owing to reduced dopamine levels. To identify the most appropriate intervention for fatigue, it is important to identify the cause. Factors that may contribute to fatigue include low mood, lack of sleep at night, and medications. If depression is a problem, potential causes should be considered and managed. Such issues may include:

- Psychological adjustment to the advancing condition. Initially this can be managed by the OT within the team but it may require a neuropsychologist for management of more severe symptoms.
- Reduction in physical abilities or increased Parkinson's symptoms. This calls for further discussion with the consultant or PDNS.
- Low mood due to other life events. Such persons can be referred to a community psychological therapy service for general counseling or to CBT programs. In the United Kingdom, these can be accessed via self-referral to Improving Access to Psychological Therapies (IAPT) programs.

Advice is given with regard to pacing during the day, making sure that the individual completes some form of physical activity daily and, if possible, goes outdoors daily.

Cognitive changes and psychosis

Memory loss, executive dysfunction, hallucinations, delusions and dementia become more prevalent with the duration of Parkinson's and with age. Confusional states may include restlessness and irrational behaviours and may vary throughout the day according to medication times or perhaps in relation to increased stress or fatigue. "Sundowner" confusion can occur in the evening hours and may be triggered by fatigue. If the confusion is related to medication times, it should be discussed with the consultant or PDNS. It is important to help the caregiver explore potential triggers (see Chapter 9).

Apathy

Although apathy may be evident throughout the condition, it can be especially bothersome in the complex stage. Caregivers in particular may find apathy frustrating. Trying to motivate someone with Parkinson's can lead to the disruption of relationships. The individual's mood can become low. Lack of dopamine contributes to the individual's reduced ability to self-motivate, so it is important to consider external motivators such as the following:

- Goal setting. This is a constructive way to manage apathy. Identify with the individual their hobbies and interests, and make a list of varied activities (both physical and cognitive) that he or she would enjoy. It is important that chores be included if they are part of the individual's role.
- A timetable. This can be used to plan activities for a week. A schedule can help motivate the individual to complete activities and tasks.
- Rewards. Encourage individuals to think about the rewards linked to different activities and tasks—for example, discussing the physical benefits from a daily walk or thinking about how they feel when they have visited friends or family.

Speech and language therapy

Swallowing difficulties

Swallowing difficulties are most prevalent in the complex stage of Parkinson's. It is considered best practice for a SLT to document the timing of Parkinson's medication in relation to a swallowing assessment and whether the individual is "on" or "off." The variability in Parkinson's, where a person has access to movement at one moment but then switches off, can be among the most challenging to manage. A person with Parkinson's must understand aspiration risk in relation to such fluctuations in order to make flexible food and drink choices. The challenge comes when individuals do not remember the consequences of aspiration and therefore require close supervision and support from people around them.

Chapter 6 describes a selection of the many different types of swallowing therapy available. Using rehabilitation strategies in the context of a progressive condition is really important for maintaining QoL and reducing the need for hospital admissions due to aspiration pneumonia. Cognition can impact the implementation of postural strategies (e.g., chin tuck and head turn). Therefore, in the complex stage, we are more likely to consider environmental or food and fluid modification as first-line strategies. Therapies such as "Expiratory Muscle Strength Training", Lee Silverman voice therapy, or choral singing therapy are also beneficial.

Kyphosis (forward curvature of the spine) can have a significant impact on swallowing. Helping the individual to find corrective strategies is crucial. People with Parkinson's report that they feel as though their voice box were displaced or that they are struggling with the increased effort required to push food vertically every time they swallow. Visual feedback in the form of videofluoroscopy can help to explain and reassure them. A modified texture may be helpful, but it is most useful to collaborate with the physiotherapist to explore whether they would benefit from custom neck support such as the head-up neck collar.

When swallowing becomes more difficult, the pros and cons of tube feeding and risk feeding should be discussed (Table 7.7). Risk feeding is the current terminology for ongoing oral feeding even though no safe oral consistency is available; that is, the risk of aspiration is acknowledged. Enteral feeding includes feeding via nasogastric (NG) tubes, percutaneous endoscopic gastrostomy (PEG) tubes, and radiologically inserted gastrostomy (RIG) tubes. NG tube feeding may be appropriate for short-term feeding when swallowing is temporarily impaired—for example, due to drowsiness or fatigue associated with infection. When long-term enteral feeding is appropriate, PEG feeding is preferred. RIG tubes are usually used only when PEG feeding is not possible. There is no randomised controlled clinical trial comparing outcomes for tube feeding and risk feeding.

All people in the complex stage should have a conversation regarding advance care planning; their views and wishes regarding non-oral feeding should

TABLE 7.7 Considerations in percutaneous endoscopic gastrostomy feeding decisions in dysphagic Parkinson's

Percutaneous endoscopic gastrostomy (PEG) is a reliable means of delivering food, fluid, and medication to the stomach.

PEG may be appropriate if mealtimes are prolonged and burdensome to the individual.

PEG may be appropriate if dysphagia results in omitted medication and a trial of nasogastric medication has led to significant improvements in Parkinson's symptoms.

PEG does not reverse neurodegeneration.

The PEG procedure is initiated under local anaesthesia and has a procedure-related mortality of less than1%.

Food delivered via tube is not tasted, but an individual may choose to accept the risk and take some food by mouth in order to enjoy the taste.

Psychosocial benefits of mealtimes may be lost.

Tube feeding does not abolish the risk of aspiration as saliva may be aspirated or feed regurgitated. Aspiration severe enough to need hospital treatment occurs in about 30% of people with Parkinson's who are fed via PEG.

PEG complications include perforated bowel, bruising or infection at the PEG site, and tube dislodgement

Thirty-day mortality among such patients is about 6% and median survival is over 400 days (in carefully selected individuals).

Around one-third of individuals formerly living in their own homes are institutionalised following PEG placement (Brown et al., 2020).

Dysphagia may be a marker of advanced disease: if dysphagia is accompanied by dementia and immobility, PEG feeding is unlikely to improve QoL in the time remaining.

be documented. Members of the MDT must work together to recognise markers of advanced disease (weight loss, chest infections, nursing home placement, dementia, worsening dysphagia) and collaborate with the individual and family to make sure that a care plan is made and documented. There is a strong recommendation that all acute and community teams engage in the seamless and timely sharing of information so as to enable quick decisions later on in hospital, when an individual is acutely ill.

Persons with Parkinson's and their families may need reminding of the challenge of multitasking and how this applies as much to eating and drinking as it does to walking. They may need to look closely at the eating environment, reduce distractions, change utensils, or alter seating. There are companies that offer equipment solutions to the greatest such challenges, including tremor mugs, weighted cuffs, pacing mugs (controlled flow mugs), or even more high-tech gadgets such as the Neater Eater or Power Drinker. An example pacing mug is the Provale cup. It is available in the US and is designed to deliver specific, predetermined small volumes of liquid in a normal drinking motion.

Communication difficulties

The complex stage of Parkinson's can see significant changes to voice, speech, and communication skills. Historically the majority of referrals to speech therapy were made in this complex stage.

Communication and interaction: Slower responses can make it harder to keep up in conversation; therefore people may gradually reduce the amount of talking they do. Reduced facial expressiveness and fewer body gestures mean that the non-verbal signals that often aid conversation flow are often not present. Families and caregivers may need training in conversation support to notice the changes and provide the kind of support and understanding that will enable maximum participation. Sometimes just raising awareness of what helps and what does not can be enough to prompt a positive change.

Speech rate: If dysfluency, speech initiation, or fast speech is affecting intelligibility, a pacing board should be considered. There are two main types of such boards: the alphabet chart or a simple line of dots. Even though there is a demand on the individual to point and talk at the same time, the board can be effective at slowing a fast rate of speech. An alternative strategy is altered auditory feedback (previously known as delayed auditory feedback), which sends a masking noise into one or both ears. Altered auditory feedback reduces sensory feedback and provides enough delay to also slow the rate of speech.

Voice: SLTs can enable the person with Parkinson's to achieve a louder voice using airflow and voice-projection exercises. Lee Silverman Voice Therapy is an approach that achieves carryover of the louder voice in a range of settings. In the complex stage, individuals may need additional time to compensate for attentional reading difficulties and slower thought processing. It is essential to practise voice tasks while multitasking, gradually adding motor and cognitive demands (Sapir at al., 2011). This prepares the individual for the demands of talking in conversation, which requires multiple mental processes to be working simultaneously (see Chapter 6, Fig. 6.4). For example, the individual can be asked to say "ah" while tapping a foot or passing a ball from hand to hand. He or she may also be asked to say "ah" while imagining words flashing up on a screen, such as days of the week, numbers or any category that seems interesting.

<u>Equipment and technology</u>: It has been suggested that when intelligibility falls below 90%, a backup to communication should be considered (Fried-Oken at al., 2015). There is now wide ownership of smartphones, iPads, and tablet computers, so using text-to-speech apps can provide an inexpensive option. If tremor is a concern, more robust devices such as the Allora 2 or Toby Churchill SL50 Lightwriter may be helpful. These devices can store phrases, larger volumes of text, and send text messages. Amplifier technology has also advanced and the Echovoice-EV6, for example, can amplify a whispered voice successfully. Older adults may also benefit from linking up with hearing support services, to explore devices that work with hearing aids, such as the Roger Pen or other personal listeners.

Dietitian

Individuals with Parkinson's may be overweight or underweight. In a community-based study, weight loss (>5% of baseline weight) at 1 year predicted dependency, dementia, and death (Cumming at al., 2017). On average, those with Parkinson's lose weight more rapidly than healthy controls. Weight loss also increases the risk of malnutrition, dyskinesia, postural hypotension, falls, and hip fracture. The mechanism of weight loss in Parkinson's is multifactorial but must involve an imbalance between food (energy) intake and energy expenditure (Bachmann & Trenkwalder, 2006). Factors that reduce food intake include:

- Anosmia
- Poor motor function or tremor leading to difficulties getting the food to mouth
- Chewing and swallowing problems (in advanced Parkinson's). Slow eating can lead to food going cold. The individual or caregiver may tire of the process before an adequate quantity of food has been taken.
- Gastroparesis—delayed gastric emptying may lead to a sense of fullness.
- Medication-induced nausea.
- Constipation.
- Dementia. Impaired executive function might lead to poor shopping decisions and may compromise meal preparation. Those living alone are at greatest risk of malnutrition, but the presence of high caregiver burden is also linked with weight loss in people with Parkinson's.
- Depression.
- Low-protein diet.

- Impaired reward processing.
- Neuroendocrine factors—reduced levels of appetite-stimulating hormones such as ghrelin and neuropeptide Y.
- Social factors—for example, not wanting to eat in front of people owing to feelings of embarrassment about drooling, dropping food or choking.

Factors that increase energy expenditure include:

- Rigidity, tremor, and dyskinesia
- Increased physical activity due to dopaminergic medication
- Increased release of growth hormone due to dopaminergic medication (Bachmann & Trenkwalder, 2006; Ma et al., 2018)

Weight should be measured at every visit. For frail individuals, a malnutrition screening tool such as the Malnutrition Universal Screening Tool (MUST) should be considered. It is important for the physician to consider causes of weight loss unrelated to Parkinson's. It is usual to ask about new symptoms, including rectal bleeding, cough, hemoptysis, hematuria, lumps, swellings, and retrosternal dysphagia. A full physical examination and simple blood tests should be done. Further investigation will depend on the results of this initial assessment as well as on patient preference and clinical judgment.

The dietitian should consider all of the mentioned factors in assessing an individual with Parkinson's who has lost weight. When anosmia is a factor, it is important for food to look appealing. Sweet, salty and spicy foods should be explored. The dietitian should work closely with the physician and PDNS to make sure that constipation and nausea are treated and motor function is optimised. If depression is present, mirtazapine should be considered, as it can stimulate appetite. Close cooperation with an SLT is advisable.

Enriching foods with cream and butter may help. Snacking can be helpful for those with early satiety or those who tire during long meals. Oral nutritional supplements should be considered. PEG feeding might be considered if there is significant dysphagia, but it is important to determine whether the weight loss and dysphagia are part of a terminal decline characterised by dementia and immobility.

Being obese (having a body mass index [BMI] > 30 kg/m^2) or overweight (BMI $= 25$–29.9 kg/m^2) may actually be more common in Parkinson's than being underweight (BMI < 20 kg/m^2) (Barichella at al., 2003). Obesity is associated with an increased risk of functional dependency and faster motor decline in Parkinson's (Kim & Jun, 2020). Weight reduction is advisable for these individuals, as there are generic health benefits. Weight reduction may also allow greater physical activity. DBS treatment is associated with weight gain, and dopamine agonist treatment can cause binge eating so these individuals need close monitoring.

There is insufficient evidence to support low-protein diets, but physicians may refer individuals with motor fluctuations for a protein redistribution diet. Individuals on this diet must restrict protein intake at breakfast and lunch but can have unrestricted protein at dinner. These diets are well tolerated in the short term, but individuals tend to drift back to their former dietary habits. Although motor symptoms often improve, some individuals have levodopa side effects. Many can maintain a stable weight on this diet, but close monitoring is required as some suffer significant weight loss.

Conclusion

Multidisciplinary work is especially important in the complex stage of Parkinson's. The combination of physical and mental health problems require the complementary skills of different disciplines working together. We find meetings of the MDT to be a valuable way of coordinating treatment for those under our care.

A personal experience of the complex stage

During a discussion with one of the team at clinic, I said, "I know that you all talk about me when I am not here."

Thank goodness we have the assurance that the team all know each one of us and will share in our care using their many disciplines to support the management of this cruel condition.

I have walked along with "the devil Parkinson's" for 19 years now and, after perhaps 17 of those years when I was quite pleased with the day-to-day management of my condition, I now feel that the devil is finding more complex and cruel ways of testing me.

Dyskinesia is crazy; sometimes I feel that I am bouncing off the walls and then it will suddenly be freezing, and this now completely debilitates me, rendering me helpless for as long as the devil wishes—10 minutes, an hour, or most of a day. In a group discussion a little while ago, I commented that sometimes there seems nothing left to do except cry. So, I do! Brian, a friend in the group, agreed.

I am also, for the first time, having difficulties balancing my medication to the best advantage. The Parkinson's specialist nurses are always a phone call away and give valuable advice with sympathy and understanding.

I remember someone saying a long time ago that this is a degenerative disease, so I know that it can only get worse—not an easy thought to live with. I have always lived by telling people that I have the disease, and now let's get on with life. Not so easy now!

It is a blessing to have such a good team to support my needs.

Carole Bagnall (March 2020)

Top tips for the multidisciplinary team in the complex stage

1. Not all Parkinson's symptoms respond to levodopa.
2. Time lines or on-off charts can help individuals investigate any relationship between timing of symptoms and medication. Wearing-off symptoms are common and there are multiple strategies available to manage this.
3. Dyskinesia may be well tolerated.
4. Consider advanced treatments for motor fluctuations.
5. Deep brain stimulation can help achieve similar motor effects to the best current motor effects on levodopa.
6. Except for tremor, deep brain stimulation will not solve problems that are not helped by levodopa.
7. Non-drug approaches can lead to significant improvements.
8. Parkinson's psychosis can lead to caregiver burden and is associated with nursing home placement.
9. Caregiver burden may be considerable; therefore regular caregiver assessments should be offered. Educational programs, social support, and cognitive behavioural therapy may be beneficial.
10. Clozapine is an effective treatment for psychosis in Parkinson's. Despite monitoring requirements, clozapine should be made available.
11. Teach strategies to manage transfers.
12. Deteriorating posture is common and should be measured and managed.

References

Arbouw, M. E., Movig, K. L., Koopmann, M., Poels, P. J., Guchelaar, H. J., Egberts, T. C., et al. (2010). Glycopyrrolate for sialorrhoea in Parkinson disease: a randomised, double-blind, crossover trial. *Neurology, 74*(15), 1203–1207.

Archibald, N. (2018). *Parkinson's Advanced Symptoms Unit (PASU) Business Case 2017/18 [online]*: South Tees Hospitals NHS Foundation Trust. Available at https://multiplesclerosisacademy.org/wp-content/uploads/sites/2/2019/07/PASU-business-case-2017.18.pdf.

Ashour, R., & Jankovic, J. (2006). Joint and skeletal deformities in Parkinson's disease, multiple system atrophy, and progressive supranuclear palsy. *Movement Disorders, 21*(11), 1856–1863.

Bachmann, C. G., & Trenkwalder, C. (2006). Body weight in patients with Parkinson's disease. *Movement Disorders, 21*(11), 1824–1830.

Balestrino, R., Baroncini, D., Fichera, M., Donofrio, C. A., Franzin, A., Mortini, P., et al. (2017). Weight gain after subthalamic nucleus deep brain stimulation in Parkinson's disease is influenced by dyskinesias' reduction and electrodes' position. *Neurological Science, 38*(12), 2123–2129.

Barbosa, P., Lees, A. J., Magee, C., Djamshidian, A., & Warner, T. T. (2017). A retrospective evaluation of the frequency of impulsive compulsive behaviours in Parkinson's disease patients treated with continuous waking day apomorphine pumps. *Movement Disorders Clinical Practice, 4*(3), 323–328.

Barichella, M., Marczewska, A., Vairo, A., Canesi, M., & Pezzoli, G. (2003). Is underweightness still a major problem in Parkinson's disease patients? *Eur J Clin Nutr, 57*(4), 543–547.

Barone, P., Antonini, A., Colosimo, C., Marconi, R., Morgante, L., Avarello, T. P., et al. (2009). The PRIAMO study: a multicentre assessment of nonmotor symptoms and their impact on quality of life in Parkinson's disease. *Movement Disorders, 24*(11), 1641–1649.

Barone, P., Santangelo, G., Amboni, M., Pellecchia, M. T., & Vitale, C. (2016). Pisa syndrome in Parkinson's disease and parkinsonism: clinical features, pathophysiology, and treatment. *Lancet Neurology, 15*(10), 1063–1074.

Borgemeester, R. W., Lees, A. J., & van Laar, T. (2016). Parkinson's disease, visual hallucinations and apomorphine: A review of the available evidence. *Parkinsonism Relat Disord, 27*, 35–40.

British Association of Dermatologists. (2019). *Iontophoresis for hyperhidrosis*. Retrieved October 6, 2020, from https://www.bad.org.uk/shared/get-file.ashx?id=3849&itemtype=document.

Broen, M. P., Braaksma, M. M., Patijn, J., & Weber, W. E. (2012). Prevalence of pain in Parkinson's disease: a systematic review using the modified QUADAS tool. *Movement Disorders, 27*(4), 480–484.

Brown, L., Oswal, M., Samra, A. -D., Martin, H., Burch, N., Colby, J., et al. (2020). Mortality and institutionalization after percutaneous endoscopic gastrostomy in Parkinson's disease and related conditions. *Movement Disorders Clinical Practice*.

Burack, M., Aldred, J., Zadikoff, C., Vanagunas, A., Klos, K., Bilir, B., et al. (2018). Implementing Levodopa-Carbidopa Intestinal Gel for Parkinson Disease: Insights from US Practitioners. *Movement Disorders Clinical Practice, 5*(4), 383–393.

Carbone, F., Djamshidian, A., Seppi, K., & Poewe, W. (2019). Apomorphine for Parkinson's Disease: Efficacy and Safety of Current and New Formulations. *CNS Drugs, 33*(9), 905–918.

Cumming, K., Macleod, A. D., Myint, P. K., & Counsell, C. E. (2017). Early weight loss in PARKINSONISM predicts poor outcomes: Evidence from an incident cohort study. *Neurology, 89*(22), 2254–2261.

Doherty, K. M., van de Warrenburg, B. P., Peralta, M. C., Silveira-Moriyama, L., Azulay, J. P., Gershanik, O. S., et al. (2011). Postural deformities in Parkinson's disease. *Lancet Neurol, 10*(6), 538–549.

Duncan, R. P., Van Dillen, L. R., Garbutt, J. M., Earhart, G. M., & Perlmutter, J. S. (2018). Physical therapy and deep brain stimulation in Parkinson's Disease: protocol for a pilot randomised controlled trial. *Pilot Feasibility Stud, 4*, 54.

Evans, J. (2006). Theoretical influences on brain injury rehabilitation. Presented at the Oliver Zangwill Centre 10th Anniversary Conference. Available at *www.ozc.nhs.uk*.

Ford, B. (2010). Pain in Parkinson's disease. *Movement Disorders, 25*(Suppl 1), S98–S103.

Fox, S., Cashell, A., Kernohan, W. G., Lynch, M., McGlade, C., O'Brien, T., et al. (2017). Palliative care for Parkinson's disease: patient and carer's perspectives explored through qualitative interview. *Palliative Medicine, 31*(7), 634–641.

Fried-Oken, M., Mooney, A., & Peters, B. (2015). Supporting communication for patients with neurodegenerative disease. *NeuroRehabilitation, 37*(1), 69–87.

Geraedts, V. J., Kuijf, M. L., van Hilten, J. J., Marinus, J., Oosterloo, M., & Contarino, M. F. (2019). Selecting candidates for Deep Brain Stimulation in Parkinson's disease: the role of patients' expectations. *Parkinsonism Relat Disord, 66*, 207–211.

Grosset, D., Antonini, A., Canesi, M., Pezzoli, G., Lees, A., Shaw, K., et al. (2009). Adherence to anti-Parkinson medication in a multicentre European study. *Movement Disorders, 24*(6), 826–832.

Hand, A. (2017). Understanding carer strain and its influence on the decision making process of care home placement for people with Parkinson's—a mixed methods study. D Nursing Thesis. Northumbria University, Newcastle-upon-Tyne. Retrieved January 20, 2021, from http://nrl.northumbria.ac.uk/id/eprint/36209/1/hand.annette_prof.doct.pdf.

Hely, M. A., Morris, J. G., Reid, W. G., & Trafficante, R. (2005). Sydney Multicentre Study of Parkinson's disease: non-L-dopa-responsive problems dominate at 15 years. *Movement Disorders, 20*(2), 190–199.

Heuft-Dorenbosch, L., Vosse, D., Landewe, R., Spoorenberg, A., Dougados, M., Mielants, H., et al. (2004). Measurement of spinal mobility in ankylosing spondylitis: comparison of occiput-to-wall and tragus-to-wall distance. *J Rheumatol, 31*(9), 1779–1784.

Kim, R., & Jun, J. S. (2020). Impact of overweight and obesity on functional and clinical outcomes of early Parkinson's disease. *J Am Med Dir Assoc, 21*(5), 697–700.

Kluger, B. M., & Friedman, J. H. (2014). Fatigue in Parkinson's disease. In K. R. Chaudhuri, E. Tolosa, A. H. V. Schapira, & W. Poewe (Eds.), *Non-motor Symptoms of Parkinson's Disease* (pp. 172–183). Oxford, United Kingdom: Oxford University Press.

Kumar, N., Van Gerpen, J. A., Bower, J. H., & Ahlskog, J. E. (2005). Levodopa-dyskinesia incidence by age of Parkinson's disease onset. *Movement Disorders*, *20*(3), 342–344.

Ma, K., Xiong, N., Shen, Y., Han, C., Liu, L., Zhang, G., et al. (2018). Weight loss and malnutrition in patients with Parkinson's disease: current knowledge and future prospects. *Front Aging Neurosci*, *10*, 1.

MacMahon, D. G., Sachdev, D., Boddie, H. G., Ellis, C. J., Kendal, B. R., & Blackburn, N. A. (1990). A comparison of the effects of controlled-release levodopa (Madopar CR) with conventional levodopa in late Parkinson's disease. *J Neurol Neurosurg Psychiatry*, *53*(3), 220–223.

Martinez-Martin, P., Rizos, A. M., Wetmore, J., Antonini, A., Odin, P., Pal, S., et al. (2018). First comprehensive tool for screening pain in Parkinson's disease: the King's Parkinson's Disease Pain Questionnaire. *Eur J Neurol*, *25*(10), 1255–1261.

Mendonca, D. A., Menezes, K., & Jog, M. S. (2007). Methylphenidate improves fatigue scores in Parkinson disease: a randomised controlled trial. *Movement Disorders*, *22*(14), 2070–2076.

Miller, N., Walshe, M., & Walker, R. W. (2019). Sialorrhoea in Parkinson's disease: prevalence, impact and management strategies. *Research and Reviews in Parkinsonism*, *9*, 17–28.

Mostile, G., & Jankovic, J. (2014). Thermoregulatory dysfunction in Parkinson's disease. In K. R. Chaudhuri, E. Tolosa, A. H. V. Schapira, & W. Poewe (Eds.), *Non-motor symptoms of Parkinson's Disease*Oxford, United Kingdom: Oxford University Press.

Muenter, M.D., & Tyce, G.M. (1971). L-dopa therapy of Parkinson's disease: Plasma L-dopa concentration, therapeutic response, and side effects. *Mayo Clin Proc* 46:231-239 National Institute for Health and Care Excellence (NICE) (2017). Parkinson's disease in adults: NICE guideline [NG71]. Retrieved June 7, 2020, from https://www.nice.org.uk/guidance/ng71/resources/parkinsons-disease-in-adults-pdf-1837629189061.

NHS Commissioning Board (2013). Clinical Commissioning Policy: Deep Brain Stimulation (DBS) In Movement Disorders (Parkinson's Disease, Tremor and Dystonia). Retrieved June 7, 2020, from https://www.england.nhs.uk/wp-content/uploads/2013/04/d03-p-b.pdf.

Olanow, C. W., Kieburtz, K., Odin, P., Espay, A. J., Standaert, D. G., Fernandez, H. H., et al. (2014). Continuous intrajejunal infusion of levodopa-carbidopa intestinal gel for patients with advanced Parkinson's disease: A randomised, controlled, double-blind, double-dummy study. *The Lancet Neurology*, *13*(2), 141–149.

Pappert, E. J., Goetz, C. G., Niederman, F., Ling, Z. D., Stebbins, G. T., & Carvey, P. M. (1996). Liquid levodopa/carbidopa produces significant improvement in motor function without dyskinesia exacerbation. *Neurology*, *47*(6), 1493–1495.

Parkinson's UK and All Party Parliamentary Group for Parkinson's Disease (2018). Mental health matters too: improving mental health services for people with Parkinson's who experience anxiety and depression. London, UK, Parkinson's UK.

Perez-Lloret, S., Dellapina, E., Pelleprat, J., Rey, M. V., Brefel-Courbon, C., & Rascol, O. (2014). Chronic pain and Parkinson's disease. In K. R. Chaudhuri, E. Tolosa, A. H. V. Schapira, & W. Poewe (Eds.), *Non-motor symptoms of Parkinson's disease* (pp. 332–341). Oxford, United Kingdom: Oxford University Press.

Poltawski, L., Edwards, H., Todd, A., Watson, T., Lees, A., & James, C. A. (2009). Ultrasound treatment of cutaneous side-effects of infused apomorphine: a randomised controlled pilot study. *Movement Disorders*, *24*(1), 115–118.

Poltawski, L., Todd, A., Edwards, H., & Watson, T. (2008). *Ultrasound in the treatment of apomorphine nodules [online]*: Electrotherapy on the Web. Retrieved May 26, 2020, from http://www.electrotherapy.org/modality/ultrasound-in-the-treatment-of-apomorphine-nodules.

Prizer, L. P., Kluger, B. M., Sillau, S., Katz, M., Galifianakis, N. B., & Miyasaki, J. M. (2020). The presence of a caregiver is associated with patient outcomes in patients with Parkinson's disease and atypical PARKINSONISMS. *Parkinsonism Relat Disord*, *78*, 61–65.

Ravina, B., Marder, K., Fernandez, H. H., Friedman, J. H., McDonald, W., Murphy, D., et al. (2007). Diagnostic criteria for psychosis in Parkinson's disease: report of an NINDS, NIMH work group. *Movement Disorders, 22*(8), 1061–1068.

Renoux, C., Dell'Aniello, S., Khairy, P., Marras, C., Bugden, S., Turin, T. C., et al. (2016). Ventricular tachyarrhythmia and sudden cardiac death with domperidone use in Parkinson's disease. *Br J Clin Pharmacol, 82*(2), 461–472.

Sapir, S., Ramig, L. O., & Fox, C. M. (2011). Assessment and treatment of the speech disorder in Parkinson disease. In D. Theodoros, & L. Ramig (Eds.), *Communication and swallowing in Parkinson disease* (pp. 89–122). San Diego, CA: Plural Publishing.

Schifitto, G., Friedman, J. H., Oakes, D., Shulman, L., Comella, C. L., Marek, K., et al. (2008). Fatigue in levodopa-naive subjects with Parkinson's disease. *Neurology, 71*(7), 481–485.

Secker, D. L., & Brown, R. G. (2005). Cognitive behavioural therapy (CBT) for carers of patients with Parkinson's disease: a preliminary randomised controlled trial. *J Neurol Neurosurg Psychiatry, 76*(4), 491–497.

Seppi, K., Ray Chaudhuri, K., Coelho, M., Fox, S. H., Katzenschlager, R., Perez Lloret, S., et al. (2019). Update on treatments for nonmotor symptoms of Parkinson's disease: an evidence-based medicine review. *Movement Disorders, 34*(2), 180–198.

Simons, G., Thompson, S. B., Smith Pasqualini, M. C., & Members of the EduPark, c. (2006). An innovative education programme for people with Parkinson's disease and their carers. *Parkinsonism Relat Disord, 12*(8), 478–485.

Stocchi, F., Hsu, A., Khanna, S., Ellenbogen, A., Mahler, A., Liang, G., et al. (2014). Comparison of IPX066 with carbidopa-levodopa plus entacapone in advanced PD patients. *Parkinsonism Relat Disord, 20*(12), 1335–1340.

Sung, S., Vijiaratnam, N., Chan, D. W. C., Farrell, M., & Evans, A. H. (2018). Pain sensitivity in Parkinson's disease: systematic review and meta-analysis. *Parkinsonism Relat Disord, 48*, 17–27.

Tassorelli, C., Buscone, S., Sandrini, G., Pacchetti, C., Furnari, A., Zangaglia, R., et al. (2009). The role of rehabilitation in deep brain stimulation of the subthalamic nucleus for Parkinson's disease: a pilot study. *Parkinsonism Relat Disord, 15*(9), 675–681.

Todd, A., & James, C. R. (2008). Apomorphine nodules in Parkinson's disease: best practice considerations. *British Journal of Community Nursing, 13*, 457–463.

Todd, D., Simpson, J., & Murray, C. (2010). An interpretative phenomenological analysis of delusions in people with Parkinson's disease. *Disabil Rehabil, 32*(15), 1291–1299.

Tyler, C. M., Henry, R. S., Perrin, P. B., Watson, J., Villasenor, T., Lageman, S. K., et al. (2020). Structural Equation Modeling of Parkinson's Caregiver Social Support, Resilience, and Mental Health: A Strength-Based Perspective. *Neurol Res Int, 2020*, 7906547.

Van Gerpen, J. A., Kumar, N., Bower, J. H., Weigand, S., & Ahlskog, J. E. (2006). Levodopa-associated dyskinesia risk among Parkinson disease patients in Olmsted County, Minnesota, 1976-1990. *Arch Neurol, 63*(2), 205–209.

Volpe, D., Giantin, M. G., Manuela, P., Filippetto, C., Pelosin, E., Abbruzzese, G., et al. (2017). Water-based vs. non-water-based physiotherapy for rehabilitation of postural deformities in Parkinson's disease: a randomised controlled pilot study. *Clin Rehabil, 31*(8), 1107–1115.

Williams, A., Gill, S., Varma, T., Jenkinson, C., Quinn, N., Mitchell, R., et al. (2010). Deep brain stimulation plus best medical therapy versus best medical therapy alone for advanced Parkinson's disease (PD SURG trial): a randomised, open-label trial. *Lancet Neurol, 9*(6), 581–591.

Worth, P. F. (2013). When the going gets tough: how to select patients with Parkinson's disease for advanced therapies. *Pract Neurol, 13*(3), 140–152.

Zoldan, J., Friedberg, G., Livneh, M., & Melamed, E. (1995). Psychosis in advanced Parkinson's disease: treatment with ondansetron, a 5-HT3 receptor antagonist. *Neurology, 45*(7), 1305–1308.

Chapter 8

Palliative care in Parkinson's

Edward W Richfield and Sarah McCracken

Introduction

Palliative care for people with Parkinson's has gained increasing attention over the last decade. It is an area that relies on multidisciplinary working, not just within the Parkinson's service but also with colleagues in specialist palliative care. In this chapter, using a broad definition and an integrated approach to care, we seek to outline the times at which palliative care could be considered. We discuss the role of medication and medication management, identify the potential roles for individual members of the multidisciplinary team (MDT), and discuss the terminal care of people with Parkinson's. It should be recognised that this is a rapidly evolving area and the following section aims to give an introduction and guidance while recognising that some of the specifics of care are likely to change in the coming years as our experience grows.

The palliative stage - what is it and when does it begin?

Parkinson's is often considered to have a palliative stage preceded by the diagnostic, maintenance, and complex stages (Thomas & MacMahon, 2004). In this model, the palliative stages is defined by any of the following: (1) onset of significant cognitive impairment; (2) need for 24-hour care (in the United Kingdom, this refers to residential or nursing care); and (3) waning response to dopaminergic medications.

This model has merit and has been useful in recognising the needs of people with Parkinson's in the later stages of the condition; however, it also presents some difficulty when modern definitions of palliative and supportive care are being applied.

The World Health Organization defines palliative care as an approach that, in seeking to alleviate suffering for people with the condition as well as caregivers and families, is applicable from the time of diagnosis and alongside active treatment (World Health Organization, 2015). This definition is now echoed in national guidance; for example, the UK National Institute for Health and Care Excellence advises practitioners to be prepared to discuss Parkinson's progression, prognosis and preparation for advanced stages from the time of diagnosis "where appropriate" (National Institute for Heath and Care Excellence, 2017).

Such an approach is clearly not possible if we stick rigidly to the four-stage model already described. Moreover, the introduction of a distinct palliative stage which was previously helpful in highlighting a role for palliative interventions, now risks defining a "cliff edge" at which individuals are defined as "palliative." In Parkinson's as with other conditions, this can lead to negative attitudes toward palliative care, a false perception that palliative interventions are suitable only for people who are dying and, by implication, that clinicians suggesting palliative interventions must think that the person is in the last stages of life. Not surprisingly, this can generate a perception among people with Parkinson's that palliative care is not open to them during the vast majority of their time living with the condition. It can also lead to resistance to being referred to palliative care specialists for fear of being defined as being at the end of life.

An alternative approach, which recognises that the latter stages of Parkinson's may pose specific palliative issues, seeks to move away from a rigid "palliative stage" and to open up the potential for palliative interventions throughout the course of the condition (Richfield, 2013). This "integrative" approach to palliative and supportive care appears well suited to chronic non-malignant conditions such as Parkinson's and has been adopted in other chronic conditions such as heart failure (Johnson, 2011; Fallon & Foley, 2012). This approach also offers advantages in terms of service configuration and managing the demand for specialist intervention.

In adopting an integrative approach, it may be helpful for professionals working with people with Parkinson's to have an understanding of the potential for unmet palliative care needs throughout the condition, as discussed in the following sections.

Diagnostic stage

Although we may be surprised to encounter palliative needs at the time of diagnosis, there are a number of factors here that it can be useful to bear in mind.

Studies of people living with Parkinson's consistently highlight the diagnostic period as a source of dissatisfaction (Habermann, 1996, 1999; Phillips, 2006). This may stem from a number of factors.

First, Parkinson's has a long "premotor" stage that is often associated with significant morbidity from non-motor features. In addition, there is often a significant delay between the onset of motor features and the receipt of specialist review and diagnosis. As such, at the time of first review and subsequent diagnosis, people with Parkinson's may have been living with significant, often unattributed symptoms for some time (Habermann, 1996).

In addition to the distress caused by the symptoms themselves, this may also lead to challenges in communication during the early consultations. Many people come to see health care professionals when they already believe themselves to have Parkinson's or are worried that this may be the case. They may have explored their symptoms on the internet or know someone with Parkinson's and thus recognise some of the symptoms in themselves. If so, their preconsultation expectations are likely to be very different from those of someone who has not considered the possibility of Parkinson's or has no idea that he or she is being assessed for this possibility.

Finally, it is important to recognise the diagnostic uncertainty that exists in the early stages of Parkinson's, with some diagnostic criteria being dependent on time, such that the diagnosis is sometimes revised (Schrag, 2002).

For members of the MDT, an understanding of the preheld expectations of the individual, the impact of undiagnosed symptom burden, and the diagnostic uncertainty that exists in the early stages of Parkinson's is important in helping people through this diagnostic period; that is, communication may have to be tailored to reflect these issues.

This may be particularly challenging where therapists have contact with individuals prior to the diagnosis; for example, when they are recognising signs of Parkinson's following an unrelated referral such as after a fall or for a swallowing issue where the underlying diagnosis has not been made.

Maintenance stage

The maintenance stage of Parkinson's is described in earlier chapters. Although it may be reasonable to assume that more palliative care needs prevail in the later stages of the condition, members of the MDT should be mindful of the possibility of unmet needs in this stage. In particular, unmet needs commonly associated with the palliative stage (such as the planning of future care) may be easier to deal with if they are identified earlier in the course of the condition. For example, given the prevalence of cognitive impairment in Parkinson's (cumulative incidents 60% at 8 years [Aarsland, 2003]), this may be an important time to consider advance care planning (ACT) in order to best preserve the patient's autonomy.

Finally, the concept of "downward comparison," whereby an individual with early-stage Parkinson's finds it difficult to meet people at later stages of the condition because they imagine their future when they may experience similar advanced symptoms, can be a barrier to people accessing support groups. When a person is being offered access to support groups, members of the MDT should consider this phenomenon.

Complex stage

The suggestion of unmet palliative care needs in the complex stage of Parkinson's is likely to be less controversial. Both qualitative and quantitative methodologies have been used to show that the burden of unmet need in late-stage Parkinson's is similar to that in malignant conditions (Hudson et al., 2006; Miyasaki et al., 2012). Further studies have compared late-stage Parkinson's with motor neuron disease and have found that the symptom burden was similar in both conditions but that people with Parkinson's were less likely to be prepared for the terminal stage, less likely to say goodbye to loved ones, and less likely to be able to make decisions about their future care during the last month of life (Goy et al., 2008). This once again highlights the importance of early consideration of ACP, where appropriate, at a time when the person with Parkinson's is able to fully participate.

Close working between members of the MDT, the person with Parkinson's, and the caregiver are key to good-quality care in this stage. It is important for the MDT to understand the role that palliative and supportive care can play in enhancing quality of life (QoL) and to integrate this into their practice. It is also important to have good links with specialist palliative care services and a venue for the discussion of difficult problems—for example, a palliative care multidisciplinary meeting or a multidisciplinary clinic where members of the therapy team, nurse specialists, and consultant are present at the same clinic to provide multifaceted care. The potential roles of team members within a palliative care service are illustrated in Figure 8.1.

During consultations it may be useful to consider the top 10 symptoms (Table 8.1) that were found to dominate the day for people with Parkinson's (Lee et al., 2007). It is noteworthy that although motor symptoms are included here, urinary symptoms also occur on three occasions. This highlights the importance of searching for non-motor symptoms (NMSs) in particular, which may not be volunteered in a clinic setting. Consultations should be structured in such a way that these symptoms are routinely reviewed. Some may find the use of screening tools such as the NMS questionnaire helpful for this purpose, facilitating the prioritisation of patient need before the clinic commences.

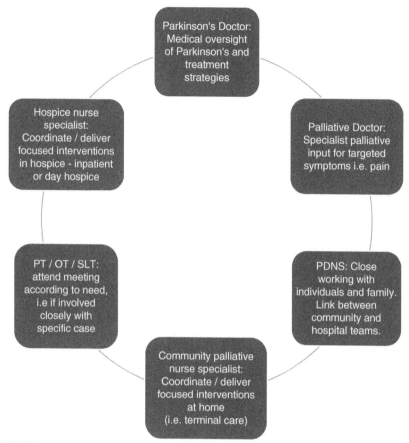

FIGURE 8.1 Members and roles of the Parkinson's palliative care multidisciplinary team

Medication management in the late stages of Parkinson's

Health and social care professionals working with older people will be familiar with the concept of polypharmacy and the movement to encourage the review and appropriate rationalisation of medications. People in the later stages of Parkinson's, even though they may not be elderly, often have features of frailty and thus may benefit from a similar approach to medication management. From a practical perspective, this may be approached in the following way.

Review in response to new symptoms

Whenever a person with Parkinson's develops a new symptom, it is useful to ask whether it could be due to medications so that this can be addressed, but we can also offer reassurance where medications are not implicated.

TABLE 8.1 Top 10 symptoms dominating the day for people with Parkinson's

Symptom	Frequency (%)
Immobility	35 (28.5)
Pain	25 (20.3)
Slowness of movement	21 (17.1)
Insomnia	19 (15.4)
Stiffness	11 (8.9)
Urinary urgency	11 (8.9)
Urinary incontinence	11 (8.9)
Anxiety	11 (8.9)
Urinary frequency	10 (8.1)
Drowsiness	9 (7.3)

Source: Adapted from Lee et al., 2007.

The simplest approach is to ask whether any new medications have recently been introduced or an existing one increased; if so, it would be appropriate to review the side-effect profile and interactions of this drug. It is important to recognise that many drugs used for other conditions may have a deleterious effect in Parkinson's, particularly (but not only) those with antidopaminergic or anticholinergic activity. Resources such as the guidelines of the Scottish Intercollegiate Guidelines Network (Scottish Government, 2018) may help to identify potential culprit medications.

It is important to note that drug-related issues can also develop without any recent changes to prescription owing to altered pharmacodynamics (the way drugs act within the body) and pharmacokinetics (the way drugs move within the body). A common and often unrecognised example is the altered volume of distribution caused by weight loss, which is common in late-stage Parkinson's (Cersosimo et al., 2018). Such a change in drug distribution results in higher levels of drug availability, which can contribute to dopa-driven side effects such as dyskinesia (Sharma & Vassallo, 2014). To address this, one can consider adjusting the dopamine dose according to weight.

Whereas changes in weight alter the action of medications, medications can themselves contribute to weight loss. For example, cholinesterase inhibitors are not uncommonly associated with anorexia (Sheffrin et al., 2015).

It is clear that the connection between weight loss, medication, and medication side effects is complex; this serves to illustrate the importance of multidisciplinary management in late-stage Parkinson's and considering the contributions of each team member in optimisation of care:

- The dietitian by providing nutritional support
- The speech and language therapist (SLT), by optimizing swallow
- The pharmacist, by offering advice on drug effects and side effects
- The physiotherapist, by preventing sarcopenia
- The occupational therapist (OT), by, for example, providing appropriate equipment and thus optimising the mechanics of eating
- The Parkinson's disease specialist nurse (PDSN), by identifying weight loss and providing appropriate referrals

More generally, as the condition progresses, people with Parkinson's may become more physically and cognitively frail, leading to a greater susceptibility to medication side effects. Health care professionals will notice the increasing neuropsychiatric side effects experienced by many individuals as the condition progresses (Hely et al., 1999), which often necessitate a reduction in dopaminergic treatments.

The reduction or withdrawal of dopaminergic medication is often required to control side effects in late-stage Parkinson's; this should always be done with caution, considering the potential negative effects on motor function (depending on residual dopaminergic responsiveness), the specific challenges of withdrawing dopamine agonists (dopamine agonist withdrawal syndrome [Pondal et al., 2013]), and the importance of avoiding abrupt cessation (risk of neuroleptic malignant-like syndrome [Keyser & Rodnitzky, 1991]).

Routine review

In caring for people with Parkinson's, health care professionals should also take the opportunity to review all other prescription and non-prescription drugs at regular intervals. Prescribers may like to incorporate one of the established tools for deprescribing in their practice (Scottish Government, 2018). Specific issue to highlight include the following:

Anticholinergic burden: Anticholinergic drugs are now rarely used as a Parkinson's treatment, but they may still be encountered in the management of resistant tremor and are more commonly used to counter bladder urgency or reduce chronic pain. Moreover, we should be mindful of the large number of medications for other conditions which, while not categorised as "anticholinergic," nevertheless contribute to the total anticholinergic burden.

The myriad side effects of anticholinergics makes them a key target for deprescribing in Parkinson's (Crispo et al., 2016). This is particularly important for people with Parkinson's, where anticholinergics have been linked with increased rates of dementia (Hong et al., 2019); they may also contribute to an increased risk of falling (Crispo et al., 2016), and will worsen common NMSs such as constipation and postural hypotension.

When anticholinergics are legitimately used (e.g., for bladder symptoms), we should seek to use the smallest effective dose and to utilise agents such as trospium that do not appear to cross the blood-brain barrier (Chancellor et al., 2012).

Concordance: The term *concordance* implies an agreement regarding medication following a discussion between people with Parkinson's and the health care team with a focus on the individual's priorities of care (Weiss & Britten, 2009). In starting or reviewing medication, we must consider whether we are using the best route (might the individual find a patch easier?), whether concordance will be possible (e.g. oral bisphosphonate in someone with antecollis or dyskinesia), and seek to discuss these issues with the individual to gain his or her approval.

Running a Parkinson's palliative care service

Over the past decade the potential for palliative care in Parkinson's has been increasingly recognised; it is now enshrined in national guidance (National Institute for Health and Care Excellence, 2017). As a result, some centres have developed Parkinson's palliative care services. However, these remain scattered and many individuals do not have access. The recent confirmation of clinical benefit to both the person with Parkinson's (improved QoL) and caregiver (reduced caregiver burden) from structured palliative care for Parkinson's in the United States is a significant step (Kluger et al., 2020) and will stimulate the expansion of services.

At the time of writing, several international collaborations are focusing on neuropalliative care; it is likely that this will lead to the development of collaborations and the establishment of standards in the coming years.

Navigating the chronic/palliative interface

This may be the key factor in successful service development. The recognition of a wider role for palliative care in the early stages of chronic incurable illness, encompassing chronic non-malignant conditions, has led to a huge increase in the numbers of people meeting the criteria for treatment. With this comes recognition that it is neither possible nor appropriate for specialist palliative care units to meet all of this demand (Murray et al., 2005). Rather, the majority of unmet needs must be addressed by existing teams (referred to as a "palliative approach" or, in the United States, as "primary palliative care"), with input from specialist palliative care for specific, focused interventions. Managing the interface between these services (referred to as the chronic/palliative interface [Lanoix, 2009]) to ensure appropriate, timely referrals and intervention is central to service development and sustainability.

Our own Parkinson's palliative care MDT runs bimonthly, with a core attendance from the Parkinson's consultant, palliative care consultant, palliative specialist nurse (hospice), palliative specialist nurse (community) and case-by-case remote attendance by the community PDNS responsible for the person with Parkinson's (see Fig. 8.1).

Measuring response to treatment

Quantification of palliative symptoms is important not only to establish the efficacy of intervention but also to guide service development (understanding which interventions are useful) and make the economic case for intervention.

A number of tools have now been developed to specifically measure palliative care needs in Parkinson's (Richfield & Johnson, 2020), which may be helpful within the integrated model of care described earlier.

Multidisciplinary team working in the palliative stage

The members of the MDT work closely together during the palliative stage to support the individual and, where present, his or her caregiver. This work is especially important in promoting independence and autonomy and, during the later stages, honouring advance decisions the individual may have made regarding care.

It is often the case that one member of the team takes a coordinating role. Traditionally this has been the PDNS, but increasingly other therapists are taking on this role, sometimes referred to as Parkinson's specialist therapists. Importantly, there is learning within and between team members, which means that individuals become highly skilled not only in their parent disciplines but also in the other therapy roles.

The Parkinson's disease nurse specialist

The PDNS's role in the palliative stage is explained here, at first hand, by an advanced practitioner:

Our specialist neurological MDT, which has evolved over 10 years, is based at a health centre in the heart of Nottingham City. Generally, caseload managers are the specialist nurses, and in addition to managing people with advanced Parkinson's, our caseload includes those with atypical Parkinsonian syndromes, Lewy body dementia with Parkinsonism, and Parkinson's disease dementia.

As a community-based Parkinson's nurse with 15 years of Parkinson's experience as well as experience in community nursing and tissue viability, I have managed cases involving advanced Parkinson's, including home visits, regular medication reviews, and prescribing. Non-medical prescribing means that I can stop non-essential medications, convert medication to syrup or patch formulations, titrate Parkinson's medications up or down, and make recommendations regarding palliative medications. Working closely with our community neurology team as well as signposting to other services, I liaise with the hospice service for day therapy support, caregiver respite, the sitting service, the through-the-night support service and day and night sitters. I run an informal MDT clinic at the local hospice and often do joint visits there with allied health professionals—SLTs, OTs, and physiotherapists. Some individuals are referred to the palliative care team in the community for a period of intervention. Communication with the general practitioner (GP) and attendance at gold standard framework meetings for palliative care is an important part of the role, being facilitated by a computer system shared with most local GPs. This means that messages, letters and prescriptions can be acted upon in a timely manner. A Parkinson's MDT clinic with our neurology SLT is also held at a local GP practice.

The role involves referring people to social care for complex care packages and attending decision-support-tool meetings (continuing health care funding). It also includes providing specialist input regarding neurological deterioration and prognosis as well as making referrals so that individuals can have a robust and timely package of care in the home.

I liaise closely with secondary care colleagues, including geriatricians, neurologists, old-age psychiatrists, hospital-based Parkinson's nurses, OTs, and physiotherapists. The ability to cross the primary/secondary interface is an important aspect of the specialist nurse role and is especially useful in the palliative stage. I can attend hospital MDT meetings for complex discharge planning or help to manage a complex safeguarding situation.

As I am community-based, meaning that most of my contact with individuals occurs in their own homes or nursing homes. I get to know them over several months or years and so can recognise the deterioration in their symptoms at the end of life. We aim to start ACP before the individual loses mental capacity and together draw up a plan that includes a documented decision regarding resuscitation using ReSPECT paperwork, which is a tool for documenting CPR decisions and goals of care in the United Kingdom. It is important here to document relevant assessments of mental capacity. Members of the MDT work together to navigate and manage the individual's journey, anticipating mobility changes, speech and swallow problems, and the need for specialist equipment. We adopt a person-centred approach (Stokes, 2017), with the person with Parkinson's and the family driving all decision making.

Outreach to nursing homes

Prior to the individual making a decision about moving into a care or nursing home, I will have a discussion with the person and his or her loved ones.

I visit care homes regularly and often work with several residents in one home, teaching the staff about Parkinson's and offering them support. We have developed excellent links with the "City care homes and dementia outreach team," which is set up to support complex residents in care homes. The links with mental health services are beneficial for this group of individuals, who may have dementia, depression, apathy, anxiety, sleep disorders, psychosis and delirium.

Working with the individual as well as the family members and care home staff, I make sure that their wishes are respected. Some people choose a hospital-admission-avoidance approach as part of their ACP, and this is often formally documented. In the absence of an ACP or lasting power of attorney, we take a best-interest approach and hold a best-interests meeting with the next of kin and the relevant clinicians. This is all documented clearly in the individual's notes and the GP records, and a copy is sent to the local hospital.

If the individual is receiving terminal care in a residential home, the local multidisciplinary care homes team will help to replenish medication if a syringe driver is in use, helping the individual to stay in the residential home environment. In nursing homes, trained nursing staff can complete this task themselves. If the individual has made an advanced decisions to donate his or her brain to the Brain Bank or to medical science and has completed the consent form and paperwork, I will help to make sure that this wish is met—for example, providing the 24-hour mobile number for the London Brain Bank or contact details for the medical school.

Physiotherapy

When Parkinson's is advanced and the individual is still able to mobilise, intervention may focus on the prevention of falls and provision of appropriate walking aids. If the individual is no longer able to mobilise, the physiotherapist, working closely with the OT can provide a referral to wheelchair services.

Managing safe transfers for both the individual and, importantly, the caregiver is also essential. Assessment can be made for manual handling equipment such as a rotunda (which can enable a safe transfer when a turn is involved) or stand aid for those who are still able to stand. In addition and where possible, therapeutic intervention will address the maintenance of muscle strength, range of movement, and avoidance of contractures. Pain management and offering support to the individual as he or she comes to terms with changes in mobility, goals, and aspirations are also key.

Respiratory management must also be considered, and the individual may require referral to a community respiratory team.

Occupational therapy

The OT's role includes assessment and the prescription of appropriate equipment to help both individuals and their caregivers to manage care needs at home. This includes assessment of seating, positioning and transfers and provision of equipment such as a riser-recliner chair or wheelchair that is suitable for the person's specific needs and environment. Where necessary, it may include major adaptations to the property, such as arranging for ramps to be installed, providing a stair lift, and adapting the bathroom by installing floor lifts, ceiling or gantry hoists and extensions. Bed transfers will also be assessed and appropriate transfer aids provided.

For individuals with reduced mobility, positioning must be addressed, particularly considering the management of pressure areas and reduction of pressure damage. It is important to minimise contractures, which may require splinting or sometimes interventions such as botulinum toxin. Consultation with a specialist rehabilitation service may also be helpful.

OT support, both practical and emotional, is particularly important when care needs change, particularly when care home placement is being considered. In such circumstances, the OT may support the assessment of mental capacity.

In the terminal stage care and death at home is often an important goal. The OT has a key role to play, alongside other MDT members, in facilitating this through rapid assessment of the individual's care needs, provision of equipment and the identification of funding streams (i.e., Continuing Health Care Fast Track funding in the United Kingdom).

Speech and language therapist

Choking and aspiration are key markers of poor prognosis in late-stage Parkinson's. SLTs can help to optimise swallow and educate individuals and caregivers on the safest swallow techniques, offering recommendations regarding food and fluid consistency to promote safe swallowing. However, in the end stages of Parkinson's, it is not uncommon for risk to be present with all consistencies; here the SLT can help to explore options including artificial feeding; for example, via a percutaneous endoscopic gastrostomy or continued oral intake with accepted risk. SLTs thus have an important role in promoting advance care planning (ACP) with regard to the management of unsafe swallowing and the exploration of alternative non-oral routes where appropriate.

In our experience, the role of the SLT in communication is often overlooked in late-stage Parkinson's. Optimised communication is life enhancing and also helps people to participate meaningfully in ACP in late stages. Expert SLT support can also help to optimise the capacity for and participation in decision making, even where verbal skills are very limited or where visual or electronic communication aids are indicated.

Dietitian

Weight loss has been associated with increased mortality in Parkinson's (Walker, Davidson, & Gray, 2012). Maintaining weight is therefore an important goal in an MDT-based approach to care. Dietitians can help to optimise nutrition, particularly when oral intake may be limited by swallow or cognitive decline.

It is important to consider the impact of protein-rich foods on medication absorption for people with Parkinson's. If significant motor fluctuations occur, particularly if these have a temporal relationship to the intake of food, it can be useful to consult a dietitian to explore dietary modification.

Advance care planning

ACP is sometimes discussed as though it were a discrete activity. In reality, however, it is an ongoing process that seeks to explore the preferences of individuals with Parkinson's and to include them in decision making about their future care. This longitudinal approach is crucial, as it recognises that people with Parkinson's may be more or less open to ACP at various times in their lives (Tuck, 2015). It also takes into account that perceptions of our future selves—and the consequent care decisions we take—may change as the condition progresses (Jordan et al., 2020). That is, symptoms or impairments that may seem unacceptable initially may appear more acceptable as the condition progresses, perhaps in response to evolving measures of self-efficacy, life story or expectations. In fact, it has been suggested that envisaging the future self during ACP may be more difficult for people with Parkinson's (Sokol et al., 2019). It is therefore a good idea to establish a system to revisit and check prior decision making.

The four strands of ACP

1. **Do not attempt cardiopulmonary resuscitation (DNACPR) orders:** At its most basic level ACP may simply constitute a discussion of cardiopulmonary resuscitation; many professionals will be involved with such discussions on a daily basis. In the United Kingdom, the introduction of the ReSPECT form (Resuscitation Council UK, 2020) expands these discussions to include wider goals of treatment and the desire for life-prolonging therapy.
2. **Lasting power of attorney:** This allows a person who retains decision-making capacity to appoint an advocate (often a relative, but not necessarily so) who will make medical decisions on their behalf if they are no longer able to do so. As with all decision making, it is essential to recognise that a person can maintain the capacity to make some decisions yet be unable to make others, and that the ability to do so may fluctuate over time. This is particularly pertinent in neurological disorders such as Parkinson's, where delirium (characterised by fluctuating alertness) is common in the later stages, often in response to reversible intercurrent illnesses. All members of the MDT should be familiar with the application of legal principles relating to capacity, specific to their area of practice (e.g. Mental Capcity Act in the UK) in order to help individuals and caregivers navigate these issues.
3. **Advance decision to refuse treatment (ADRT):** This is a legally binding document that sets out in advance specific interventions refused by the individual. Such an order is most appropriate when discrete interventions and the setting in which they may be used can be anticipated; for example, PEG feeding or mechanical ventilation. Although accurate data are not available, anecdotally these documents are seldom used in the United Kingdom by people with Parkinson's.

4. **Advance statement of wishes and preferences:** This is a non–legally binding document and as such allows greater flexibility, enabling individuals to state their treatment goals, values, and preferences with regard to a wide range of clinical interventions. It is perhaps best used to ensure that the individual has a voice in decision making, to guide but not predetermine the process. In our experience, it is often helpful to work with the individual and caregiver to discuss a number of common issues, such as the following which describe our practice in the UK:

> *Swallow.* A full exploration is beyond the scope of this chapter, but it may be helpful to discuss both acute dysphagia, where swallow may be temporarily impaired by intercurrent illness, as well as the chronic dysphagia due to progression of the condition, where there is no reversibility. For example, some individuals with Parkinson's would be willing to accept temporary nasogastric tube (NGT) feeding to enable nutrition and administration of medication during an acute illness in the hope of later recovery of the ability to swallow. However, this does not imply that they would countenance long-term PEG feeding with its implied reduction or loss of oral intake and the pleasure derived from eating, which should be explored separately.

> *Life-prolonging treatment.* It may be useful to consider any circumstances under which the individual would no longer wish to receive life-prolonging treatment (because this is not an ADRT, it may not be necessary to define such interventions strictly). For example, is there a level of impairment or dependency that, if irreversible, would mark a point at which the individual would wish to receive care focused on symptom management, rather than life prolongation?

> *Hospital admission.* Many people express a wish to avoid hospital admission. In our experience, it is often helpful to supplement this with an exploration of any exceptional circumstances when admission might be acceptable. For example, if an individual no longer wishes to receive life-prolonging interventions and sees home as the preferred place of care, would he or she accept hospital admission for symptomatic treatment in specific reversible circumstances such as urinary retention or following a fracture?

These examples are drawn from our own practice, but the scope of discussion should not be limited and should be directed by the priorities of the person with Parkinson's and the caregiver.

On occasion, it may be appropriate to combine a statement of wishes and preferences alongside an LPA. This can be helpful for family advocates making difficult decisions, particularly when they are declining interventions on their relative's behalf, by providing a record of the individual's previously held wishes. As mentioned earlier, it may also be reassuring for individuals to know that they continue to have a presence within this decision-making process.

In order for ACP to be a part of their practice, professionals must consider how documents will be held and shared with the relevant organisations. Only this way can the individual's priorities of care to be met. It is therefore essential to be familiar with local practice in data sharing across organisations, including community and secondary care partners.

Terminal care for Parkinson's

Much of our approach to the terminal care for people with Parkinson's is based on personal experience and opinion drawn from experts in the field, as there are currently very few peer reviewed publications in this area. We have highlighted areas for future development, some of which are being actively addressed by current research. This is an area that is likely to evolve rapidly.

Dopaminergic medication at end of life

Rapid cessation of dopaminergic medication should be avoided and can be dangerous, with risk of neuroleptic malignant-like syndrome. When asked to review an individual who is considered to be at the end of life (EoL), health care professionals should be certain that the presentation is not the result of "off state" from missed medication or reduced responsiveness to medications secondary to acute illness. In this situation, due consideration should be given to replacing dopaminergic medication, either via NGT or using a rotigotine patch (off label) before starting EoL care.

Once EoL care has been started, it is generally good practice to continue dopaminergic medication if possible. Where individuals are able to take medication orally, this is relatively simple, either continuing previous medications or converting to the dopa-equivalent dose of dispersible levodopa. Tools to aid conversion are readily available online, with the OPTIMAL calculator an online tool to help clinicians convert medication into a dopa-equivalent dispersible form, (http://www.parkinsonscalculator.com/index.html) having been approved by the British Geriatric Society.

Where use of the oral route is no longer possible, the balance of risk and benefit is less clear. Use of a NGT will rarely, if ever, be appropriate at EoL. The dopamine agonist rotigotine is available as a transdermal patch and can be used off license to continue dopaminergic medication, although published evidence is limited to case report and service description (Hindmarsh et al., 2019). There are, however, theoretical concerns regarding rotigotine at EoL. First, it will often be impossible to achieve dopa equivalence even at the top dose of rotigotine (16mg). Second, agonists are felt to promote delirium more than levodopa, and this is a concern at EoL, especially in people who are have never previously received an agonist. A recent publication reported terminal agitation in about 25% of people with Parkinson's on rotigotine at EoL (Ibrahim et al., 2020). While the reported range for the general population at EoL is extremely wide (Hosie et al., 2013), a retrospective review of terminal symptoms suggested that where rotigotine was used, lower than equivalent dopaminergic doses resulted in less delirium, with no deterioration in other symptoms. (Hindmarsh, Hindmarsh & Lee, 2021).

Why continue dopaminergic medication at the end of life?

If people remain responsive to dopa, there is concern that missed medication at EoL will result in both physical discomfort (such as terminal stiffness) and psychological discomfort in the form of the non-motor 'off' state.

A pragmatic approach could consider three important questions before starting patch replacement at EoL:

1. Is the individual likely to have significant dopa responsiveness?
2. Was the individual previously on an agonist, and if so, was it tolerated?
3. Is the person at significant risk for delirium? (The default answer is yes.)

Once a person has been started on rotigotine, we can consider adopting one of three approaches, with the appropriate choice guided by the answers to the previous questions:

1. Start at the lowest dose and titrate to response.
2. Start at a modified "delirium risk" dose (i.e., using the OPTIMAL calculator, discussed earlier).
3. Start at a dopa-equivalent dose (rarely advised).

Determining dopa responsiveness will require liaison with the caregiver, family, and MDT members involved in recent care. If medications were being reduced owing to waning effect (see definition of the palliative stage earlier) without any adverse reactions, this may suggest reduced dopa responsiveness. Alternatively, if the individual is dying because of another pathology with no suggestion of waning response, dopa responsiveness should be assumed.

Symptom management at the end of life

Nausea: Once again, the evidence-base for positive intervention in people with Parkinson's is limited. To a large extent, advice is focused on what not to do and the way in which care for people with Parkinson's differs from routine approaches. First, it is important to emphasise the need to avoid dopa-blocking medication. This primarily precludes the use of drugs such as metoclopramide and haloperidol; there may also be the need for caution with levomepromazine, although a case study using the latter successfully has been published (Hindmarsh et al., 2019). Although not a dopa blocker, cyclizine has been reported to rarely have antiparkinsonian effects (King et al., 2003); it may be used with caution.

Members of the MDT caring for people with Parkinson's at EoL could consider using ondansetron first line for centrally mediated nausea and domperidone for gastric stasis. This may, of course, be more of a problem in people with Parkinson's owing to autonomic dysfunction. Where symptoms are not responsive to a single medication, the need for cautious use of cyclizine and levomepromazine should be evaluated, and there should be a low threshold for liaison with colleagues from the specialist palliative care team.

Agitation: There are a number of potential causes of terminal agitation at EoL, which may be more common in people with Parkinson's; for example, motor stiffness due to dopaminergic withdrawal, higher risk of pressure sores due to reduced mobility, and agitation due to constipation. Therefore agitation at EoL should prompt a thorough search for potential triggers. In the absence of an identifiable trigger, we should consider the possibility that agonist therapy at EoL may be contributing, and this should be reviewed (see earlier).

When reversible causes have been excluded, midazolam may be helpful, and it is imperative that traditional antipsychotic-type medications such as haloperidol be avoided.

Terminal stiffness: There are few case reports of this in the literature, but it remains a concern. It may be that terminal stiffness is more common in people who have residual dopaminergic responsiveness (see earlier). With stiffness, there should also be further review of the need for dopaminergic therapy in the terminal stage. Once dopaminergic therapy has been optimised, consensus supports the use of midazolam (Irish Palliative Care in Parkinson's Disease Group, 2016).

Supporting caregiver and family: several studies highlight the challenges faced by caregivers and families, both before and after bereavement. Terminal decline often comes as a surprise, and some people may feel unprepared for the death of their loved one (Hasson et al., 2010). Members of the MDT should be mindful of this and give consideration to caregiver and family support in advance of the terminal stage. This may be a simple as addressing the possibility of dying, but it may also involve accessing specialist services—for example, via the hospice team—to provide caregiver support and pre- or post bereavement counselling. The need for improved support for family and caregivers, both before and after bereavement, has been identified as an important area for development (Fox et al., 2020); it should be actively considered where people are approaching the terminal stages of Parkinson's.

Conclusions

Palliative and supportive care for Parkinson's should not be restricted to the traditional palliative stage but rather considered throughout the course of the condition according to the needs of the individual. The MDT is central to enacting this modern, integrative interpretation of palliative care. Team members should be open to the possibility of palliative need, aware of common palliative problems and interventions, and empowered to trigger specialist palliative care referral where appropriate.

The importance of openness to ACP and the skills to facilitate this should never be underestimated. Opportunities should be found to engage people with Parkinson's in this process at the time that suits their needs and preserves their autonomy.

In the terminal stage of Parkinson's, members of the MDT will have to provide advice to professionals who do not specialise in the condition; they should mutually develop a working knowledge of common issues in terminal care. They are ideally placed to promote a patient-centred model of care that prioritises the needs of the person with Parkinson's as well as the caregiver.

Top tips for the multidisciplinary team in Parkinson's palliative care

Timing of palliative interventions
- Throughout all stages of Parkinson's, be alert to unmet palliative need.
- "Milestones" may be specific to the condition or person; unmet needs should be considered when milestones are evaluated. Members of the MDT are often the first to identify person specific milestones.
- Have a strategy for approaching ACP so that you can be open to verbal and non-verbal cues.

Advance care planning
- Consider ACP to be an ongoing process, not "one stop."
- Check ACP over time—it can be difficult to envisage our future selves.
- Statement of wishes may be useful, alongside the Lasting Power of Attorney (LPA), to reduce strain on the advocate.
- Consider SLT support to optimise capacity and participation.

Opimisation of medication
- Total anticholinergic burden can be estimated using an anticholinergic burden score.
- Discuss and negotiate medication changes with the individual to optimise concordance.
- Try converting oral rivastigmine to transdermal patch formulation where weight loss is an issue (causes less anorexia).
- Consider specialist pharmacist support for medication reviews.

Terminal care
- Consider the likely degree of dopa responsiveness.
- Seek drivers of agitation before treating with drugs.
- Share decision making with the MDT and palliative colleagues—this is a rapidly evolving area of expertise.
- Consider specialist physiotherapy input for positioning or turning to relieve pressure areas.
- Early OT involvement may facilitate care at home where desired.

Abbreviations: ACP, advance care planning; MDT, multidisciplinary team; OT, occupational therapist; SLT, speech and language therapist

---

References

Aarsland, D., Anderson, K., Larsen, J. P., Lolk, A., & Kragh-Sorensen, P. (2003). Prevalence and characteristics of dementia in Parkinson's disease: an 8-year prospective trial. *Archives of Neurology*, *60*(3), 387–392.

Cersosimo, M. G., Raina, G. B., Pellene, L. A., Micheli, F. E., Calandra, C. R., & Maiola, R. (2018). Weight loss in Parkinson's disease: the relationship with motor symptoms and disease progression. *BioMed Research International*, vol. 9, Article ID 9642524, 6 pages, 2018. https://doi.org/10.1155/2018/9642524.

Chancellor, M. B., Staskin, D. R., Kay, G. G., Sandage, B. W., Oefelein, M. G., & Tsao, J. W. (2012). Blood-brain barrier permeation and efflux exclusion of anticholinergics used in the treatment of overactive bladder. *Drugs Aging*, *29*, 259–273.

Crispo, J. A. G., Willis, A. W., Thibault, D. P., Fortin, Y., Hays, H. D., Mcnair, D. S., et al. (2016). Associations between anticholinergic burden and adverse health outcomes in Parkinson disease. *PloS one*, *11*, e0150621–e1150621.

Fallon, M., & Foley, P. (2012). Rising to the challenge of palliative care for non-malignant disease. *Palliat Med*, *26*, 99–100.

Fox, S., Azman, A., & Timmons, S. (2020). Palliative care needs in Parkinson's disease: focus on anticipatory grief in family carers. *Annals of Palliative Medicine*, S34–S43.

Goy, E. R., Carter, J., & Ganzini, L. (2008). Neurologic disease at the end of life: caregiver descriptions of Parkinson disease and amyotrophic lateral sclerosis. *J Palliat Med*, *11*, 548–554.

Habermann, B. (1996). Day-to-Day Demands of Parkinson's Disease. *Western Journal of Nursing Research*, *18*, 397–413.

Habermann, B. (1999). Continuity challenges of Parkinson's disease in middle life. *J Neurosci Nurs*, *31*, 200–207.

Hasson, F., Kernohan, W. G., McLaughlin, M., Waldron, M., McLaughlin, D., Chambers, H., & Cochrane, B. (2010). An exploration into the palliative and end-of-life experiences of carers of people with Parkinson's disease. *Palliat Med*, *24*, 731–736.

Hely, M. A., Morris, J. G. L., Traficante, R., Reid, W. G. J., O'sullivan, D. J., et al. (1999). The Sydney multicentre study of Parkinson's disease: progression and mortality at 10 years. *J Neurol Neurosurg Psychiatry*, *67*, 300–307.

Hindmarsh, J., Hindmarsh, S., & Lee, M. (2021). Idiopathic Parkinson's disease at the end of life: a retrospective evaluation of symptom prevalence, pharmacological symptom management and transdermal rotigotine dosing. *Clin Drug Investig*, *41*(8), 675–683.

Hindmarsh, J., Hindmarsh, S., Lee, M., & Telford, R. (2019). The combination of levomepromazine (methotrimeprazine) and rotigotine enables the safe and effective management of refractory nausea and vomiting in a patient with idiopathic Parkinson's disease. *Palliat Med*, *33*, 109–113.

Hong, C. T., Chan, L., Wu, D., Chen, W. T., & Chien, L. N. (2019). Antiparkinsonism anticholinergics increase dementia risk in patients with Parkinson's disease. *Parkinsonism Relat Disord*, *65*, 224–229.

Hosie, A., Davidson, P. M., Agar, M., Sanderson, C. R., & Phillips, J. (2013). Delirium prevalence, incidence, and implications for screening in specialist palliative care inpatient settings: a systematic review. *Palliat Med*, *27*, 486–498.

Hudson, P. L., Toye, C., & Kristjanson, L. J. (2006). Would people with Parkinson's disease benefit from palliative care? *Palliative Medicine*, *20*, 87–94.

Ibrahim, H., Woodward, Z., Pooley, J., & Richfield, E. W. (2020). Rotigotine patch prescription in inpatients with Parkinson's disease: evaluating prescription accuracy, delirium and end-of-life use. *Age and Ageing*.

Irish Palliative Care in Parkinson's Disease Group. (2016). *Palliative care in people with Parkinson's disease: Guidelines for professional healthcare workers on the assessment and management of palliative care needs in Parkinson's disease and related parkinsonian syndromes*. Cork: University College Cork.

Johnson, M. J., & Gadoud, A. (2011). Palliative care for people with chronic heart failure: when is it time? *J Palliat Care*, *27*, 37–42.

Jordan, S. R., Kluger, B., Ayele, R., Brungardt, A., Hall, A., Jones, J., et al. (2020). Optimizing future planning in Parkinson disease: suggestions for a comprehensive roadmap from patients and care partners. *Annals of Palliative Medicine*, S63–S74.

Keyser, D. L., & Rodnitzky, R. L. (1991). Neuroleptic malignant syndrome in Parkinson's disease after withdrawal or alteration of dopaminergic therapy. *Arch Intern Med*, *151*, 794–796.

King, H., Corry, P., Wauchob, T., & Barclay, P. (2003). Probable dystonic reaction after a single dose of cyclizine in a patient with a history of encephalitis. *Anaesthesia*, *58*, 257–260.

Kluger, B. M., Miyasaki, J., Katz, M., Galifianakis, N., Hall, K., Pantilat, S., et al. (2020). Comparison of integrated outpatient palliative care with standard care in patients with Parkinson disease and related disorders: a randomised clinical trial. *JAMA Neurology*, e194992.

Lanoix, M. (2009). Palliative care and Parkinson's disease: managing the chronic-palliative interface. *Chronic Illn*, *5*, 46–55.

Lee, M. A., Prentice, W. M., Hildreth, A. J., & Walker, R. W. (2007). Measuring symptom load in idiopathic Parkinson's disease. *Parkinsonism Relat Disord*, *13*, 284–289.

Miyasaki, J. M., Long, J., Mancini, D., Moro, E., Fox, S. H., Lang, A. E., et al. (2012). Palliative care for advanced Parkinson disease: an interdisciplinary clinic and new scale, the ESAS-PD. *Parkinsonism Relat Disord*, *18*(Suppl 3), S6–9.

Murray, S. A., Boyd, K., & Sheikh, A. (2005). Palliative care in chronic illness: We need to move from prognostic paralysis to active total care. *BMJ*, 611–612.

National Institute For Health and Care Excellence 2017. Parkinson's disease in Adults. July https://www.nice.org.uk/guidance/NG71.

Phillips, L. J. (2006). Dropping the bomb: the experience of being diagnosed with Parkinson's disease. *Geriatric Nursing*, *27*, 362–369.

Pondal, M., Marras, C., Miyasaki, J., Moro, E., Armstrong, M. J., Strafella, A. P., et al. (2013). Clinical features of dopamine agonist withdrawal syndrome in a movement disorders clinic. *J Neurol Neurosurg Psychiatry*, *84*, 130–135.

Resuscitation Council UK 2020. Retrieved January 13, 2021, from https://www.resus.org.uk/respect.

Richfield, E., Alty, J., & Jones, E. (2013). Palliative care for Parkinson's disease: a summary of evidence and future directions. *Palliative Medicine*, *27*, 805–810.

Richfield, E., & Johnson, M. (2020). Palliative care in parkinson's disease: review of needs assessment tools. *Ann Palliat Med*, S6–S15.

Schrag, A., Ben-Shlomo, Y., & Quinn, N. (2002). How valid is the clinical diagnosis of Parkinson's disease in the community? *Journal of Neurology, Neurosurgery & Psychiatry*, *73*, 529–534.

Scottish Government Polypharmacy Model of Care Group. 2018. Polypharmacy Guidance, Realistic Prescribing. 3rd ed.

Sharma, J. C., & Vassallo, M. (2014). Prognostic significance of weight changes in Parkinson's disease: the Park-weight phenotype. *Neurodegener Dis Manag*, *4*, 309–316.

Sheffrin, M., Miao, Y., Boscardin, W. J., & Steinman, M. A. (2015). Weight Loss Associated with Cholinesterase Inhibitors in Individuals with Dementia in a National Healthcare System. *Journal of the American Geriatrics Society*, *63*, 1512–1518.

Sokol, L. L., Young, M. J., Paparian, J., Kluger, B. M., Lum, H. D., Besbris, J., et al. (2019). Advance care planning in Parkinson's disease: ethical challenges and future directions. *NPJ Parkinson's disease*, *5*, 24–124.

Stokes G. (2017) Challenging behaviour in Dementia. A Person-centred approach. Routledge.

Thomas, S., & Macmahon, D. (2004). Parkinson's disease, palliative care and older people. *Nurs Older People*, *16*, 22–27.

Tuck, K. K., Brodd, L., Nutt, J., & Fromme EK (2015). Preferences of patients with Parkinson's disease for communication about advanced care planning. *Am J Hosp Palliat Care*, *32*, 68–77.

Walker, R., Davidson, M., & Gray, W. (2012). Gender differences in 1-year survival rates after weight loss in people with idiopathic Parkinson's disease. *International Journal of Palliative Nursing*, *18*.

Weiss, M., & Britten, N. (2009). *The Pharmaceutical Journal*, *271*, 493.

World Health Organization, 2015. WHO definition of palliative care [Online]. Retrieved September 9, 2015, from http://www.who.int/cancer/palliative/definition/en/.

Chapter 9

Parkinson's Disease Dementia and Dementia With Lewy Bodies

Sabina Vatter, Clare Johnson and Rob Skelly

Chapter outline

Introduction

James Parkinson described "the senses and intellects being uninjured," but we now know that dementia and neuropsychiatric symptoms occur frequently in Parkinson's (Weintraub & Burn, 2011). Cognitive deficits have been identified at all stages of Parkinson's. These deficits are usually subtle at the time of diagnosis but, as time passes, progression to dementia may occur. Indeed, the point prevalence of dementia in those with Parkinson's is 30% and the risk of developing dementia is at least 75% in those who survive 10 years from Parkinson's diagnosis (Aarsland & Kurz, 2010). The impact of dementia on the individual and caregiver should not be underestimated. For the person with Parkinson's, dementia heralds reduced life expectancy, increased dependency, and risk of institutionalisation (Aarsland et al., 2000). Dementia also brings increased caregiver burden and depression (Leroi et al., 2012a).

The multidisciplinary team should provide information, advice, and support for people with Parkinson's disease dementia and their caregivers. In this chapter we discuss:

- Mild cognitive impairment in Parkinson's
- Parkinson's disease dementia
- Dementia with Lewy bodies
- The impact of Lewy body spectrum disorders on the individual, caregivers and society
- Medical and pharmacological management
- Intervention by the multidisciplinary team for non-pharmacological management

Cognitive impairment in Parkinson's

Three stages of cognitive dysfunction have been postulated in Parkinson's: (1) no cognitive impairment (which may include subjective cognitive impairment); (2) Parkinson's disease with mild cognitive impairment (PD-MCI); and (3) Parkinson's disease dementia (PDD). Additionally, if cognitive symptoms predate motor symptoms or occur within the first 12 months following the onset of motor symptoms, dementia with Lewy bodies (DLB) may be diagnosed (Mrak & Griffin, 2007). Specific guidelines have been developed for diagnosing PD-MCI, PDD, and DLB (see Table 9.1), which are jointly referred to as "Lewy body spectrum disorders" (Aarsland, 2016) because intracytoplasmic eosinophilic collections containing α-synuclein (called Lewy bodies) can be seen in all of these conditions. PDD and DLB can be regarded as ends of a spectrum and the term *Lewy body dementia* covers both PDD and DLB. In this book we are principally concerned with PDD but we also address DLB, as many Parkinson's services also see individuals with that condition.

TABLE 9.1 diagnostic criteria for Parkinson's disease with mild cognitive impairment, Parkinson's disease dementia, and dementia with Lewy bodies

	PD-MCI	PDD	DLB
Core features required to diagnose	• Diagnosis of PD (according to Brain Bank Criteria, Gibb & Lees, 1988) and gradual decline in cognitive ability in context of established PD. • Cognitive deficits on either formal neuropsychological testing or a global cognitive abilities scale. • Cognitive deficits do not interfere with functional independence but subtle difficulties on complex functional tasks may be present.	• Diagnosis of PD (according to Brain Bank criteria, Gibb & Lees, 1988) and dementia syndrome with insidious onset and slow progression in context of established PD. • Diagnosed by history, clinical and mental examination; defined as: impairment in more than one cognitive domain; represents a decline from premorbid level; deficits severe enough to impair daily life (social, occupational, personal care), independent of the impairment ascribable to motor or autonomic symptoms.	• Dementia: progressive cognitive decline sufficient to interfere with normal social, occupational or daily functioning. • Prominent or persistent memory impairment may not necessarily occur in the early stages but is usually evident with progression. • Deficits on tests of attention, executive function, and visuoperceptual ability may be especially prominent and occur early.
Associated clinical features	**Level I:** Impairment on a scale of global cognitive abilities. **Level II:** Neuropsychological testing that includes at least two of five tests that measure attention and working memory, executive functioning, language, memory, or visuospatial abilities *or* impairment on neuropsychological tests (if performance is 1 to 2 SDs below the norms or decline is seen on serial cognitive testing).	**Probable:** Two or more cognitive with or without behavioural. **Possible:** One or more atypical (e.g., prominent or receptive-type aphasia, pure amnesia with no benefit from cueing, preserved attention) cognitive symptoms with or without behavioural. **Cognitive:** impairment in attention, executive functions, memory, visuospatial functions, but language largely preserved. **Behavioural:** apathy, changes in personality and mood (i.e., depression, anxiety), excessive daytime sleepiness, hallucinations, delusions.	**Probable:** Two or more core clinical features with or without indicative biomarkers or one core feature with one or more indicative biomarkers. **Possible:** One core clinical feature without an indicative biomarker or one or more indicative biomarkers with no core clinical features for possible. **Core clinical:** fluctuating cognition (with pronounced variations in attention and alertness), recurrent detailed and well-formed visual hallucinations, REM sleep behaviour disorder, spontaneous cardinal features of Parkinsonism (i.e., bradykinesia, rest tremor or rigidity).

(Continued)

TABLE 9.1 diagnostic criteria for Parkinson's disease with mild cognitive impairment, Parkinson's disease dementia, and dementia with Lewy bodies (*Cont.*)

	PD-MCI	PDD	DLB
Supportive features		**Features** that make the diagnosis uncertain (if both absent, probable diagnosis of PDD, if one absent, possible diagnosis): coexistence of other abnormality that by itself may cause cognitive impairment but judged not to be the cause of dementia and/or time interval between motor and cognitive symptoms unknown. **Features** suggesting other conditions or diseases as cause of mental impairment, making it impossible to reliably diagnose PDD must be absent, such as acute confusion, major depression, features compatible with vascular dementia according to NINDS-AIREN criteria.	**Supportive clinical:** Severe sensitivity to antipsychotic agents, postural instability, repeated falls, syncope or other transient episodes of unresponsiveness, severe autonomic dysfunction, hypersomnia, hyposmia, hallucinations in other modalities; systematised delusions, apathy, anxiety and depression. **Supportive biomarkers:** Relative preservation of medial temporal lobe structures on CT/MRI; generalised low uptake on SPECT/PET perfusion/metabolism scan with reduced occipital activity & the cingulate island sign on FDG-PET imaging; prominent posterior slow-wave activity on EEG with periodic fluctuations in the pre-alpha/theta range.

Abbreviations: CT, computed tomography; DLB, dementia with Lewy bodies; EEG, electroencephalography; FDG-PET, fluorodeoxyglucose positron emission tomography; MRI, magnetic resonance imaging; NINDS-AIREN, National Institute of Neurological Disorders–Stroke and Association Internationale pour la Recherche et l'Enseignement en Neurosciences; PD-MCI, Parkinson's disease and mild cognitive impairment; PDD, Parkinson's disease dementia; PET, positron emission tomography; REM, rapid eye movement; SPECT, single-photon emission computed tomography
Adapted from Fields, 2017; Litvan et al., 2012; Emre et al., 2007; and McKeith et al., 2017.

Parkinson's with mild cognitive impairment

Mild cognitive impairment (MCI) represents a change in cognition, which falls between normal cognitive functioning and early dementia. MCI extraneous to movement disorders is diagnosed in the presence of a subjective memory complaint (preferably corroborated by an informant), an objective memory impairment relative to age and education, normal general cognitive function, intact or minimal decline in functional activities of daily living (ADLs) and absence of dementia (Petersen, 2004). Amnestic-type MCI, where memory loss is predominant, has a high risk of transforming into Alzheimer's disease (AD), whereas non-amnestic MCI, where impairments occur in domains other than memory, is more likely to convert into other types of dementia, such as frontotemporal dementia, vascular dementia or DLB.

Over the last two decades, researchers have increasingly recognised that cognitive impairment may occur during the early stages of Parkinson's. Nearly 25% of newly diagnosed people with Parkinson's without dementia have been found to present with cognitive impairment (Aarsland et al., 2009). Diagnostic criteria for PD-MCI are shown in Table 9.1. PD-MCI is associated with older age, male gender and depression as well as the duration and severity of Parkinson's (Litvan et al., 2011). Goldman and colleagues (2018) have proposed that PD-MCI can remain as PD-MCI, progress to PDD, or revert back to normal cognition. The authors also argue that a stage of "pre-PD-MCI" can be identified when an individual with Parkinson's is experiencing some cognitive symptoms that do not yet meet diagnostic criteria for PD-MCI.

Parkinson's disease dementia

Each year about 11% of people with Parkinson's develop dementia (Hobson & Meara, 2015). It is possible that the number of people with PDD could triple by 2060 (Savica et al., 2018). Furthermore, by the time PD-MCI is diagnosed, the chances of advancing to PDD are fourfold as compared with Parkinson's without cognitive impairment (Hobson & Meara, 2015).

The main risk factors for developing PDD are:

- Having a limited cognitive reserve (Emre et al., 2007)
- Having MCI at baseline (Emre et al., 2007)
- Experiencing hallucinations (Aarsland et al., 2003)
- Being of older age (Emre et al., 2007)
- Having more severe Parkinson's (Emre et al., 2007)
- Experiencing mainly gait dysfunction (Emre et al., 2007)
- Being of older age at diagnosis (Emre et al., 2007)
- Having rapid-eye-movement (REM) sleep behaviour disorder (Kim et al., 2018)

Genetic risk factors for the development of dementia in Parkinson's have also been described. For example, presence of the apolipoprotein E ε4 allele increases PDD risk modestly (odds ratio 1.5) (Sun et al., 2019). Mutations in the glucocerebrosidase gene (GBA) increase the risk of PD-MCI or PDD 5.8-fold (Alcalay, 2012). Although no specific treatment is currently available for GBA-associated Parkinson's, it is possible that specific treatments could be developed in the future, and direct-to-consumer testing for GBA and other mutations is already available.

In a person with Parkinson's, if cognitive decline is sufficient to impair daily functioning (social interactions, personal care), a diagnosis of PDD should be considered (see Table 9.1 for PDD diagnostic criteria).

Cognitive profile in Parkinson's disease dementia

PDD is characterised by a deterioration in attention, visuospatial function and executive function. Decline in memory may occur but is a less prominent feature than in AD, and recall may be aided by prompts. Cognitive assessment tools such as the Montreal Cognitive Assessment (MoCA) can be used to document cognitive deficits. Executive dysfunction and visuospatial deficits may lead to problems with personal care. Activities may be poorly planned. Individuals may get lost in all but the most familiar surroundings. They may struggle with ADLs—for example, with shopping, cooking, driving, washing and dressing.

Behavioural and neuropsychiatric features of Parkinson's disease dementia

Neuropsychiatric symptoms in PDD and DLB include apathy, hallucinations, delusions, anxiety, depression, agitation, REM-sleep behaviour disorder and excessive daytime somnolence. At least one neuropsychiatric symptom is reported in 64% of those with PDD (Aarsland et al., 2007). Although hallucinations and delusions can occur in Parkinson's in the absence of dementia, these symptoms are more common in PDD. Hallucinations are usually visual, well-formed and dynamic, typically consisting of anonymous people or animals. Often the hallucinations are not threatening or frightening, but they may be so. Tactile, auditory, and olfactory hallucinations may occur but are less common. Delusions are less common than hallucinations in PDD but may be very troublesome when they occur. Delusional jealousy (Othello syndrome) and delusional misidentifications syndromes (such as Capgras syndrome, when the sufferer believes an individual has been replaced by an imposter) may occur and put caregivers at risk. Where caregivers are thought to be at risk, referral to specialist mental health services for expert risk assessment should be prompt. Apathy, anxiety and depression are common.

Dementia with Lewy bodies

DLB represents the second most common type of neurodegenerative dementia (following AD), with a prevalence of 4.2% to 4.6% of all dementia cases (Kane et al., 2018). Pathologically, the distinctive feature of DLB is the appearance of Lewy bodies, which occur in the central, peripheral and autonomic nervous system. Unlike PDD, which is diagnosed within firmly established Parkinson's, the clinical diagnosis of DLB takes place when cognitive impairment precedes or occurs alongside the motor symptoms of Parkinsonism within 12 months of motor symptom onset. "Pure DLB" is less common than "DLB with concurrent Alzheimer pathology" owing to the overlap of Lewy bodies and neurofibrillary tangles specific to AD (Mueller et al., 2017). However, comparative studies have demonstrated that cognitive decline is faster in DLB than in AD (Rongve et al., 2016), confirming that DLB is a separate condition.

Diagnosing dementia with Lewy bodies

McKeith et al. (2017) established consensus criteria for the diagnosis of DLB. The central feature of DLB is a dementia syndrome—a progressive cognitive decline that interferes with normal social and occupational functioning as well as activities of daily living (ADLs).

In addition to the cognitive symptoms, core clinical features include:

- Marked fluctuations in attention and alertness
- Visual hallucinations, recurrent and well formed
- REM sleep behaviour disorder, which includes acting out in dreams, shouting out, moving and even hitting out while asleep
- Parkinsonism

Supportive clinical features include

- Postural instability and falls
- Syncope or other transient episodes of unresponsiveness
- Autonomic dysfunction (constipation, postural hypotension, detrusor instability)
- Excessive daytime somnolence
- Loss of sense of smell
- Hallucinations in other modalities
- Delusions
- Apathy, anxiety and depression
- Sensitivity to neuroleptics

The guidelines of the National Institute for Health and Care Excellence (2018a) for dementia support use of imaging to help define the dementia subtype. Indicative biomarkers for DLB include:

- Reduced dopamine transporter uptake in basal ganglia demonstrated by single photon emission computed tomography (SPECT) or positron emission tomography (PET)
- Abnormal (low) uptake of [123]iodine-meta-iodobenzylguanidine on myocardial scintigraphy
- Polysomnographic confirmation of REM sleep disorder without atonia

Supportive biomarkers include:

- Computed tomography (CT) or magnetic resonance imaging (MRI) brain scans showing generalised atrophy without predominant medial temporal atrophy
- Generalised low uptake on SPECT perfusion scanning (including the occipital lobes)

Marked fluctuations in cognitive function are typical of DLB. Cognitive function can vary throughout the day. Assessment tools such as the Mayo Fluctuations Questionnaire can be used to establish the presence of fluctuations (Ferman et al., 2004). A quite distinctive symptom of early DLB is a state of anxiety with some agitation. Individuals can become agitated during clinic or therapy sessions, being unable to sit still or to concentrate. This can be very distressing for the caregiver.

As with PDD, cognitive difficulties in DLB include reduced attention and executive skills. There may be evidence of delayed mental processing, particularly with more complex tasks.

The progressive cognitive decline will result in

- Poor problem solving and difficulty learning new skills
- Impaired decision making
- Problems with attention and spatial awareness

Significant memory loss may not develop until later.

Delusions and hallucinations in DLB are similar in nature to those found in PDD, described earlier. Motor symptoms are similar to those in Parkinson's. These include a shuffling gait, freezing of gait (FOG) and stooped posture. In DLB, these physical changes may occur up to a year before the dementia, concurrently with the dementia, or after the cognitive difficulties have emerged.

Comparison of Parkinson's disease with dementia and dementia with Lewy bodies

Owing to the overlap in cognitive, motor and neuropsychiatric features, researchers have debated whether PDD and DLB are the same condition (McKeith et al., 2017). Likewise, the 1-year window that differentiates between PDD and DLB may be arbitrary, as there is no strong pathological or clinical evidence to demonstrate its validity (Taylor & O'Brien, 2012). Some researchers have concluded that PDD and DLB do not differ in regard to cognitive, attentional, and neuropsychiatric profiles; sleep and autonomic dysfunction; Parkinson's type and severity; neuroleptic sensitivity; and responsivity to cholinesterase inhibitors (Aldridge et al., 2018). However, this has been challenged by further studies undertaken with both populations (see Table 9.2). Furthermore, a comparative study including people with PDD, DLB, and AD concluded that the neuropsychiatric symptom presentation in PDD is more similar to that of AD than of

TABLE 9.2 Differentiating Parkinson's disease dementia and dementia with Lewy bodies

Features	PDD	DLB
Age of onset	60 to 70 years	65 to 75 years
Gender	More common in men	More common in men
Dementia onset in regard to Parkinson's	Later	Earlier (65-75)
Dementia progression	More rapid compared with Parkinson's; dementia increases mortality	Dementia at diagnosis; either rapid (1-5 years) or moderate annual decline
Parkinson's motor symptoms	100% More asymmetrical	25% to 50%, less tremor More symmetrical
Average survival following diagnosis	3 to 15 years	6.5 to 7.5 years
Motor and non-motor symptom progression	Slower	Faster
Cognitive functioning and fluctuations (e.g., attention)	Moderate to severe	Severe
Memory deficits	Deficit in recall but not learning	Recall and learning
Psychiatric symptoms (e.g., visual hallucinations, delusions)	Common, onset often after levodopa	Very common, spontaneous onset, often at presentation
Other neuropsychiatric symptoms (e.g., depression, apathy, anxiety)	Common	Common
REM sleep behaviour disorder	Common	Common
Response to levodopa	Common	Variable

Abbreviations: DLB, dementia with Lewy bodies; PDD, Parkinson's disease dementia; REM, rapid eye movement.
Adapted from Buter et al., 2008; Fields, 2017; and McShane, 2008.

DLB (Chiu et al., 2016), suggesting that PDD and DLB are separate clinical conditions but share a common underlying pathology. Despite the contradictory findings about similarities and differences between PDD and DLB, it has been recommended that when a clinical diagnosis is being made, the 12-month rule separating DLB from PDD should be followed because of its convenience (McKeith et al., 2017) and that clinicians should verify the diagnosis via an individual clinical assessment of each person.

Impact of Lewy body spectrum disorders

A formal diagnosis of DLB may take time owing to the fluctuating and differing symptoms of DLB that can be experienced. Furthermore, health professionals may have a poor understanding of the LBDs. This can contribute to higher levels of stress for both the individual and the caregiver, especially when information and postdiagnostic support are lacking. The Lewy Body Society (www.lewybody.org) offers useful information, advice, and support. Compared with those with Alzheimer's, individuals with DLB are at greater risk for hospital admission, and they have longer lengths of hospital stay (Mueller et al., 2018). Poor physical health early on appears to be the main driver for high rates of hospital admission, whereas neuropsychiatric symptoms, such as hallucinations, may lead to longer stays.

The presence of dementia in a person with Parkinson's leads to a significantly greater caregiver burden and reduced quality of life (QoL) compared with those who have Parkinson's without dementia or PD-MCI (Leroi et al., 2012b; Vatter et al., 2020). Also, caregivers to those with PDD have a greater burden than caregivers to those with AD. In PDD, neuropsychiatric symptoms, particularly visual hallucinations and apathy, are an important cause of caregiver burden (Leroi et al., 2012a; Shin et al., 2012). Other factors, such as the following, also contribute to caregiver burden:

- Increasingly compromised functional abilities, including driving, in the person with dementia
- A poor level of support services (Connors et al., 2019)

Assessment by the multidisciplinary team (MDT) may help to identify sources of caregiver burden. Both pharmacological and non-pharmacological interventions to improve functional ability and address depression and agitation should be considered. Referral to social services for additional support or respite care should be offered. Provision of education and information (direction to websites, directories of specialist care providers, research information) and referral to support groups may be helpful (Galvin et al., 2010).

Cognitive impairment in Parkinson's significantly raises the likelihood of institutionalisation (Aarsland et al., 2000) and increases healthcare costs and mortality (Larsson et al., 2018). The emergence of cognitive impairment can also significantly decrease the QoL of people with Parkinson's and increase emotional stress.

Similarly to Parkinson's and PDD, a diagnosis of DLB can also escalate healthcare costs, shorten time to death (Price et al., 2017), and accelerate the rate of admission to care homes and hospitals (Zweig & Galvin, 2014). Mueller and colleagues (2018) estimate that approximately 80,000 people with DLB in the United Kingdom will incur over 27,000 hospital admissions and spend over 300,000 days in hospital, which will exceed £35 million in hospitalisation costs in just 1 year. This is higher per capita than is the case with AD.

Assessment by the multidisciplinary team

Medical assessment

The neurologist or geriatrician in the Parkinson's clinic is well placed to make the diagnosis of PDD (based on the diagnostic criteria in Table 9.1) and prescribe appropriate medication. In case of uncertainty or according to local practice, referral to local mental health services may take place. Poor communication between physical and mental health services is a source of dissatisfaction both for clinicians and people with Parkinson's (Parkinson's UK and All Party Parliamentary Group for Parkinson's Disease, 2018). More joined-up computer systems, better training in mental health for neurologists and geriatricians, better training in Parkinson's for psychiatrists, flexible access to support services and good communication are all needed. Inclusion of a psychiatrist in the Parkinson's MDT can improve communication and the experience of care (Taylor et al., 2020), but institutional barriers to integrated work may be difficult to overcome.

The doctor should exclude reversible causes of cognitive decline by doing simple blood tests, including urea and electrolytes, liver function tests, thyroid function tests and vitamin B12 level. Brain imaging should be considered. Medication should be reviewed and anticholinergic medications such as oxybutynin and trihexyphenidyl should be withdrawn. Parkinson's medications should be reviewed and simplified. Dopamine agonists and amantadine, for example, may contribute to confusion and hallucinations in people with Parkinson's; therefore, generally speaking, these should be reduced or withdrawn. Motor symptoms should be controlled with L-dopa preparations if possible. Depression can sometimes mimic dementia; thus, it should be identified and treated.

Measuring psychiatric and cognitive manifestations

A significant body of literature has specifically focused on assessing the psychiatric and cognitive manifestations of Parkinson's through self-reported, informant-reported and/or clinician-rated scales. Comprehensive clinical assessment should be carried out for each individual (Jankovic, 2008) and symptoms closely monitored over time.

Cognition

A full cognitive assessment should be completed. The Mini Mental State Examination (MMSE) is recommended by the International Parkinson and Movement Disorder Society (Dubois et al., 2007). Scores below 26/30 are evidence of decreased global cognitive efficiency. However, the MMSE may fail to detect executive dysfunction, and there are issues around copyright. The MoCA is a good screening tool, but more comprehensive assessments can provide greater detail regarding cognitive impairment. These assessments include Addenbrooke's Cognitive Assessment and the Edinburgh Cognitive Assessment, both of which are validated for use in Parkinson's. The PDD-Short Screen includes tests of immediate and delayed recall, verbal fluency, the clock drawing test and a five-item informant questionnaire. It takes about 5 to 7 minutes to complete (Pagonabarraga et al., 2010). The American Association of Neurologists recommends annual cognitive screening for people with Parkinson's (Zesiewicz et al., 2010).

Mood and mental well-being

A variety of scales are available for screening and monitoring mood disorders in Parkinson's; these have been reviewed and critiqued by Schrag and colleagues (2007). The Hospital Anxiety & Depression Scale is a self-reported tool that we recommend for use in the clinic. However, clinicians should be aware that cognitively impaired individuals may struggle to complete it. The Short Warwick-Edinburgh Mental Wellbeing Score is also useful and free to use. The Neuropsychiatric Inventory (NPI) is a useful observer-rated tool that assesses twelve neuropsychiatric symptoms separately and considers the frequency and severity of each symptom. The Parkinson's Disease Questionnaire (PDQ-39) is a self-reported QoL scale that assesses a variety of symptoms, not just mental health. Whatever scale is used, it is important that the assessment leads to appropriate therapeutic intervention.

Caregiver strain

Caregiver strain assessments such as the Caregiver Strain Index (Robinson, 1983) and the Zarit Burden Interview (Vatter et al., 2018; Zarit et al., 1980) can ascertain the physical, mental and financial impact of supporting an individual living with a chronic illness such as PDD or DLB.

Multidisciplinary interventions for Parkinson's disease dementia and dementia with Lewy bodies

General principles of care for people with Parkinson's disease dementia and dementia with Lewy bodies

MDT management is focussed on maintaining function for as long as possible, improving QoL and reducing caregiver burden and stress. Increasing dopaminergic (dopamine stimulating) medications may help motor symptoms at the expense of worsening cognition and psychotic symptoms. Therefore, pharmacological treatment aims to alleviate motor, cognitive and psychiatric symptoms with a particular focus on the most distressing symptoms for the individual at the time.

All members of the MDT are involved in offering a holistic approach to the individual's needs, with the consultant or Parkinson's disease nurse specialist (PDNS) taking a lead in management and other team members offering non-pharmacological interventions. The MDT should implement strategies such as giving only one instruction to the individual at a time, as people with dementia may struggle to process two or more instructions given in the same sentence or within a task-specific instruction. In a Parkinson's MDT the role of the occupational therapist (OT) is especially important in offering management strategies for cognition-related as well as physical problems. The OT has a role in advising on practical solutions to physical problems as well.

Post-diagnostic care

When dementia is diagnosed in a person with Parkinson's, it is advisable to run through a checklist (see Table 9.3). People with Parkinson's, PDD, or DLB and their caregivers may receive appropriate support from services such as Parkinson's UK, the Lewy Body Society, Carers UK, or the Alzheimer's Society, which offer support to people with any type of dementia.

It is important to explore whether wills and lasting powers of attorney are in place or whether they can be arranged following a capacity assessment. In the United Kingdom, a lasting power of attorney may apply to health and welfare and/or finances and property. Without a will and lasting power of attorney and

TABLE 9.3 Postdiagnostic checklist for dementia
Make sure that the diagnosis has been communicated to the individual and their caregiver
Offer a referral to the Alzheimer's Society, Parkinson's UK, Making Space, or Lewy Body Society
Supply printed information (e.g., from Parkinson's UK or the Parkinson's Foundation)
Reassess functional abilities and care needs, including the ability to manage medication
Make sure that the person has a will and power of attorney in place
Refer to a "Living Well With Dementia" course or similar
Review driver safety
Assess for caregiver burden, strain and stress

if the individual lacks testamentary capacity and is unable to manage his or her own financial affairs, a referral should be made to the Court of Protection in England and Wales. That court will appoint a guardian to look after the person's financial affairs. Usually, the application is made by a solicitor, and both the solicitor and the Court of Protection charge fees.

A diagnosis of dementia should also prompt a review of the person's care needs, which are usually assessed by an OT. If an OT finds that the individual has increasing difficulties with ADLs, he or she should advise on strategies that increase the chance of successful task completion. The OT should also consider referral to social services for help with personal care if the caregiver's help is insufficient or if the caregiver is overburdened. Additionally, instrumental ADLs—such as managing finances and medication as well as driving safely— should be reviewed and assessed.

"Living well with dementia" or similar courses may be available locally and referral should be offered when possible. Also, Parkinson's UK and the Lewy Body Society run support groups. People with Parkinson's, PDD and DLB and their caregivers can receive helpful advice, tips and support from these charities, courses and groups.

Medical and pharmacological treatment of Parkinson's disease dementia and dementia with Lewy bodies

Several medications are available for the treatment of cognitive impairment related to PDD and DLB. The findings from meta-analyses have determined that cholinesterase inhibitors such as rivastigmine and donepezil are beneficial in terms of cognition, behavioural disturbances and global functioning in people with PDD and DLB (Rolinski et al., 2012; Stinton et al., 2015). Oral rivastigmine commonly causes gastrointestinal side effects (nausea, vomiting, anorexia), but transcutaneous rivastigmine, delivered via a patch, is better tolerated. Other adverse effects of rivastigmine include tremor, drooling, urinary symptoms, slow heart rate, syncope and wheezing. Rivastigmine may be unsuitable for those who already have a poor appetite or are underweight. Cholinesterase inhibitors should be used with caution in those with a history of chronic obstructive airways disease or peptic ulceration. A pretreatment electrocardiogram (ECG) is advisable to document the resting heart rate and look for evidence of heart block. As a rule, we advise against cholinesterase inhibitors if the resting heart rate is less than 50. If the heart rate is between 50 and 60, we advise against cholinesterase inhibitors if the person has syncope (fainting) or presyncope. If the bradycardia is due to beta blockers or other rate-limiting drugs, consider whether these drugs can be reduced or withdrawn. The oral dose of rivastigmine used in clinical trials was 6 mg twice daily. However, if symptoms have improved on a lower dose, a case can be made for maintaining the lower dose. In any case, it is important to review effects of the treatment after a few weeks to decide whether to stop the treatment, continue or increase the dose.

Memantine, an N-methyl D-aspartate receptor antagonist, can also improve global clinical status and neuropsychiatric symptoms in people with mild to moderate DLB but not in people with PDD (Emre et al., 2010). However, when people with PDD were taking memantine, it was found that the burden among caregivers appeared to be reduced (Leroi et al., 2014). Memantine is generally well tolerated but can worsen constipation. It should be used with caution in seizure disorders and should not be used with amantadine. Dose reduction may be required in the presence of chronic kidney disease. Memantine should be considered for PDD and DLB when cholinesterase inhibitors are contraindicated or not tolerated.

Medications also have a role in the management of neuropsychiatric symptoms of PDD and DLB. The management of many of these symptoms is described in Chapters 6 and 7 and summarised in Table 9.4.

TABLE 9.4 Management of neuropsychiatric symptoms in Parkinson's disease and dementia with Lewy bodies

Problem	Management approaches
Depression/anxiety (see Chapter 6)	Provide meaningful activity.
	CBT is unlikely to be beneficial if dementia is advanced.
	Consider medical causes and contributors (hypothyroidism, anemia).
	SSRIs are better tolerated than TCAs.
	Choice of antidepressants may depend on other factors. For example, mirtazapine may aid sleep and stimulate appetite.
Apathy (see Chapter 6)	Suggest using a diary and planning activities into the week. Thinking about rewards can help with motivation.
	Consider depression and treat if present.
	Rivastigmine may be helpful.
Hallucinations and delusions (see Chapter 7)	Optimise vision and hearing. Arrange for optician consultation.
	Reduce visual distraction. Highly patterned carpets, cushions and curtains may exacerbate visual hallucinations; therefore plainer decor is advised.
	Consider physical causes (e.g., metabolic problem, infection, constipation).
	Review medications: stop anticholinergics, reduce or wean off dopamine agonists, amantadine, and MAOIs. Aim to manage motor symptoms with co-careldopa or co-beneldopa alone.
	Consider rivastigmine, other AChIs, and/or memantine.
	Consider an antipsychotic such as quetiapine or clozapine.

(Continued)

TABLE 9.4 Management of neuropsychiatric symptoms in Parkinson's disease and dementia with Lewy bodies (*Cont.*)

Problem	Management approaches
Agitation/resistance to care (Cankurtaran, 2014; Volicer & Hurley, 2003)	Consider antecedents, behaviours and consequences.
	Consider physical causes: metabolic, infective, medication, constipation.
	Determine whether agitated behaviour is an expression of an unmet need (e.g., for food, drink, toileting, company, meaningful activity).
	Assess for pain and consider regular analgesia.
	Adjust the way in which care is offered. For example, getting up earlier or later than average may suit certain individuals, or a bed bath may be preferred to a shower.
	Optimise rivastigmine, other AChIs and/or memantine.
	Consider a cognitive intervention, such as CST.
	Consider stimulant-based therapies such as reminiscence therapy, music, aromatherapy, massage, pet therapy.
	Consider depression and treat if present.
	Consider sedation if non-drug methods are not helping and person is a danger to self or others. Preferred options include benzodiazepines or quetiapine (increased falls risk with both).
Sleep disturbance (see Chapter 6)	Exercise can improve nighttime sleep (Amara et al., 2020).
	Offer sleep hygiene advice and information sheet (see Table 6.4).
	Consider depression.
	Consider melatonin.
	Consider clonazepam for REM sleep behaviour disorder.
Sexual disinhibition	Wean off dopamine agonist.
	Consider an SSRI as first line if drug therapy is required (Guay, 2008).
	Consider an antiandrogen such as medroxyprogesterone or leuprorelin (limited evidence base).

AChI, acetylcholinesterase inhibitor (rivastigmine, donepezil, galantamine); CBT, cognitive behavioural therapy; CST, cognitive stimulation therapy; MAOIs, monoamine oxidase inhibitors; REM, rapid eye movement; SSRI, selective serotonin reuptake inhibitor; TCA, tricyclic antidepressant

Drug-based treatments are often the first suggested treatment choice for cognitive and neuropsychiatric symptoms in PDD and DLB owing to their evidence base and efficacy. However, medication can be expensive, may not suit each individual, have modest effects, cause side effects and can even result in the worsening of motor and cognitive symptoms in Parkinson's. Therefore it is also essential to look beyond simply providing pharmacological treatment.

Non-pharmacological intervention for cognitive and neuropsychiatric symptoms

Cognitive intervention

There are three specific types of cognitive intervention (Table 9.5), all of which are evidence-based and appropriate for people with Parkinson's and cognitive impairment:

- Cognitive training (Orgeta et al., 2020), specific exercises aimed at improving cognitive ability
- Cognitive rehabilitation (Hindle et al., 2018), a more holistic approach to daily cognitive function
- Cognitive stimulation (Leroi et al., 2019), aiming to stimulate and engage individuals

Cognitive training

Cognitive training includes guided and repeated practice of selected standardised tasks addressing specific cognitive domains such as memory, attention, executive function, language and speed of processing. These tasks encourage remembering, planning, the focusing of attention or organising of information (Bahar-Fuchs et al., 2013; Orgeta et al., 2020). The intervention can be facilitated using either a pen-and-pencil method or a computer (e.g., exergames, virtual reality) and delivered in a group, individually or guided by a family member with support from a therapist. Depending on the stage of the cognitive impairment, some people are also keen to do cognitive tasks such as crosswords, processing of information, planning and reading. Positive results have been found for people with Parkinson's, where working memory, executive function and processing speed improved with cognitive training (Leung et al., 2015). However, cognitive training is not supported by the National Institute for Health and Care Excellence (2018a), and there are no studies supporting its use among people with PDD and DLB.

Cognitive rehabilitation

Cognitive rehabilitation aims to support people with cognitive decline by improving their daily functioning through the setting of goals and implementation of a tailored plan to address the goals using evidence-based strategies (Bahar-Fuchs et al., 2013). The intervention is highly individual and tailored according to each person's symptoms, impairments, needs, situational factors and preferences (Clare et al., 2010). Participants' goals may relate to everyday functioning, ADLs, personal care, language or social interaction; they are discussed with a trained therapist who works closely with each individual. Although, traditionally, cognitive rehabilitation has been classified as one of the cognition-based interventions, the focus more recently has been on considering

TABLE 9.5 Comparisons of cognitive stimulation, cognitive training, and cognitive rehabilitation

	Cognitive stimulation	Cognitive training	Cognitive rehabilitation
Aim	Enhance cognition and social function	Maintain and enhance cognitive functioning	Improve daily functioning and enhance well-being
Focus of intervention	A range of generic mentally stimulating activities and discussion	Guided practice on standardised tasks of cognitive memory, attention and executive function	Set goals to identify functional needs (required to perform everyday tasks) & develop techniques to address these needs
Context	Cognitive tasks in a social setting	Structured tasks and environments	Real-world setting
Format	Individualised or group	Individualised or group	Individualised
Goals	Improvements in cognition and behavioural symptoms	Improved or maintained ability in specific cognitive domains	Performance & functioning in relation to collaboratively set goals
Evidence-based in dementia and in Parkinson's	Improves global cognition, quality of life, communication and social interaction in people with dementia No trials in Parkinson's	Improves executive functioning, working memory and processing speed in people with dementia and those with Parkinson's	Can improve self-rated competence, quality of life and memory capacity in people with dementia and people with Parkinson's
Evidence-based in Parkinson's-related dementia	One trial in PD-MCI (Farzana et al., 2015) and one pilot trial in PDD and DLB (Leroi et al., 2019)	Two trials in PD-MCI (Costa et al., 2014; Reuter et al., 2012)	One pilot trial in PDD and DLB (Hindle et al., 2018)

Abbreviations: DLB, dementia with Lewy bodies; PDD, Parkinson's disease dementia; PD-MCI, Parkinson's disease with mild cognitive impairment
Adapted from Bahar-Fuchs et al., 2013; Clare & Woods, 2004.

this intervention as targeting functional disability associated with cognitive impairment (Clare, 2017). To date, some evidence for the effectiveness of cognitive rehabilitation has been found in people with Parkinson's (Alzahrani & Venneri, 2018) and PDD/DLB (Hindle et al., 2018); however, the number of studies is limited.

Cognitive stimulation

Cognitive stimulation is a manualised psychosocial therapy that can improve QoL for those diagnosed with mild to moderate dementia, including DLB (Lobbia et al., 2019). Individual cognitive stimulation therapy can improve QoL for the caregivers too (Orrell et al., 2017). It is recommended in The National Institute for Health and Care Excellence (2018b) guidelines for mild to moderate dementia, although not specifically for Parkinson's.

Cognitive stimulation therapy (CST) is most commonly provided in a group setting and was initially set up as an intervention within mental health settings. However, in the first major study for its use with people with PD-MCI, PDD, and DLB, the intervention was carried out in individuals' own homes and was delivered by a trained caregiver (Leroi et al., 2019). Although the therapy and control groups did not differ following adapted individual CST, the caregivers' burden and stress were reduced and QoL significantly improved among those in the therapy group (Leroi et al., 2019).

CST was developed by psychology researchers and uses specific materials to enable trained therapists to provide a standardised programme. Group CST consists of 14 or more sessions focused on different stimulating topics and themed activities aimed at encouraging conversation, but it also encourages learning and reminiscence. Therapists fully trained in the principles of CST adapt the intervention to meet the needs of the individuals involved, and topics are chosen by group members.

The process takes a biopsychosocial approach, using mental stimulation, the "use it or lose it" theory that mental activity can lead to new learning and improved cognitive functioning in dementia. It may also lead to the formation of new neural pathways, a process called neuroplasticity (Swaab, 1991).

The social aspect of the intervention involves letting the subjects take responsibility for the programme and the contents of the sessions. Intervention takes a person-centred approach, aiming to empower the participants.

Groups should be small so as to encourage conversation (up to about 8 or 10 people). It is also important to consider the stage of dementia, making sure that those in the group have similar levels of cognitive functioning so that activities can be pitched accordingly. Different groups can be offered to individuals at different stages. Gender mix can promote interaction within the group.

Reality orientation should be completed at the start of each session. The topics are chosen from the CST manual to suit the needs and wishes of each individual group. Key principles of the intervention are shown in Table 9.6 (Spector et al., 2003).

Interventions for memory changes

Mild memory impairment is the most common form of cognitive decline in Parkinson's. Individuals may have conversations with their caregivers yet soon after have no recollection of them. Individuals may be unable to memorise appointments or social engagements. Table 9.7 lists strategies for managing

TABLE 9.6 Components of cognitive stimulation therapy

Mental stimulation
New thoughts, ideas and associations
Using orientation sensitively and implicitly
Opinions rather than facts
Using reminiscence as an aid to the here and now
Providing triggers to aid recall
Continuity and consistency between sessions
Implicit learning
Stimulating the use of language
Stimulating the use of executive function
Person centred
Respect
Involvement
Inclusion
Choice
Fun
Maximising potential
Building/strengthening relationships

memory difficulties. The MDT should make sure that caregivers are aware of these strategies and understand why they are used.

Non-drug interventions for neuropsychiatric symptoms

Interventions for neuropsychiatric symptoms in PDD and DLB are summarised in Table 9.4.

Making use of the senses

The optimisation of vision and hearing may help to reduce hallucinations (Hamedani, 2021), social isolation and behavioural disturbance while also improving QoL and relationship satisfaction (Leroi et al., 2020). Caregivers should make sure that spectacles and hearing aids are available, up to date, and in working order. In our experience, reminiscing with the person with dementia and involving the senses (hearing, seeing and touching) can be useful in moderating anxiety, depression and apathy. For example, listening to music that the person used to enjoy and touching objects or seeing photos that carry memories of past may be beneficial. This type of sensory stimulation can be incorporated into a cognitive stimulation therapy programme. Simple interventions can be surprisingly effective. In a study of Alzheimer's disease, a "placebo"

TABLE 9.7 Strategies to deal with memory problems

Strategy	Impact
Encourage individuals and caregivers to make daily/weekly plans together	Reduces stress for individuals and caregivers
Write reminders on a white board (or similar) and display it in a frequently accessed area	The individual may get into the habit of looking at such reminders and is more likely to remember the issues
Use a phone or alarm system for medication reminders	Can help to avoid missed medications
Use sticky notes around the home to give instructions	Reminds the person to switch off appliances
Encourage the individual to put items such as keys always in the same place	Helps to avoid losing or mislaying items
Encourage individuals to reduce multitasking and ask their caregivers to ensure this	Enables the individual to concentrate on one task at a time
Use cue cards listing strategies for transfers (e.g., from chair to bed)	Reminds the individual of the stages of transfer and can thus facilitate transfer

intervention of touch and interaction and an active intervention of aromatherapy both led to a 37% improvement in NPI (Burns et al., 2011).

Consider triggers for agitation

Confusional states may include restlessness and irrational behaviours and may vary throughout the day according to medication times or in relation to increased stress or fatigue. "Sundown" confusion can occur in the evenings and may be triggered by fatigue. It is important to help the caregiver explore potential triggers. If confusion appears to fluctuate in relation to levodopa doses, this should be discussed with the consultant or PDNS. Table 9.8 lists some triggers and suggested management strategies. Agitation may also arise from unmet needs such as hunger, thirst, cold, pain, boredom or loneliness.

Caregiver education

A discrepancy between the individual's capabilities and the caregiver's expectations can be stressful for both. By educating caregivers about dementia and triggers for agitation, behavioural disturbances and negative reactions on the part of the caregiver can be reduced.

Occupational therapy

The OT has an important role in assessment and intervention for people with dementia. In addition to the cognitive interventions already described, the OT

TABLE 9.8 Triggers for confusional states and strategies to reduce their impact

Trigger	Management Strategies
Fatigue	Implement a daily routine that improves function of the circadian rhythm, ensuring regular rests and the pacing of physical activities during the day.
Stress	Aim to reduce stressful situations where possible.
	Reduce multitasking during activities.
	Make sure that the individual is focusing on one task at a time.
	Reduce the number of people in a social situation, as conversation can become more difficult with larger numbers of participants.
	Consider using music to reduce stress and promote calmness. It can also be used regularly to maintain a calm environment.
Disorientation	Make sure that the person's orientation to current day and date is maintained daily.
	Clocks and calendars should be clearly visible.

should also offer advice regarding the management of stress, the individual's daily routine and his or her home environment.

Stress management

Increased stress can exacerbate symptoms of dementia such as hallucinations and agitation. A degree of stress is a normal part of daily living, so it can only be reduced rather than removed. A conversation with the individual and caregiver about any life stresses that may be occurring and considering how these can be dealt with is recommended. Discussions of the condition and the provision of regular support may be all that is required for some, but others may need referral to external services. Strategies to manage such stress include the following:

- Keep calm in the situation. Try not to correct any delusional thoughts. However, this does not necessarily mean going along with them or accepting them as real. Move the conversation on to topics that are not contentious.
- Provide comfort and support.
- Think about the current situation; is there anything happening or in the individual's visual field that could be exacerbating the symptom? For example, if the individual describes seeing someone sitting on the sofa and there are cushions on the sofa, removing the cushions may help.
- Use distractions to change the situation.
- Music can be used to reduce stress. It is important to use music that is familiar and liked by the individual. A daily routine that includes letting the individual spend time quietly listening to relaxing music can be helpful and

for those experiencing agitation. Relaxing music can be used to distract and calm the situation (Raglio, 2015).

Routine management

People with Parkinson's as well as those with PDD or DLB respond well to routine. From the outset, medication is prescribed in a regimen that should be followed daily. The circadian rhythm involved in the sleep/wake cycle also responds well to a daily routine.

Even for those with more advanced dementia, a daily routine is encouraged. The following strategies are recommended:

- Getting up at the same time every day.
- Always getting washed and dressed and having breakfast before starting any activity.
- Getting outdoors daily or whenever possible, even if only into a garden.
- Adhering to regular mealtimes.
- Having at least one daytime nap or rest before 4 p.m. (See the section on sleep hygiene in Chapter 6.)
- Making sure that plans for every day include some type of physical and mental activity.
- Follow sleep hygiene guidelines.

Environment

Where possible, advice regarding adjustments in the home environment can help to reduce excess stimulation for the individual and ensure a peaceful environment. This might include lighting and decor (for instance, a heavily patterned carpet or wallpaper may exacerbate hallucinations or increase anxiety by inducing FOG). The individual can also be encouraged to adopt a daily routine, including a healthy diet and regular exercise.

Physiotherapy

Exercise in Parkinson's improves executive function (Cruise, 2011) and may have a role in preventing dementia (Safarpour & Willis, 2016). Physiotherapy intervention for people with DLB and PDD is not dissimilar to that offered for Parkinson's, although the individual's level of cognition may present challenges and affect the outcome of some interventions. In conjunction with the individual and his or her caregiver, the MDT should work to assess physical and cognitive function and their impact on ADLs; that is, they should agree on shared goals and plan appropriate interventions.

Strength and flexibility should be targeted early, as well as gait training, balance and the prevention of falls. Exercise, particularly aerobic, should be encouraged as early as possible to maintain cardiovascular fitness, which may also improve non-motor symptoms such as sleep and fatigue (Physiopedia

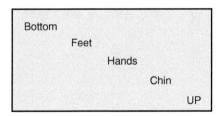

Bottom
       Feet
            Hands
                Chin
                    UP

FIGURE 9.1   Cue card for sit to stand transfer.

contributors, 2020). In a study by Sondell and colleagues (2019), a high-intensity functional exercise programme improved balance in individuals with dementia despite progression of the condition. Cognitive symptoms can also benefit from physical exercise. In a systematic review of the effects of exercise on cognition in people with Parkinson's, significant improvements were found in global cognitive function, processing speed, sustained attention and mental flexibility (Da Silva et al., 2018). Another systematic review (Stuckenschneider et al., 2019) found that all exercise modes in nine studies improved executive function and that aerobic activity had the greatest impact on memory.

However, it should be remembered that home exercise programmes may have to be adapted as the condition progresses, and the caregiver may have to supervise such a programme to make sure that they are carried out safely and correctly. The impact of this extra responsibility should be considered in terms of potentially increasing caregiver stress.

FOG is more common in DLB than in Parkinson's (Palermo, 2019), and the success of cueing techniques depends on the cognitive ability of the individual. As the condition progresses, external cues (visual and auditory) are more likely to be successful than internal ones, which rely on the ability to self-generate the cue. Cue cards with different-colored single words written in a descending diagonal can help to prompt transfer strategies. Figure 9.1 shows an example for the key words of the stages of a sit-to-stand transfer. This could be placed in front of the individual's chair as a prompt for standing.

In considering the provision of a walking aid, the individual's cognitive burden should be taken into account; an unfamiliar aid may increase the risk of falling if the individual cannot learn (and remember) how to use it.

Conclusion

There is considerable overlap between PDD and DLB. Both conditions shorten life expectancy, heighten the chances of institutionalisation, and increase caregiver burden. Although cholinesterase inhibitors can improve cognitive function and reduce hallucinations, non-pharmacological interventions delivered by the MDT or trained therapists are of great importance. Assessment of self-care abilities and caregiver strain should be undertaken and may prompt referral to social services for help with personal care or respite care. Advice and strategies formerly taught to individuals may have to be adapted and taught to caregivers. A diagnosis of dementia should lead to consideration of what the future holds and an exploration of treatment preferences toward the end of life. Although the timing of such conversations must be individualised, there is a risk of putting off discussions for too long, so that the capacity to participate in such planning may be lost before preferences have been established. Life can still be enjoyable despite dementia, and the MDT should promote activities that are fun and improve QoL.

Top tips for Parkinson's disease dementia and dementia with Lewy bodies

1. *Lewy body dementia* is an umbrella term covering both PDD and DLB.
2. The main cognitive symptoms of PDD are deterioration in memory, attention, visuospatial function, and executive function.
3. Behavioural symptoms are common in PDD and include visual hallucinations and apathy.
4. In order to detect PDD at an early stage, cognition should be assessed regularly in people with Parkinson's. We recommend annual screening in those over the age of 70 years.
5. A diagnosis of PDD should not be made on the basis of a cognitive score alone. Cognitive decline must be severe enough to impair personal care or social functioning.
6. Core features of DLB are
   - Marked fluctuations of symptoms
   - Visual hallucinations
   - Parkinsonism
   - REM sleep behaviour disorder
7. Useful sources of information, advice, and support for individuals, caregivers and health professionals include:
   - The Lewy Body Society (www.lewybody.org)
   - Parkinson's UK (www.parkinsons.org.uk)
   - Parkinson's Australia (www.parkinsons.org.au)
   - Parkinson's Foundation (www.parkinson.org)
   - Other national Parkinson's charities
8. "Sundown" confusion can occur in the evenings and may be triggered by fatigue. It is important to help the caregiver explore potential triggers.
9. Consider stimulant-based therapies such as reminiscence therapy, music, aromatherapy, massage and pet therapy to reduce stress and agitation.
10. Cognitive stimulation therapy can improve quality of life for those diagnosed with dementia, including PDD.
11. Exercise, particularly aerobic, should be encouraged as early as possible.
12. Improvements achieved in vision and hearing may reduce hallucinations, behavioural disturbance and social isolation.
13. Use of a postdiagnostic checklist is recommended to make sure that information and support are offered.
14. Wills and power of attorney should be discussed at an early stage.
15. For those with declining cognition, an ECG should be kept on file and thus available should treatment with rivastigmine be considered.

Abbreviations: DLB, dementia with Lewy bodies; ECG, electrocardiogram; PDD, Parkinson's disease dementia; REM, rapid eye motion

Conflict of interest

Sections of this chapter are based on the doctoral thesis of Vatter, 2018.

References

Aarsland, D. (2016). Cognitive impairment in Parkinson's disease and dementia with Lewy bodies. *Parkinsonism & Related Disorders*, *22*(1), S144–S148.

Aarsland, D., Andersen, K., Larsen, J. P., Lolk, A., & Kragh-Sørensen, P. (2003). Prevalence and characteristics of dementia in Parkinson disease: an 8-year prospective study. *Archives of Neurology*, *60*(3), 387–392.

Aarsland, D., Bronnick, K., Ehrt, U., De Deyn, P. P., Tekin, S., Emre, M., et al. (2007). Neuropsychiatric symptoms in patients with Parkinson's disease and dementia: frequency, profile and associated care giver stress. *Journal of Neurology, Neurosurgery & Psychiatry*, *78*(1), 36–42.

Aarsland, D., Brønnick, K., Larsen, J. P., Tysnes, O. B., & Alves, G. (2009). Cognitive impairment in incident, untreated Parkinson disease: the Norwegian ParkWest study. *Neurology*, *72*(13), 1121–1126.

Aarsland, D., Brønnick, K., Williams-Gray, C., Weintraub, D., Marder, K., Kulisevsky, J., & Emre, M. (2010). Mild cognitive impairment in Parkinson disease: a multicentre pooled analysis. *Neurology*, *75*(12), 1062–1069.

Aarsland, D., & Kurz, M. W. (2010). The Epidemiology of Dementia Associated with Parkinson's Disease. *Brain Pathology*, *20*(3), 633–639.

Aarsland, D., Larsen, J. P., Tandberg, E., & Laake, K. (2000). Predictors of nursing home placement in Parkinson's disease: a population-based, prospective study. *Journal of the American Geriatrics Society*, *48*(8), 938–942.

Alcalay, R. N., Caccappolo, E., Mejia-Santana, H., Tang, M., Rosado, L., Orbe Reilly, M., et al. (2012). Cognitive performance of GBA mutation carriers with early-onset PD: the CORE-PD study. *Neurology*, *78*(18), 1434–1440.

Aldridge, G. M., Birnschein, A., Denburg, N. L., & Narayanan, N. S. (2018). Parkinson's disease dementia and dementia with Lewy bodies have similar neuropsychological profiles. *Frontiers in Neurology*, *9*, 123.

Alzahrani, H., & Venneri, A. (2018). Cognitive rehabilitation in Parkinson's disease: a systematic review. *Journal of Parkinson's Disease*, *8*(2), 233–245.

Amara, A. W., Wood, K. H., Joop, A., Memon, R. A., Pilkington, J., Tuggle, S. C., et al. (2020). Randomised, Controlled Trial of Exercise on Objective and Subjective Sleep in Parkinson's Disease. *Movement Disorders*, *35*(6), 947–958.

Bahar-Fuchs, A., Clare, L., & Woods, B. (2013). Cognitive training and cognitive rehabilitation for mild to moderate Alzheimer's disease and vascular dementia. *Cochrane Database of Systematic Reviews*, *6*. CD003260.

Burns, A., Perry, E., Holmes, C., Francis, P., Morris, J., Howes, M., et al. (2011). A Double-Blind Placebo-Controlled Randomised Trial of *Melissa officinalis* oil and donepezil for the treatment of agitation in Alzheimer's disease. *Dement Geriatr Cogn Disord*, *31*, 158–164.

Buter, T. C., van den Hout, A., Matthews, F. E., Larsen, J. P., Brayne, C., & Aarsland, D. (2008). Dementia and survival in Parkinson disease: a 12-year population study. *Neurology*, *70*(13), 1017–1022.

Cankurtaran, E. S. (2014). Management of Behavioural and Psychological Symptoms of Dementia. *Noro Psikiyatri Arsivi*, *51*(4), 303–312.

Chiu, P. -Y., Tsai, C. -T., Chen, P. -K., Chen, W. -J., & Lai, T. -J. (2016). Neuropsychiatric symptoms in Parkinson's disease dementia are more similar to Alzheimer's disease than dementia with Lewy bodies: a case-control study. *PLoS One, 11*(4), e0153989.

Clare, L. (2017). Rehabilitation for people living with dementia: a practical framework of positive support. *PLoS Medicine, 14*(3), e1002245.

Clare, L., Linden, D. E., Woods, R. T., Whitaker, R., Evans, S. J., Parkinson, C. H., & Rugg, M. D. (2010). Goal-oriented cognitive rehabilitation for people with early-stage Alzheimer disease: a single-blind randomised controlled trial of clinical efficacy. *American Journal of Geriatric Psychiatry, 18*(10), 928–939.

Clare, L., & Woods, R. T. (2004). Cognitive training and cognitive rehabilitation for people with early-stage Alzheimer's disease: a review. *Neuropsychological Rehabilitation, 14*(4), 385–401.

Connors, M. H., Seeher, K., Teixeira-Pinto, A., Woodward, M., Ames, D., & Brodaty, H. (2020). Dementia and caregiver burden: A three-year longitudinal study. *International Journal of Geriatric Psychiatry, 35*(2), 250–258.

Costa, A., Peppe, A., Serafini, F., Zabberoni, S., Barban, F., Caltagirone, C., & Carlesimo, G. A. (2014). Prospective memory performance of patients with Parkinson's disease depends on shifting aptitude: evidence from cognitive rehabilitation. *Journal of the International Neuropsychological Society, 20*(7), 717–726.

Cruise KE, Bucks RS, Loftus AM, Newton RU, Pegoraro R, Thomas MG. (2011). Exercise and Parkinson's: benefits for cognition and quality of life. Acta Neurol Scand, 123(1), 13-19.

Da Silva, F. C., Iop, R. D. R., De Oliveira, L. C., Boll, A. M., De Alvarenga, J. G. S., Gutierres Filho, P. J. B., et al. (2018). Effects of physical exercise programmes on cognitive function in Parkinson's disease patients: A systematic review of randomised controlled trials of the last 10 years. *PLoS One, 13*(2), e0193113.

Dubois, B., Burn, D., Goetz, C., Aarsland, D., Brown, R. G., Broe, G. A., et al. (2007). Diagnostic procedures for Parkinson's disease dementia: Recommendations from the movement disorder society task force. *Movement Disorders, 22*(16), 2314–2324.

Emre, M., Aarsland, D., Brown, R., Burn, D. J., Duyckaerts, C., Mizuno, Y., & Dubois, B. (2007). Clinical diagnostic criteria for dementia associated with Parkinson's disease. *Movement Disorders, 22*(12), 1689–1707.

Emre, M., Tsolaki, M., Bonuccelli, U., Destée, A., Tolosa, E., Kutzelnigg, A., & Jones, R. (2010). Memantine for patients with Parkinson's disease dementia or dementia with Lewy bodies: a randomised, double-blind, placebo-controlled trial. *Lancet Neurology, 9*(10), 969–977.

Farzana, F., Sreekanth, V., Mohiuddin, M. K., Mohan, V., Balakrishna, N., & Ahuja, Y. R. (2015). Can individual home-based cognitive stimulation therapy benefit Parkinson's patients with mild to moderate cognitive impairment? *International Journal of Geriatric Psychiatry, 30*(4), 433–435.

Ferman, T. J., Smith, G. E., Boeve, B. F., Ivnik, R. J., Petersen, R. C., Knopman, D., et al. (2004). DLB fluctuations: specific features that reliably differentiate DLB from AD and normal aging. *Neurology, 62*(2), 181–187.

Fields, J. A. (2017). Cognitive and neuropsychiatric features in Parkinson's and Lewy body dementias. *Archives of Clinical Neuropsychology, 32*(7), 786–801.

Galvin, J. E., Duda, J. E., Kaufer, D. I., Lippa, C. F., Taylor, A., & Zarit, S. H. (2010). Lewy Body Dementia: Caregiver Burden and Unmet Needs. *Alzheimer Disease & Associated Disorders, 24*(2), 177–181.

Gibb, W. R. G., & Lees, A. J. (1988). The relevance of the Lewy body to the pathogenesis of idiopathic Parkinson's disease. *Journal of Neurology, Neurosurgery, and Psychiatry, 51*(6), 745–752.

Goldman, J. G., Holden, S. K., Litvan, I., McKeith, I., Stebbins, G. T., & Taylor, J. -P. (2018). Evolution of diagnostic criteria and assessments for Parkinson's disease mild cognitive impairment. *Movement Disorders*, *33*(4), 503–510.

Guay, D. R. (2008). Inappropriate sexual behaviours in cognitively impaired older individuals. *The American journal of geriatric pharmacotherapy*, *6*(5), 269–288.

Hamedani, A. G. (2021). Vision loss and hallucinations: perspectives from neurology and ophthalmology. *Curr Opin Neurol*, *34*(1), 84–88.

Hindle, J. V., Watermeyer, T. J., Roberts, J., Brand, A., Hoare, Z., Martyr, A., & Clare, L. (2018). Goal-oriented cognitive rehabilitation for dementias associated with Parkinson's disease – A pilot randomised controlled trial. *International Journal of Geriatric Psychiatry*, *33*(5), 718–728.

Hobson, P., & Meara, J. (2015). Mild cognitive impairment in Parkinson's disease and its progression onto dementia: a 16-year outcome evaluation of the Denbighshire cohort. *International Journal of Geriatric Psychiatry*, *30*(10), 1048–1055.

Jankovic, J. (2008). Parkinson's disease: clinical features and diagnosis. *Journal of Neurology. Neurosurgery, and Psychiatry*, *79*(4), 368–376.

Kane, J. P. M., Surendranathan, A., Bentley, A., Barker, S. A. H., Taylor, J. P., Thomas, A. J., & O'Brien, J. T. (2018). Clinical prevalence of Lewy body dementia. *Alzheimer's Research & Therapy*, *10*(1), 19.

Kim, Y., Kim, Y. E., Park, E. O., Shin, C. W., Kim, H. -J., & Jeon, B. (2018). REM sleep behaviour disorder portends poor prognosis in Parkinson's disease: A systematic review. *Journal of Clinical Neuroscience*, *47*, 6–13.

Larsson, V., Torisson, G., & Londos, E. (2018). Relative survival in patients with dementia with Lewy bodies and Parkinson's disease dementia. *PLoS One*, *13*(8), e0202044.

Leroi, I., Harbishettar, V., Andrews, M., McDonald, K., Byrne, E. J., & Burns, A. (2012a). Carer burden in apathy and impulse control disorders in Parkinson's disease. *International Journal of Geriatric Psychiatry*, *27*(2), 160–166.

Leroi, I., McDonald, K., Pantula, H., & Harbishettar, V. (2012b). Cognitive impairment in Parkinson disease: impact on quality of life, disability, and caregiver burden. *Journal of Geriatric Psychiatry & Neurology*, *25*(4), 208–214.

Leroi, I., Atkinson, R., & Overshott, R. (2014). Memantine improves goal attainment and reduces caregiver burden in Parkinson's disease dementia. *International Journal of Geriatric Psychiatry*, *29*(9), 899–905.

Leroi, I., Vatter, S., Carter, L. -A., Smith, S. J., Orgeta, V., Poliakoff, E., et al. (2019). Parkinson's-adapted cognitive stimulation therapy: a pilot randomised controlled clinical trial. *Therapeutic Advances in Neurological Disorders*, *12*. 175628641985221.

Leroi, I., Simkin, Z., Hooper, E., Wolski, L., Abrams, H., Armitage, C. J., et al. (2020). Impact of an intervention to support hearing and vision in dementia: The SENSE-Cog Field Trial. *International Journal of Geriatric Psychiatry*, *35*(4), 348–357.

Leung, I. H. K., Walton, C. C., Hallock, H., Lewis, S. J. G., Valenzuela, M., & Lampit, A. (2015). Cognitive training in Parkinson's disease: a systematic review and meta-analysis. *Neurology*, *85*(21), 1843–1851.

Litvan, I., Aarsland, D., Adler, C. H., Goldman, J. G., Kulisevsky, J., Mollenhauer, B., & Weintraub, D. (2011). MDS task force on mild cognitive impairment in Parkinson's disease: critical review of PD-MCI. *Movement Disorders*, *26*(10), 1814–1824.

Litvan, I., Goldman, J. G., Tröster, A. I., Schmand, B. A., Weintraub, D., Petersen, R. C., & Emre, M. (2012). Diagnostic criteria for mild cognitive impairment in Parkinson's disease: Movement Disorder Society Task Force guidelines. *Movement Disorders*, *27*(3), 349–356.

Lobbia, A., Carbone, E., Faggian, S., Gardini, S., Piras, F., Spector, A., et al. (2019). The Efficacy of Cognitive Stimulation Therapy (CST) for People With Mild-to-Moderate Dementia. *European Psychologist*, *24*(3), 257–277.

McKeith, I. G., Boeve, B. F., Dickson, D. W., Halliday, G., Taylor, J. -P., Weintraub, D., & Kosaka, K. (2017). Diagnosis and management of dementia with Lewy bodies: fourth consensus report of the DLB consortium. *Neurology*, *89*(1), 88–100.

McShane, R. (2008). Clinical aspects of dementia: dementia in Parkinson's disease and dementia with Lewy bodies. In R. Jacoby, C. Oppenheimer, T. Dening, & A. Thomas (Eds.), *Old age Psychiatry (fourth edition)* (pp. 453–459). New York, NY, USA: Oxford University Press.

Mrak, R. E., & Griffin, W. S. T. (2007). Dementia with Lewy bodies: definition, diagnosis, and pathogenic relationship to Alzheimer's disease. *Neuropsychiatric Disease and Treatment*, *3*(5), 619–625.

Mueller, C., Ballard, C., Corbett, A., & Aarsland, D. (2017). The prognosis of dementia with Lewy bodies. *Lancet Neurology*, *16*(5), 390–398.

Mueller, C., Perera, G., Rajkumar, A. P., Bhattarai, M., Price, A., O'Brien, J. T., & Aarsland, D. (2018). Hospitalisation in people with dementia with Lewy bodies: frequency, duration and cost implications. *Alzheimer's Dementia: Diagnosis, Assessment & Disease Monitoring*, *10*, 143–152.

National Institute for Health and Care Excellence [NICE]. (2018a). Dementia: assessment, management and support for people living with dementia and their carers. NICE Guideline [NG97].

National Institute for Health and Care Excellence [NICE]. (2018b, February). Parkinson's disease. Quality standard. Retrieved June 28, 2020, from www.nice.org.uk/guidance/qs164.

Orgeta, V., McDonald, K. R., Poliakoff, E., Hindle, J. V., Clare, L., & Leroi, I. (2020). Cognitive training interventions for dementia and mild cognitive impairment in Parkinson's disease. *Cochrane Database of Systematic Reviews*, *2*doi: 10.1002/14651858.CD011961.pub2. CD011961.

Orrell, M., Yates, L., Leung, P., Kang, S., Hoare, Z., Whitaker, C., & Orgeta, V. (2017). The impact of individual Cognitive Stimulation Therapy (iCST) on cognition, quality of life, caregiver health, and family relationships in dementia: a randomised controlled trial. *PloS Medicine*, *14*(3), e1002269.

Pagonabarraga, J., Kulisevsky, J., Llebaria, G., García-Sánchez, C., Pascual-Sedano, B., Martinez-Corral, M., et al. (2010). PDD-Short Screen: A brief cognitive test for screening dementia in Parkinson's disease. *Movement Disorders*, *25*(4), 440–446.

Palermo, G., Frosini, D., Corsi, A., Giuntini, M., Mazzucchi, S., Del Prete, E., et al. (2019). Freezing of gait and dementia in parkinsonism: A retrospective case-control study. *Brain Behav*, *9*(6), e01247.

Parkinson's UK and All Party Parliamentary Group for Parkinson's Disease. (2018). *Mental health matters too: improving mental health services for people with Parkinson's who experience anxiety and depression*. London, UK: Parkinson's UK.

Petersen, R. C. (2004). Mild cognitive impairment as a diagnostic entity. *Journal of Internal Medicine*, *256*(3), 183–194.

Physiopedia contributors. (2020). Lewy Body Disease. Physiopedia, from https://www.physiopedia.com/index.php?title=Lewy_Body_Disease&oldid=246010. [Accessed January 5, 2021].

Price, A., Farooq, R., Yuan, J. -M., Menon, V. B., Cardinal, R. N., & O'Brien, J. T. (2017). Mortality in dementia with Lewy bodies compared with Alzheimer's dementia: a retrospective naturalistic cohort study. *BMJ Open*, *7*(11), e017504.

Raglio, A. (2015). Music Therapy Interventions in Parkinson's Disease: The State-of-the-Art. *Frontiers in Neurology*, *6*.

Reuter, I., Mehnert, S., Sammer, G., Oechsner, M., & Engelhardt, M. (2012). Efficacy of a multimodal cognitive rehabilitation including psychomotor and endurance training in Parkinson's disease. *Journal of Aging Research*, 235765.

Robinson, B. C. (1983). Validation of a Caregiver Strain Index. *Journal of Gerontoogy*, *38*(3), 344–348.

Rolinski, M., Fox, C., Maidment, I., & McShane, R. (2012). Cholinesterase inhibitors for dementia with Lewy bodies, Parkinson's disease dementia and cognitive impairment in Parkinson's disease. *Cochrane Database of Systematic Reviews*, *3*. CD006504.

Rongve, A., Soennesyn, H., Skogseth, R., Oesterhus, R., Hortobagyi, T., Ballard, C., & Aarsland, D. (2016). Cognitive decline in dementia with Lewy bodies: a 5-year prospective cohort study. *BMJ Open*, *6*(2), e010357.

Safarpour, D., & Willis, A. W. (2016). Clinical epidemiology, evaluation, and management of dementia in Parkinson disease. *American Journal of Alzheimer's Disease and Other Dementias*, *31*(7), 585–594.

Savica, R., Grossardt, B. R., Rocca, W. A., & Bower, J. H. (2018). Parkinson disease with and without dementia: a prevalence study and future projections. *Movement Disorders*, *33*(4), 537–543.

Schrag, A., Barone, P., Brown, R. G., Leentjens, A. F. G., Mcdonald, W. M., Starkstein, S., et al. (2007). Depression rating scales in Parkinson's disease: critique and recommendations. *Movement Disorders*, *22*(8), 1077–1092.

Shin, H., Youn, J., Kim, J. S., Lee, J. -Y., & Cho, J. W. (2012). Caregiver Burden in Parkinson Disease With Dementia Compared to Alzheimer Disease in Korea. *Journal of Geriatric Psychiatry and Neurology*, *25*(4), 222–322.

Sondell, A., Littbrand, H., Holmberg, H., Lindelöf, N., & Rosendahl, E (2019). Is the effect of a high-intensity functional exercise programme on functional balance influenced by applicability and motivation among older people with dementia in nursing homes? *The Journal of Nutrition, Health & Aging*, *23*, 1011–1020.

Spector, A., Thorgrimsen, L., Woods, B., Royan, L., Davies, S., Butterworth, M., et al. (2003). Efficacy of an evidence-based cognitive stimulation therapy programme for people with dementia. *British Journal of Psychiatry*, *183*(3), 248–254.

Stinton, C., McKeith, I., Taylor, J. P., Lafortune, L., Mioshi, E., Mak, E., & O'Brien, J. T. (2015). Pharmacological management of Lewy body dementia: a systematic review and meta-analysis. *American Journal of Psychiatry*, *172*(8), 731–742.

Stuckenschneider, T., Askew, C. D., Menêses, A. L., Baake, R., Weber, J., & Schneider, S. (2019). The Effect of Different Exercise Modes on Domain-Specific Cognitive Function in Patients Suffering from Parkinson's Disease: A Systematic Review of Randomised Controlled Trials. *Journal of Parkinson's disease*, *9*(1), 73–95.

Sun, R., Yang, S., Zheng, B., Liu, J., & Ma, X. (2019). Apolipoprotein E Polymorphisms and Parkinson Disease With or Without Dementia: A Meta-Analysis Including 6453 Participants. *J Geriatr Psychiatry Neurol*, *32*(1), 3–15.

Swaab, D. F. (1991). Brain aging and Alzheimer's disease, "Wear and tear" versus "Use it or lose it". *Neurobiology of Aging*, *12*(4), 317–324.

Taylor, J. -P., & O'Brien, J. T. (2012). Parkinson's disease with dementia. In K. P. Ebmeier, J. T. O'Brien, & J. -P. Taylor (Eds.), *Psychiatry of Parkinson's Disease. Advances in Biological Psychiatry* (pp. 103–124). (27). Basel, Switzerland: Karger.

Taylor, C., Johnson, C., Marsh, J., Brown, L., Silverwood, A., Stringer, R., et al. (2020). Mental Health Matters Too – Integration of physical and mental health in a multidisciplinary Parkinson's Clinic [abstract]. *Movement Disorders*, *35*.

Vatter, S. (2018). *The impact of Parkinson's-related dementia on life partner outcomes [thesis].* Manchester: University of Manchester.

Vatter, S., McDonald, K. R., Stanmore, E., Clare, L., & Leroi, I. (2018). Multidimensional care burden in Parkinson-related dementia. *Journal of Geriatric Psychiatry & Neurology, 31*(6), 319–328.

Vatter, S., Stanmore, E., Clare, L., McDonald, K. R., McCormick, S. A., & Leroi, I. (2020). Care burden and mental ill health in spouses of people with Parkinson disease dementia and Lewy body dementia. *Journal of Geriatric Psychiatry & Neurology, 33*(1), 3–14.

Volicer, L., & Hurley, A. C. (2003). Review Article: Management of Behavioural Symptoms in Progressive Degenerative Dementias. *The Journals of Gerontology Series A: Biological Sciences and Medical Sciences, 58*(9), M837–M845.

Weintraub, D., & Burn, D. J. (2011). Parkinson's disease: The quintessential neuropsychiatric disorder. *Movement Disorders, 26*(6), 1022–1031.

Xie, Y., Meng, X., Xiao, J., Zhang, J., & Zhang, J. (2016). Cognitive changes following bilateral deep brain stimulation of subthalamic nucleus in Parkinson's disease: a meta-analysis. *Biomed Research International,* 3596415.

Zarit, S. H., Reever, K. E., & Bach-Peterson, J. (1980). Relatives of the impaired elderly: correlates of feelings of burden. *Gerontologist, 20*(6), 649–655.

Zesiewicz, T. A., Sullivan, K. L., Arnulf, I., Chaudhuri, K. R., Morgan, J. C., Gronseth, G. S., et al. (2010). Practice Parameter: treatment of nonmotor symptoms of Parkinson disease: report of the Quality Standards Subcommittee of the American Academy of Neurology. *Neurology, 74*(11), 924–931.

Zweig, Y. R., & Galvin, J. E. (2014). Lewy body dementia: the impact on patients and caregivers. *Alzheimer's Research & Therapy, 6*(2), 21.

Chapter 10

Falls and Bone Health in Parkinson's

Danielle Brazier, Lily Scourfield, Veronica Lyell, Victoria J Haunton and Emily J. Henderson

Chapter outline

Introduction

Emergence of the tendency to fall in Parkinson's represents a milestone in the progress of the condition. Falls have significant physical and psychological sequelae for people with Parkinson's as well as their caregivers. This negative impact was reflected in a research priority-setting partnership—undertaken by the James Lind Alliance and Parkinson's UK— whereby dealing with falls and balance problems in Parkinson's was identified as the number-one priority by people with Parkinson's, caregivers and healthcare professionals (Deane et al., 2014).

This chapter reviews the epidemiology of falls in Parkinson's and related conditions, detailing the risk factors for falls and presenting an approach whereby multidisciplinary clinicians working in the field can deal with them.

Because hip fracture is one of the most devastating consequences of a fall, the assessment of fracture risk and optimisation of bone health are outlined.

The epidemiology of falls

The emergence and evolution of postural instability is the principal determinant of stage in Parkinson's as quantified using the Hoehn and Yahr scale (Hoehn & Yahr, 1967). The first meta-analysis of prospective studies of falling, published in 2007, demonstrated that 46% (95%CI 38%-54%) of people with Parkinson's fell over a 3-month period (Pickering et al., 2007). The majority of fallers with Parkinson's do so recurrently; that is, they have experienced more than one fall in a 12-month period (Allen et al., 2013). The rate of recurrent falls is high, with a meta-analysis reporting a rate of 20.8 falls per recurrent faller per year (Allen et al., 2013). It is important to note, however, that the range (4.7-67.6 falls per recurrent faller) is wide. Several studies have described individuals who experience extremely high rates of falls (Ashburn et al., 2019; Henderson et al., 2013), and extreme outliers may artificially skew the reporting of mean fall rate, thus requiring specific consideration clinically.

Falls risk varies with severity of condition and peaks at Hoehn and Yahr stage 3 (Bloem et al., 2001). This is a point at which gait and balance are significantly impaired but individuals are still sufficiently mobile to be at risk of falling. Risk of falling likely diminishes in the later stages of the condition, but epidemiologic data to support this are more scarce as the completion of falls diaries and enrolment into trials becomes more complex (Domingos et al., 2015). Furthermore, stage of condition is associated with the circumstances in which falls occur. In early stages, people with Parkinson's are more likely to fall during walking activities, whereas later on falls tend to occur during transfers (Mactier et al., 2015).

The epidemiology of falls in atypical Parkinson's disorders such as progressive supranuclear palsy (PSP) and multiple-system atrophy (MSA) is less well described (Brown et al., 2020; Wielinski et al., 2005). The reported incidence of falls is high but data-collection methods vary (Smith et al., 2019). The mechanism of falls in PSP is secondary to the accumulation of tau protein in the indirect locomotor pathway, which is involved in controlling ambulatory movements and turning; it results in impairment of the pedunculopontine nucleus, which is partly responsible for motor control (Bluett et al., 2017). Accumulation of tau within the subthalamic nucleus and striatum can lead to behavioural inhibition; its accumulation within the substantia nigra, dentate nucleus, red nucleus and pallidum can affect motor planning (Bohnen & Jahn, 2013). Thus individuals typically demonstrate motor recklessness (Bloem & Bhatia, 2004; Nutt et al., 2011b) and frequently get up out of a chair "like a rocket" (Burn & Lees, 2002).

MSA is rarer than idiopathic Parkinson's, with a prevalence of approximately 4 to 5 per 100,000 (Vanacore et al., 2001). Dysautonomia is a diagnostic feature and contributes to the risk of falling (Testa et al., 2001). A clinicopathological study comparing idiopathic Parkinson's with MSA and PSP showed that median latency in the months after diagnosis to first fall was longest in idiopathic Parkinson's (73 [range 8-137]), followed by MSA (24 [range 0-97]); it was shortest in PSP (6 [range 0-156]). The Incidence of Cognitive Impairment Longitudinal in Cohorts Evaluation—Parkinson's with Disease (ICICLE-PD) cohort study suggested, however, that about 25% of people with idiopathic Parkinson's at diagnosis will already have fallen (Lord et al., 2017). The temporal relationship between falls and stage of condition is useful to potentially target interventions in activities that frequently precipitate falling. Although the presence of falls in early Parkinson's should prompt the clinician to consider other diagnoses, it should not preclude a diagnosis of idiopathic Parkinson's.

Factors that contribute to falls in Parkinson's

Multiple factors contribute to the risk of falling; these frequently coexist and interact. For the purposes of clinical assessment, they can be functionally divided into those that are specific to the condition and those that are generic (van der Marck et al., 2014). They are summarised in Figure 10.1. Modifiable risk factors that augment the risk include dyskinesia (Duncan et al., 2015),

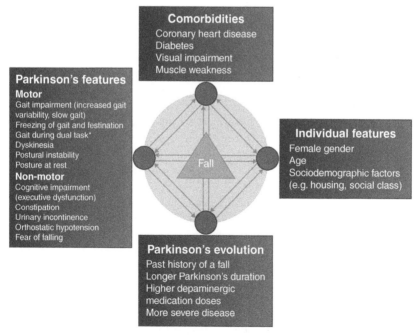

FIGURE 10.1   Factors associated with falls in Parkinson's and individual factors associated with falls in Parkinson's. The diagram illustrates the likely interactions between domains and the variability of risk that is likely to emerge and progress as the condition evolves. *Dual task* is defined as two simultaneous tasks that require information processing capacity.

gait and balance impairment (Thaut et al., 2019), and freezing of gait (Thaut et al., 2019). Non-motor aspects of Parkinson's that confer further falls risk include orthostatic hypotension (Duncan et al., 2015), fear of falling (Gervasoni et al., 2015), and cognitive impairment (Lindholm et al., 2019), particularly when manifesting as executive dysfunction (Lindholm et al., 2015). Generic factors that have been identified in Parkinson's-specific studies include muscle weakness (Henderson et al., 2016), visual impairment (Almeida et al., 2015), diabetes (Paul et al., 2014) and ischaemic heart disease (Paul et al., 2014).

Gait changes

Gait changes emerge and progress as the condition advances (Bloem et al., 2001). Alterations in gait can usefully be categorised into those that affect gait on a continuous basis (i.e., from one step to the next) versus those that occur episodically, such as freezing of gait (FOG) (Giladi et al., 2013). Slow walking is a manifestation of bradykinesia, wherein the primary deficit is the inability to generate normal step length (Morris et al., 1994). The ability to increase cadence (frequency of stepping) is maintained and is therefore employed as a compensatory strategy (Morris et al., 1996). Variability in gait is a measure of arrhythmicity and is a proxy marker for falls risk in Parkinson's as well as other neurodegenerative conditions (Balasubramanian et al., 2009; IJmker & Lamoth, 2012; Rosano et al., 2008). Increased variability of stride time is higher in Parkinson's fallers compared with non-fallers and, interestingly, is a potentially useful predictor of future cognitive decline (Savica et al., 2017).

Episodic gait impairment includes FOG and festination (Giladi et al., 2013). *Festination* is defined as "a tendency to move forwards with increasingly rapid but ever smaller steps, associated with the centre of gravity falling forward over the stepping feet" (Nutt et al., 2011a); individuals describe that the phenomena feels like being pushed from behind (Giladi et al., 2013). FOG is defined as "a brief episodic absence or marked reduction of forward progression of the feet despite the intention to walk" (Nutt et al., 2011a) or as the feet feeling "glued to the floor" (Bloem et al., 2004; Giladi & Nieuwboer, 2008). Episodic gait impairments are strongly associated with falls risk, as their unpredictability makes it difficult to utilise adaptive strategies successfully (Giladi et al., 2013). Freezing can be elicited during walking that requires precise regulation of stepping; for example, during initiation of movement, on turning or on approaching a destination (Nutt et al., 2011a). There is a strong association between executive impairment and FOG, whereby FOG is affected significantly by cognitive load. That is, FOG occurs more frequently during the execution of more complex motor behaviours that draw on more cognitive resources, during dual tasking, or when an individual is fatigued or anxious (Lord et al., 2020; Rochester et al., 2004; Spildooren et al., 2019; Witt et al., 2019). Therefore negotiating obstacles during a gait trajectory present difficulties owing to the cognitive burden of set shifting, where a change in the motor programme is required (Naismith et al., 2010; Pieruccini-Faria et al., 2014).

Balance and postural changes

Postural changes in Parkinson's are characterised by a narrow stance and stooped posture, with thoracic kyphosis and flexion of the hips and knees (Parkinson, 1817). This posture reduces trunk control during walking (Jehu & Nantel, 2018) and is prevalent particularly as Parkinson's progresses.

Postural sway worsens with progression and is important during transitions (e.g., from sitting to walking), where a change in base of support is coordinated to keep the centre of mass within the limits of stability so as to avoid falling (Contin et al., 1996; Frenklach et al., 2009). To maintain upright posture, proprioceptive, visual and vestibular information must be integrated. The relative weighting of these modalities can alter depending on sensory conditions and, although this process may remain intact, the time taken to switch can be prolonged (Contin et al., 1996; Feller et al., 2019). In Parkinson's, proprioception is reduced, causing a reliance on visual input and contributing to falls (Feller et al., 2019; Vaugoyeau & Azulay, 2010). In response to postural perturbation, individuals tend to use ankle strategy (movement around the ankle joint, keeping the head in line with the hips) owing to reduced proprioception and increased stiffness, thus limiting the normal use of hip strategy (Baston et al., 2014; Horak et al., 1992). When a person is initiating gait, he or she may rely on anticipatory postural adjustments, or movements that precede voluntary actions (Mancini et al., 2009). These are abnormal in Parkinson's, causing abnormal loading and unloading of the legs. This may, in turn, contribute to the FOG seen on gait initiation (Mancini et al., 2009).

Cognitive impairment

There is increasing recognition of the role of cognitive impairment in exacerbating the risk of falls (Camicioli & Majumdar, 2010). Mild cognitive impairment is often present in early Parkinson's and is not of a severity to warrant a diagnosis of dementia. However, when dysfunction manifests in the executive function domain, it has considerable bearing on falls risk (Lindholm et al., 2015). Functionally, cognitive impairment or dementia effectively limit the degree to which an individual can compensate for gait dysfunction (Rochester et al., 2014).

Visual changes

Parkinson's is associated with impairments in vision as well as hallucinations. Visual changes result from impairment in acuity, contrast sensitivity and abnormal colour vision, which are at least in part due to retinal dopamine deficiency (Weil et al., 2016). Oculomotor changes are common in PSP with supranuclear gaze palsy (Kleinschmidt-DeMasters, 1989). Hallucinations which often emerge in parallel with cognitive impairment can impact an individual's ability to process their environment when ambulating (Armstrong, 2017; Ekker et al., 2017).

Orthostatic hypotension

Orthostatic hypotension (OH) is defined as a fall of equal to or greater than 20 mm Hg systolic or equal to or greater than 10 mm Hg diastolic blood pressure (BP) within 3 minutes of active standing or head-up tilt (The Consensus Committee of the American Autonomic Society and the American Academy of Neurology, 1996). It is common in people with Parkinson's, with a pooled prevalence of approximately 30% (Velseboer et al., 2011), although higher rates have also been reported (Matinolli et al., 2009; Senard et al., 1997). It is thought that degeneration of the peripheral nervous system in Parkinson's is causative. Specific mechanisms are thought to include the presence of Lewy bodies within the autonomic nervous system, inadequate release of noradrenalin, cardiac sympathetic degeneration, and decreased baroreflex sensitivity (Isaacson & Skettini, 2014). OH is more common in older individuals, those who have had Parkinson's for a longer time or have a more severe form of it, and those taking higher doses of dopaminergic medications (Ha et al., 2011).

Symptoms of OH are variable. In addition to the classic symptoms of dizziness or light-headedness on standing, individuals may also report blurred vision, nausea, weakness and fatigue, difficulty concentrating and "a coat-hanger type of discomfort," with occipital headache as well as neck and shoulder pain (Low et al., 1995). OH is also associated with a reduced quality of life (QoL), cognitive decline, and specific deficits in sustained attention, verbal episodic memory, and visuospatial abilities (McDonald et al., 2016). Importantly, 38% of individuals who have confirmed OH on testing do not have symptoms but have similar rates of functional impairments and falls (Merola et al., 2016). Syncope is perhaps the most significant complication of OH and frequently occurs without a prodrome (Merola et al., 2016).

The prediction of falls

The ability to accurately forecast the likelihood of a fall offers opportunities to target interventions efficiently. Many Parkinson's fall intervention studies have recruited individuals who have already fallen, as a prior history of falls has been consistently shown to predict future falling (Gervasoni et al., 2015; Kataoka & Ueno, 2015; Pickering et al., 2007). However, this approach risks exposing individuals to secondary physical and psychological morbidities (e.g., fear of falling and injury), which risks fueling a vicious cycle of progressive functional impairment that in turn further augments risk.

Assessments of gait and balance have been widely evaluated. Clinical rating scales with established utility include the Activities-Specific Confidence Scale

16, Mini-Balance Evaluation Systems Test, Timed Up and Go test, Berg Balance Scale, and Falls Efficacy Scale International. Assessment of gait is useful in predicting falls risk and may suggest goals for rehabilitation. A meta-analysis has shown that during walking at both a preferred and fast pace, features such as slower walking speed, lower cadence (the number of steps per minute), and shorter and slower steps predict future falls (Creaby & Cole, 2018). Emerging evidence supports the supplemental use of technology-captured variables to predict falls. A study using individuals from the Oxford Discovery cohort showed that machine-learning algorithms could accurately (AUC .88) predict falls from a 7-minute smartphone test.

Management

In our practice, people with Parkinson's are asked about falls and near falls during all Parkinson's outpatient consultations. This should be performed at least annually, recognising that the risk, nature and circumstances of falls will vary as the condition evolves. Although we have presented falls interventions largely by domain, in clinical practice the implementation of a single strategy is rarely effective. Hence a comprehensive, multifaceted approach delivered by a multidisciplinary team is required. The fall-prevention strategy that we advocate seeks to treat motor dysfunction along with contributory non-motor symptoms. In parallel, treatment of generic risk factors, including medication optimisation, should occur in conjunction with strategies that include the assessment of bone health (Fig. 10.2).

Treatment of motor dysfunction

Drug treatment

Bradykinesia, including the gait dysfunction already described, is largely responsive to levodopa in the early phase of Parkinson's; this medication is gratifyingly effective in maintaining function and minimising disability. As the condition progresses, the therapeutic window narrows. The emergence of dyskinesia can increase falls risk as an individual's centre of gravity is displaced outside the base of support. In later stages, the higher doses of medication required to maintain motor control pose the risk of exacerbating OH and confusion, both of which are potent contributors to falls risk.

Surgical strategies

Deep brain stimulation (DBS) has proven effective for the relief of treatment-resistant hypokinetic motor fluctuations in Parkinson's (Fasano et al., 2015). Studies measuring its benefit in axial stability, gait balance and falls outcomes, however, have failed to produce as promising results (Follett et al., 2010; House et al., 2009; Karachi et al., 2019; Nilsson et al., 2011; Okun et al., 2012). There

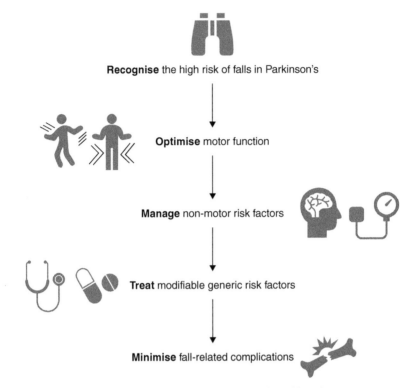

Recognise the high risk of falls in Parkinson's

Optimise motor function

Manage non-motor risk factors

Treat modifiable generic risk factors

Minimise fall-related complications

FIGURE 10.2   Overview of a falls risk management strategy in Parkinson's

is a lack of consensus in the literature: at best, DBS is reported to reduce falls and FOG in up to one-third of people with Parkinson's (Karachi et al., 2019); however, follow-up from randomised controlled trials (RCTs) has shown that individuals in DBS groups fall more often, with postural stability particularly declining in the year following stimulation of the subthalamic nucleus (STN), the traditional anatomic target (House et al., 2009; Okun et al., 2012; St George et al., 2012). A retrospective study also showed worsening scores from baseline at 10-year follow-up of STN-DBS (Castrioto et al., 2011). Stimulation of the globus pallidus pars interna lacks robust evidence on falls, although it may supersede STN-DBS in managing brittle dyskinesia (Ramirez-Zamora & Ostrem, 2018). At present, the choice of DBS target is made on the basis of clinical judgment and goals of surgery. RCTs of DBS often report falls as a secondary outcome, as part of the Unified Parkinson's Disease Rating Scale or as adverse events rather than in accordance with the established Prevention of Falls Network Europe guidelines (Lamb et al., 2005), thus limiting their reliability in this context. Novel targets of DBS such as the pedunculopontine nucleus have shown more promise in falls prevention, but this is experimental, with small sample sizes (Thevathasan et al., 2018; Moro et al., 2010) of 6 and 8 respectively.

Extrapolating from these studies is challenging owing to their to small sample sizes, confounding, and the lack of prospective falls reporting. Falls are not an indication for surgery per se, but improved motor control and lower dopaminergic requirements may mitigate falls risk. Paradoxically, improvements in ambulation and gait speed secondary to reduction in bradykinesia and improved QoL may increase the risk of falls. As DBS is generally offered only to people under the age of 70 years who have no cognitive impairment (Antonini et al., 2018), the generalisability of findings is limited.

Non-invasive stimulation

Non-invasive methods of stimulation to tackle gait dysfunction are attractive strategies. A meta-analysis of 14 studies of repetitive transcranial magnetic stimulation versus sham showed improvements in walking speed but not FOG. The lack of FOG efficacy may reflect insensitivity of the outcome (FOG questionnaire) measure (Creaby & Cole, 2018). Transcranial direct current stimulation delivers a weak electrical current to the scalp via small electrodes. There have been sustained benefits for FOG in a small (n = 10) Parkinson's study (Lee et al., 2019) as well as improved functional locomotion over the short term (Creaby & Cole, 2018).

Cueing is used to overcome FOG by providing auditory (Chang et al., 2019), visual (Barthel et al., 2018), or tactile input (Ivkovic et al., 2016; van Wegen et al., 2006); it can be used for stepping, speech or freezing of the upper limb (Nieuwboer et al., 2009; Vercruysse et al., 2014) and to facilitate repetitive movement (Nieuwboer, 2015). Visual cues can act on motor blocks, assisting effective scaling of motor amplitude, whereas auditory cues can help to reduce asymmetry during turning by facilitating FOG motor rhythm generation (Miller et al., 2019; Nieuwboer, 2008). FOG rehabilitation is thought to be mediated via two potential pathways (Delgado-Alvarado et al., 2020): a transient effect utilises a shift to spared motor pathways (i.e., anterior putamen) and longer-term effect via the modulation of corticostriatal and thalamocortical circuits. Multiple interventions appear to be necessary to reduce episodes of FOG, as evidence suggests that there is little carryover from short-term cueing interventions and a beneficial effect has not been demonstrated (Fietzek et al., 2014; Martin et al., 2015).

Physical activity and exercise

In conjunction with targeted approaches and person-centred goals, physiotherapy enables people with Parkinson's to optimise their level of function, mobility, and independence as well as to maximise QoL (Tomlinson et al., 2012). Table 10.1 summarises RCTs in this area. The terms *physical activity* and *exercise* are often used interchangeably (Bouça-Machado et al., 2020). Physical activity has been defined as any movement of the body that results in energy expenditure (Caspersen & Christenson, 1985). Physical activity (e.g., low-intensity activity such as gardening) has been shown to have beneficial effects

TABLE 10.1 Randomised controlled trials with physiotherapy interventions since 2014

Study	Year	Type of study	Blinding	Total number	Age	Duration of Parkinson's	Falls as primary or secondary outcome
Gao (Gao et al., 2014)	2014	RCT	Single	76	70 ± 7 (int); 68 ± 9 (con)	9.15 ± 8.58 (int); 8.37 ± 8.24 (con)	Primary
Canning (Canning et al., 2015)	2015	Prospective RCT	Single (assessor)	231	71 ± 8 (int); 70 ± 9 (con)	7.5 ± 5.8 (int); 8.3 ± 6.0 (con)	Primary
Martin (Martin et al., 2015)	2015	Parallel, delayed, or immediate start RCT	None	21	72 ± 5.3	11 ± 6.6	Secondary
Morris (Morris et al., 2015)	2015	RCT	Single	210	68 ± 10	6.7 ± 5.6	Primary
Shen (Shen & Mak, 2015)	2015	RCT	Single (assessor)	51	63 ± 8 (int); 65 ± 9 (con)	8.1 ± 4.3 (int); 6.6 ± 4.0 (con)	Primary
Morris (Morris et al., 2017)	2017	RCT	Single (concealed allocation & assessor blind)	133	71 ± 9	Not reported	Primary
Chivers (Chivers Seymour et al., 2019)	2019	Multi-centre, pragmatic RCT	Single (investigator)	474	71 ± 8 (int); 73 ± 8 (con)	8 ± 6.6 (int); 8 ± 5.8 (con)	Primary

Exercise intervention	Dose	Follow-up	Control intervention	p-value	Effect size
Tai Chi	3x 60 min per week, 12 weeks	6 months	Usual care	<0.05	Not reported
Resistance Training - PD-WEBB (Sherrington et al., 2008)	3x 40-60 min per week, 6 months	6 months	Usual care	0.18	IRR = 0.73 (95% CI 0.45-1.17)
Home-based specific cueing exercise + education programme	4 x 30-60 min, during first 6 weeks	6 months	Usual care	0.70	Relative rate RR = 1.22 (95% CI 0.45-3.26) * * Outlier excluded
Movement strategy or progressive resistance strengthening	1 x 120 min per week (clinic) + 1 x 120 min per week (home), 8 weeks	12 months	Life skills	Movement <0.12; Strength= <0.001	Movement – IRR = 0.385 (95% CI 0.184-0.808); Strength – IRR = 0.151 (95% CI 0.071-0.322)
Technology assisted balance and gait training	3 x 60 min per week, 12 weeks	15 months	Strength exercises	<0.05 at 3 and 6 months, 0.057 at 15 months	3 months – IRR = 0.111 (95%CI 0.013-0.956); 6 months – IRR = 0.188 (95%CI 0.047-0.740); 15 months – IRR = 0.407 (95%CI 0.161-1.028)
Home exercise programme resistance exercise + movement strategy + Falls education	2 x 60 min per week, 6 weeks	12 months	Life skills	Not reported	IRR = 1.58 (95%CI 0.73-3.43)
Resistance training - PDSAFE (Ashburn et al., 2019)	12 x 60-90 mins within 6 months, + 7 x 30 min per week (home), 6 months	6 months	Usual care + Parkinson's DVD	0.824	OR = 0.98 (95%CI 0.80-1.19)

TABLE 10.1 Randomised controlled trials with physiotherapy interventions since 2014 (*Cont.*)

Study	Year	Type of study	Blinding	Total number	Age	Duration of Parkinson's	Falls as primary or secondary outcome
Gandolfi (Gandolfi et al., 2019)	2019	RCT	Single (examiner)	27	72 ± 6	7.31 ± 5.16	Secondary
Wong-Yu (Wong-Yu & Mak, 2019)	2019	RCT	Single (assessor)	83	61 ± 9.0	Not reported	Primary
Van der Kolk (Van der Kolk et al., 2019)	2019	RCT	Double	125	59 ± 8.3 (int); 59 ± 9.3	41 (int); 38 (con)	Secondary

Abbreviations: con, control group; int, intervention group; IRR, incidence rate ratio; OR, odds ratio; RCT, randomised controlled trial; sig. diff., significant difference;

Exercise intervention	Dose	Follow-up	Control intervention	p-value	Effect size
Active self-correction exercises, with visual and proprioceptive feedback, passive and active trunk stabilisation, and functional task	2 x 60 min per week, 4 weeks	4 weeks	Joint mobilisation, strengthening, stretching	Intervention reduced falls (p < 0.05) but no sig. diff. between groups (p = 0.29)	Not reported
Indoor flexibility & strength training, balance dance, modified Wing Chun[a], square stepping exercise. Outdoor – advanced balance tasks, gait and functional training	3 x 60 min per week, 8 weeks (indoor– 4 weeks; outdoor– 4 weeks), continuing at home for 6 months	12 months	Seated upper limb exercises	=0.025	OR = 7.2 (95%CI 1.35-38.33)
Aerobic exercise – stationary cycling, with exergame	3x 30-45 min (minimum)	6 months	Stretching, flexibility and relaxation exercises 3x per week for 30 min plus motivational app and coaching	=0.76	IRR= -1.3 (95%CI -12.9 to 0.1)

[a]Wing Chun, a concept-based traditional Southern Chinese Kung fu style and a form of self-defense

on well-being and can be a good way to engage someone who has not previously been active or has a low level of baseline fitness (Ehlen et al., 2018). However, it does not offer the stimulation required to improve symptom severity or reduce the number of falls (Morris et al., 2017). Exercise, however, differs in that it is planned or structured, involves repetitive bodily movements, and has the aim of improving or maintaining one of the domains of physical fitness (Caspersen & Christenson, 1985). There is positive evidence of benefit from regular exercise at a moderate to high intensity in people with Parkinson's, showing that symptom severity and falls rate can be reduced with exercise of sufficient intensity (van der Kolk et al., 2019). New methods of training people with Parkinson's are emerging, and individuals subjectively find exercise and activity invaluable. Commercial programmes offering activities such as boxing and dance are popular not just for their physical benefits but also for the social interactions they provide (Sheehy et al., 2017).

Tai chi comprises a series of slow, flowing movements and has been practised in China since the 13th century (Tai Chi Health Institute, 2018); it has been shown to be effective in reducing falls (Li et al., 2012; Marjama-Lyons et al., 2002). A study in China randomised 76 people to 60 minutes of tai chi three times a week for 12 weeks. During the 6-month follow-up, 8 of 37 (22%) participants in the active arm fell compared with 19 of 39 (49%) (P <.05) in the control arm (Gao et al., 2014). Dose is important; a further study found that twice-weekly tai chi had no beneficial effect on reducing the rate of falls (IRR 0.88; 95% CI 0.68-1.16; $P = .37$) (Taylor et al., 2012).

Balance training may improve balance-specific neural pathways and muscular activation, but the evidence is mixed. One study of 37 participants with an average Parkinson's duration of 7 years demonstrated a reduction in the mean rate of falls (1.63 versus 0.42 per month, P <.05) following 4 weeks of two 60-minute balance exercises with visual feedback, trunk stabilisation, and functional tasks. However, the difference between groups did not reach statistical significance (Gandolfi et al., 2019). A trial with 83 participants, average Hoehn and Yahr stage 2.5, found that compared with an intervention group who received indoor and outdoor balance and functional training twice a week for 60 minutes over 8 weeks, the control group had a 72% (OR 7.2, 95% CI 1.35-38.33, $P = .02$) greater likelihood of experiencing an injurious fall at 12-month follow-up (Wong-Yu and Mak, 2019). Intensive gait and balance rehabilitation appear to be effective. A small RCT delivered intensive training three to five times a week for 12 weeks. One group received training augmented by a technologic dance programme whereas the control intervention targeted strength alone. The intervention was most effective in the technology-facilitated group, but the effect waned over time (RR was .19 at 3 months, .29 at 6 months, and .48 at 12 months; P <.05) (Shen & Mak, 2015).

Studies investigating resistance training designed to improve muscle strength have reported mixed findings. Three studies enrolled individuals with moderate-stage Parkinson's, and PDSAFE is one of the largest physical activity intervention trials published to date. Seymour et al. (2019) randomised 474 people with an 8-year average duration of Parkinson's to either a physiotherapy programme or a single session offering information and advice about Parkinson's. At 6 and 12 months, the difference in fall rates between groups was not significantly different. However, a prespecified subgroup analysis demonstrated that the intervention was beneficial to those with moderate Parkinson's, although it increased the risk of falling in those with the most severe Parkinson's. Overall, functional measures of balance and falls self-efficacy improved (Chivers Seymour et al., 2019). Positive findings also resulted from a study comprising a population with similar Parkinson's duration, whereby either movement strategy training or progressive resistance training for 8 weeks reduced the falls rate by 85% at the 12-month follow-up (IRR .15, 95% CI 0.07-0.32, P <.001). Resistance training and movement strategies training reduced falls by 62% (IRR .39, 95% CI 0.18-0.81, P = .01). The control group performed life skills (Morris et al., 2015). Another RCT, by Canning (2015), enrolled 231 participants, average Parkinson's duration 8 years, and randomised participants to three 30- to 40-minute sessions per week of weight-bearing exercise for better balance (PD-WEBB) resistance training. This consisted of cueing training for participants reporting FOG as well as balance and strengthening exercises, whereas the control group received usual care alongside a falls prevention booklet. At 6 months there was a 27% reduction in fall rate, which may have occurred by chance (IRR .73, 95% CI 0.45–1.17, P = .18) (Canning et al., 2015). Interestingly, a prespecified subgroup with less severe Parkinson's had a larger and significant 69% reduction in fall rate (IRR 0.31, 95% CI 0.15-0.62, P <.001), suggesting that the intervention may be most beneficial for those with early Parkinson's (Canning et al., 2015). Smaller studies have failed to find a difference. A study by Morris et al. (2017) recruited 133 individuals with Parkinson's and found no significant difference (RR 1.58, 95% CI 0.73-3.43) between an intervention group receiving two 60-minute resistance exercises and movement strategy sessions and a control group that performed life skills (Morris et al., 2017).

In a single-blind RCT comprising 34 people with Parkinson's who had fallen at least twice in the preceding year, Volpe et al (2014) compared 60 minutes of either hydrotherapy or land-based rehabilitation 5 days a week. At 1-week follow-up after 2-month of intervention, both groups improved, but the aquatic based exercise was more effective and included a reduction in falls. This phase II trial is supportive of hydrotherapy being feasible and efficacious, but future studies should determine whether the benefit for falls is reproducible and sustained in the longer term (Volpe et al., 2014).

Van der Kolk (2019) conducted an RCT with 125 relatively inactive participants with early Parkinson's. The trial intervention consisted of 30 minutes of stationary cycling combined with an "exergame" delivered at least three times a week, which were targeted at improving heart rates. The control intervention was a stretching, flexibility and relaxation exercises performed for 30 minutes three times a week for 6 months (van der Kolk et al., 2019). In addition, all participants received a motivational app and coaching support. The intervention arm experienced fewer falls at 6 months, but this may have occurred by chance (van der Kolk et al., 2019). Other evidence is more supportive of the feasibility and effectiveness of adding cognitive elements to a physical therapy intervention. A RCT that (a treadmill training programme augmented by virtual reality to decrease fall risk in older adults) examined treadmill training with non-immersive virtual reality versus treadmill training alone (V-TIME) and showed that the virtual reality–augmented group had a lower incidence of falls; this was sustained for 6 months (Mirelman et al., 2016). Combined interventions are promising, with further trials under way.

Physical activity summary

Individuals with Parkinson's should undertake an ongoing programme of physical activity and exercise to help ameliorate symptoms starting as soon as possible after diagnosis and continuing throughout the condition. Additionally, a full falls assessment should be undertaken in accordance with National Institute of Care Excellence (NICE) Guidelines to establish the circumstances surrounding falls. Table 10.1 summarises the RCT evidence in this area.

Educational strategies include making sure that suitable footwear is worn, trip hazards such as rugs are removed, and other environmental factors are addressed, including optimising lighting. It is also essential to ensure that each participant's vision has been optimised.

Specific exercises should be tailored to the individual depending on his or her risk profile. Individuals who are falling during episodes of freezing will benefit from cueing strategies; strength and balance interventions can tackle deficits in those areas. Strategies to help people reach help when needed and/or to get up off the floor are important for those who live alone; psychologist specialist input where specific risks are identified should be sought.

Targeting non-motor fall factors

The loss of cholinergic function in frontocortical and mesencephalic locomotor areas can result in cognitive (Yarnall et al., 2013) and gait (Karachi et al., 2010) impairments, which can subsequently lead to a propensity to fall. On this basis, three phase II trials established the potential efficacy of cholinesterase inhibitors for falls prevention in Parkinson's. A small (n = 23) crossover trial reported that donepezil reduced the falls rates by 50% ($0.25 \pm .08$ falls per day on placebo and $0.13 \pm .03$ on donepezil, $p < .05$) (Chung et al., 2010). Li et al. reported a reduced odds ratio of falling (0.31, 95% CI 0.12, 0.77, $p < .01$) in 89 people with Parkinson's treated with rivastigmine (Li et al., 2015). A larger (n = 130) RCT demonstrated that 8 months of treatment with rivastigmine improved gait variability (a proxy marker of falls risk), walking speed, and balance, leading to a 45% (95% CI 19%-62%, $p = .002$) reduction in the rate of falls per month (Henderson et al., 2016). The effectiveness and cost-effectiveness of using cholinesterase inhibitors as a fall-prevention strategy is now being evaluated in a phase III multicentre trial. Transcranial direct current stimulation (tDCS) is effective in improving executive function in people with Parkinson's (Boggio et al., 2006; Doruk et al., 2014), but positive cognitive benefits have yet to be translated to a reduction in fall rate.

All people with Parkinson's should be routinely screened for OH at outpatient appointments (National Institute for Health and Care Excellence [NICE], n.d.), and home BP monitoring may also be helpful in select cases. Management of OH includes correcting aggravating factors and implementing non-pharmacological measures and medications. In terms of aggravating factors, contributory medications such as antihypertensives, diuretics, tricyclic antidepressants and alpha blockers should be reviewed and discontinued where possible. All individuals should have a careful review of their dopaminergic medications and doses to ensure that these are appropriate; also concomitant health conditions—such as anaemia, which may worsen OH—should be treated as necessary. Non-pharmacological measures that may be helpful include advising individuals to drink plenty of fluid (2-2.5 L/d), add additional salt to meals (at least 1-2 teaspoons per day), take laxatives to avoid straining at defecation, and exercise regularly (Mathias & Kimber, 1998). Because upright exercise may increase the orthostatic drop in BP, training in a supine or sitting position (e.g., swimming, recumbent biking) is advisable. Abdominal binders, bolus water drinking and physical countermaneuvers (such as leg crossing and fist clenching) may also be of benefit, but compression stockings have not been shown to be helpful, and individuals may find them cumbersome to put on (Newton & Frith, 2018). Caffeine, alcohol, sugary beverages, large meals, hot environments and sudden postural changes can all worsen OH (Mathias and Kimber, 1998) and should be avoided. Non-pharmacological interventions for OH are summarised in Table 10.2.

TABLE 10.2 Non-pharmacological interventions for orthostatic hypotension.

Preventive strategies

Avoid alcohol

Avoid large meals

Avoid hot environments

Avoid sudden postural changes

Avoid prolonged standing

Lifestyle interventions

Increase fluid intake: drink 2 to 2.5 liters of fluid per day.

Increase salt intake: at least 1 to 2 teaspoons per meals.

Ensure that bowel movements are regular so as to avoid straining at stool.

Physical measures

Exercise regularly, with consideration of training in the supine or sitting position.

Use an abdominal binder during waking hours.

Drink boluses of cold water regularly.

Utilise physical countermaneuvers such as leg crossing or fist clenching.

There is no good-quality evidence for the pharmacological management of OH.

In the United Kingdom, the NICE recommends the use of midodrine (an alpha-receptor agonist) or—if midodrine is contraindicated, not tolerated or not effective—fludrocortisone (a synthetic mineralocorticoid). Midodrine is contraindicated in various conditions including cardiac conduction disturbances, hyperthyroidism, narrow-angle glaucoma, diabetic retinopathy and serious prostatic disorders; it can also cause urinary retention and itching. Fludrocortisone is notably not licenced for the treatment of OH and can cause bloating, ankle edema, and hypokalemia. Droxidopa has a licence for treating OH in the United States and Japan, but again the evidence base is limited. Medications that are sometimes used as third-line treatments include domperidone and pyridostigmine. There are several ongoing studies evaluating the effects of some newer pharmacological agents, but further research in this area is urgently needed.

Environmental modification

As most people with Parkinson's fall at home and face more functional limitations than age-matched controls (Ashburn et al., 2008; Slaug et al., 2013), UK National guidelines recommend referral to occupational therapists (OTs) to determine what interventions and modifications may be beneficial (National Institute for Health and Care Excellence, 2018; Scottish Intercollegiate Guidelines Network, 2010). Although this is an intuitive and pragmatic approach, there is little reliable evidence supporting environmental modifications for falls prevention in Parkinson's (Bhidayasiri et al., 2015). Physiotherapy intervention studies have embedded self-management strategies, but the efficacy of each component has not been evaluated (Owen et al., 2019). Likewise, occupational therapy has rarely been examined in isolation from other therapies, particularly as crossover skills such as cueing, mobility and cognitive aspects of rehabilitation are often included in a larger management intervention. large RCT comparing physiotherapy and occupational therapy to no therapy in mild to moderate disease (PD REHAB) trial recruited 762 individuals with mild to moderate Parkinson's and randomised them to physiotherapy and occupational therapy versus no therapy. The intervention arm receiving approximately 4 hours of intervention over the 8-week period. At 3 months, difference in Nottingham Extended Activities of Daily Living (NEADL) scale did not differ between intervention groups. This may have been a function of the instrument's insensitivity to change or the fact that in those recruited it was uncertain whether therapy would be beneficial (Clarke et al., 2016).

Minimising complications

The consequences of falls include direct physical injuries such as fractures (Low et al., 2015) and soft tissue injuries (Gazibara et al., 2014). However, activities can be further restricted by negative psychological sequelae such as fear of falling (Bloem & Bhatia, 2004) and of hospitalisation (Koller & Glatt, 1989), which are frequently associated with delirium (Lawson et al., 2020) and physical deconditioning. Pooled data from seven studies demonstrate that in those with Parkinson's, falls account for 30% of acute admissions to general wards (Koay et al., 2018). For individuals with Parkinson's residing in care homes, falls are the most common reason for emergency department admission (Walker et al., 2014).

Because people with Parkinson's often fall "like a log," hip fractures are three times more likely to occur (Bloem & Bhatia, 2004) and can be particularly devastating. Parkinson's individuals are more prone to complications such as delirium, postoperative infection and pressure ulcers (Enemark et al., 2017; Walker et al., 2013) and more likely to require reoperation; or they may have surgical complications such as non-union or fixation failure (Karadsheh et al., 2015; Walker et al., 2013). Postoperative pneumonia is a common complication due to respiratory neuromuscular dysfunction (Critchley et al., 2015). There are also long-term implications for mobility, with Parkinson's individuals being less likely to be discharged directly home (Walker et al., 2013) and more likely to experience loss of mobility (Enemark et al., 2017). Time to discharge is longer owing to slower rehabilitation times (Critchley et al., 2015), with people with Parkinson's unlikely to return home within 30 days (Lisk et al., 2017). As a result of these complications, the 5-year survival rate post fracture for people with Parkinson's is lower than that for age matched controls (10% vs. 30%).

(Karadsheh et al., 2015).

Bone health and fracture prevention

Compared with age-matched peers, people with Parkinson's are at substantially increased risk for osteoporosis (Torsney et al., 2014), a condition characterised by fragile bones. Contributing factors are lower levels of activity (bone mass in promoted by load bearing exercise), lower levels of vitamin D (Evatt et al., 2008), poorer nutritional status (affecting weight as well as calcium and vitamin D intake); osteoporosis may also be an indirect effect of some Parkinson's medication on collagen crosslinking and bone strength (Van Den Bos et al., 2013).

Osteoporosis is defined by bone mineral density, which is measured by dual-energy x-ray absorptiometry (DXA scan). A T-score below the threshold of -2.5 is classified as osteoporosis and a T-score between -1 and -2.5 as osteopenia. Almost all fractures arise as the result of a fall. However, low trauma can also cause a fracture, a fragility fracture being defined as resulting from a fall from standing height or less. It is the interplay between bone fragility and falls risk that generates fracture risk.

In recent years there has been a greater focus on the assessment of fracture risk, beyond the simple identification of osteoporosis (Curtis et al., 2017). This enables interventions to be delivered to those at higher risk even when a DXA scan is not performed. Given their dual risk of falls and osteoporosis, people with Parkinson's are prime candidates for fracture risk assessment to enable the appropriately targeted management of their bone health.

There are a number of fracture risk assessment tools. Two of these, FRAX and Qfracture (ClinRisk Ltd., 2019; Kanis and University of Sheffield, 2008), have been endorsed by NICE for use in the general population. Qfracture specifically incorporates idiopathic Parkinson's in its assessment questions, although it may overestimate fracture risk. The FRAX fracture risk assessment tool is country-specific and incorporates data regarding age, sex, height and weight as well as answers to questions about personal and family fracture history, smoking, alcohol, steroid history, and rheumatoid arthritis. It will incorporate bone density where known, but this is not needed to calculate risk. After calculation of both major osteoporotic fracture (clinical spine, forearm, hip, proximal humerus) and hip fracture probability over 10 years, it provides a direct link to treatment recommendations developed by (Compston et al., 2017). It does not specifically incorporate idiopathic Parkinson's in its algorithm. However, it calculates increased probabilities in those with a condition associated with osteoporosis ("secondary osteoporosis"). Given the double prevalence of osteoporosis in people with Parkinson's compared with controls, it is appropriate to select yes to secondary causes of osteoporosis in FRAX.

The National Osteoporosis Guidelines Group recommendations sort individuals into those appropriate for lifestyle advice only, those in whom further assessment with a DXA scan is recommended, and those in whom treatment is appropriate even without quantification of bone density. There are two caveats to the application of these recommendations to Parkinson's; first, the recommendations are based solely on the probability of major osteoporotic fracture, whereas people with Parkinson's are disproportionately at risk for hip fracture (Pouwels et al., 2013); second, there is no adjustment for the effect of falls on fracture probability, although an augmentation of 30% per fall in the previous year (to a maximum of 150% augmentation) is reasonable (Masud et al., 2011). Clinicians managing bone health should use clinical their judgment and consider using a 5% (after augmentation for falls) 10-year probability of hip fracture as a threshold for pharmacological intervention (Henderson et al., 2019).

There are many effective strategies to mitigate fracture risk, and all those managing Parkinson's should be aware of the possible interventions. Managing falls risk is of course a cornerstone addressed in the rest of this chapter.

The management of bone health has three main pillars: lifestyle factors, intake of vitamin D and calcium and pharmacological intervention. The UK Royal Osteoporosis Society has excellent online and printed resources to support the individual in self-management and understanding (Royal Osteoporosis Society, n.d.). Lifestyle factors should be addressed in primary or secondary care. Smoking, though less common among individuals with Parkinson's, has a damaging effect on bone mineral density (BMD), and smokers should be supported to stop. Alcohol also has a direct impact on BMD; it also increases falls risk. Therefore individuals should be given information about cessation/reduction, with specialist referral if needed (Compston et al., 2019). Exercise has a good effect both on falls risk and bone density, with weight-bearing exercise being particularly important in improving bone density (Kemmler et al., 2017). Underweight individuals are at increased fracture risk, particularly at the hip, in part owing to lack of soft tissue protection; thus advice regarding nutrition can be important. Hip protectors can improve confidence and reduce fracture risk if worn at the time of a fall, although overall evidence for their effectiveness is limited (Gillespie et al., 2010).

Vitamin D levels tend to be low in people with Parkinson's, possibly even before the onset of symptoms (Evatt et al., 2008); this deficiency is certainly compounded by reduced activity and insufficient sunlight exposure. Adequate levels of vitamin D and calcium—acquired by lifestyle and nutrition as well as by supplementation if needed—are essential to bone health and are a prerequisite for the pharmacological management of low bone density (Scientific Advisory Committee on Nutrition, 2016).

The mainstay of medication for bone fragility is bisphosphonate therapy. These drugs reduce osteoclast activity, lowering bone turnover and attenuating the reduction in bone mineral density over time. They are effective and cost-effective, reducing relative fracture risk by as much as half, and they are generally well tolerated (Compston et al., 2017). Oral medication (alendronic acid, risedronate) can, however, pose difficulties for individuals with Parkinson's who may have swallowing or cognitive issues. Adherence is often suboptimal (Siris et al., 2009), although clear information and counselling can support it effectively. If oral medication is not suitable, parenteral treatments exist. Intravenous zoledronic acid (National Institute for Health and Care Excellence, 2017) given yearly or, in frailer people with Parkinson's, only once (Reid et al., 2013) may be particularly appropriate for some. Denosumab—a monocloncal antibody with a suppressive effect on bone-resorbing osteoclasts—can be given every 6 months; it can be useful and is suitable even for those with poor renal function (Cummings et al., 2009). These and other parenteral treatments are generally provided within secondary care, although their availability is expanding.

Conclusion

Falls are an almost universal feature of Parkinson's and remain among the most disabling and burdensome features of the condition. Falls risk will be affected by an individual's Parkinson's phenotype, comorbidities, pharmacotherapy, sociodemographic factors, physical function, physical activity and environment. The complex interplay of these factors necessitates an individualised approach to mitigating both falls and fracture risk.

Top tips for the prevention of falls and fractures

1. Ask all people with Parkinson's whether they have fallen or experienced a near fall at least annually.
2. Recognise that falls in Parkinson's are multifactorial and that the influence of each risk factor will vary as the condition evolves.
3. Gait dysfunction and cognitive impairment are interrelated and the presence of each increases the risks of falls.
4. Postural blood pressures should be routinely recorded and inquiry made as to the presence of associated symptoms.
5. Each modifiable risk factor should be proactively treated and the response to intervention reevaluated.
6. Do not overlook comorbidities, polypharmacy and other risk factors that are indirectly related or unrelated to Parkinson's but are contributing to the risk of falling.
7. Management of falls risk is best done within the context of a skilled multidisciplinary team.
8. Physical activity is a potentially complex intervention and input of a physiotherapist should be sought early after diagnosis to improve conditioning, balance, and strength.
9. To prevent secondary harms, evaluate fracture risk in people with early, maintenance, or complex stage Parkinson's.
10. Treat fracture risk by addressing the three pillars: lifestyle factors, vitamin D and calcium intake; consider pharmacological intervention.
11. If adherence or tolerability limits oral bisphosphonate use, consider parenteral therapy.

References

Allen, N. E., Schwarzel, A. K., & Canning, C. G. (2013). Recurrent falls in Parkinson's disease: a systematic review. *Parkinson's Disease*, 2013.

Almeida, L. R. S., Sherrington, C., Allen, N. E., Paul, S. S., Valenca, G. T., Oliveira-Filho, J., et al. (2015). Disability is an independent predictor of falls and recurrent falls in people with Parkinson's disease without a history of falls: a one-year prospective study. *J. Parkinson's Disease*, 5, 4, 855–864.

Antonini, A., Stoessl, A. J., Kleinman, L. S., Skalicky, A. M., Marshall, T. S., Sail, K. R., et al. (2018). Developing consensus among movement disorder specialists on clinical indicators for identification and management of advanced Parkinson's disease: a multi-country Delphi-panel approach. *Current Medical Research and Opinion, 34*, 2063–2073.

Armstrong, R. A. (2017). *Visual dysfunction in Parkinson's disease. International Review of Neurobiology*. 134, 921–946.

Ashburn, A., Stack, E., Ballinger, C., Fazakarley, L., & Fitton, C. (2008). The circumstances of falls among people with Parkinson's disease and the use of falls diaries to facilitate reporting. *Disability and Rehabilitation, 30*, 16, 1205–1212.

Ashburn, A., Pickering, R., McIntosh, E., Hulbert, S., Rochester, L., Roberts, H. C., et al. (2019). Exercise and strategy-based physiotherapy-delivered intervention for preventing repeat falls in people with Parkinson's: The PDSAFE RCT. *Health Technol. Assess. (Rockv).*, *23*, 36, 1–147.

Balasubramanian, C. K., Neptune, R. R., & Kautz, S. A. (2009). Variability in spatiotemporal step characteristics and its relationship to walking performance post-stroke. *Gait Posture*, *29*, 3, 408–414.

Barthel, C., Nonnekes, J., Van Helvert, M., Haan, R., Janssen, A., Delval, A., Weerdesteyn, V., Debû, B., Van Wezel, R., Bloem, B. R., & Ferraye, M. U. (2018). The laser shoes. *Neurology*, *90*, 2, e164–e171.

Baston, C., Mancini, M., Schoneburg, B., Horak, F., & Rocchi, L. (2014). Postural strategies assessed with inertial sensors in healthy and Parkinsonian subjects. *Gait Posture*, *40*, 1, 70–75.

Bhidayasiri, R., Jitkritsadakul, O., Boonrod, N., Sringean, J., Calne, S. M., Hattori, N., & Hayashi, A. (2015). What is the evidence to support home environmental adaptation in Parkinson's disease? A call for multidisciplinary interventions. *Park. Relat. Disord.*, *21*, 10, 1127–1132.

Bloem, B. R., & Bhatia, K. P. (2004). Gait and balance in basal ganglia disorders. *Clin. Disord. Balanc. posture gait*, *2*, 173–206.

Bloem, B. R., Grimbergen, Y. A. M., Cramer, M., Willemsen, M., & Zwinderman, A. H. (2001). Prospective assessment of falls in Parkinson's disease. *J. Neurol.*, *248*, 11, 950–958.

Bloem, B. R., Hausdorff, J. M., Visser, J. E., & Giladi, N. (2004). Falls and freezing of Gait in Parkinson's disease: A review of two interconnected, episodic phenomena. *Mov. Disord.*, *19*, 8, 871–884.

Bluett, B., Litvan, I., Cheng, S., Juncos, J., Riley, D. E., Standaert, D. G., Reich, S. G., Hall, D. A., Kluger, B., Shprecher, D., Marras, C., & Jankovic, J. (2017). Understanding falls in progressive supranuclear palsy. *Park. Relat. Disord.*, *35*, 75–81.

Boggio, P. S., Ferrucci, R., Rigonatti, S. P., Covre, P., Nitsche, M., Pascual-Leone, A., & Fregni, F. (2006). Effects of transcranial direct current stimulation on working memory in patients with Parkinson's disease. *J. Neurol. Sci.*, *249*, 1, 31–38.

Bohnen, N. I., & Jahn, K. (2013). Imaging: What can it tell us about Parkinsonian gait? Mov. *Disord.*, *28*, 11, 1492–1500.

Bouça-Machado, R., Rosário, A., Caldeira, D., Castro Caldas, A., Guerreiro, D., Venturelli, M., Tinazzi, M., Schena, F., & Ferreira, J. (2020). Physical activity, exercise, and physiotherapy in parkinson's disease: Defining the Concepts. *Mov. Disord. Clin. Pract.*, *7*, 1, 7–15.

Brown, F. S., Rowe, J. B., Passamonti, L., & Rittman, T. (2020). Falls in Progressive Supranuclear Palsy. *Mov. Disord. Clin. Pract.*, *7*, 1, 16–24.

Burn, D. J., & Lees, A. J. (2002). Progressive supranuclear palsy: Where are we now? *Lancet Neurol.*, *1*, 6, 359–369.

Camicioli, R., & Majumdar, S. R. (2010). Relationship between mild cognitive impairment and falls in older people with and without Parkinson's disease: 1-Year Prospective Cohort Study. *Gait Posture*, *32*, 1, 87–91.

Canning, C. G., Sherrington, C., Lord, S. R., Close, J. C. T., Heritier, S., Heller, G. Z., Howard, K., Allen, N. E., Latt, M. D., Murray, S. M., O'Rourke, S. D., Paul, S. S., Song, J., & Fung, V. S. C. (2015). Exercise for falls prevention in Parkinson disease: A randomised controlled trial. *Neurology*, *84*, 3, 304–312.

Caspersen, C. J., & Christenson, G. M. (1985). Physical Activity, Exercise, and Physical Fitness: Definitions and Distinctions. *Public Heal. Rep.*, *100*, 2, 126–131.

Castrioto, A., Lozano, A. M., Poon, Y. Y., Lang, A. E., Fallis, M., & Moro, E. (2011). Ten-year outcome of subthalamic stimulation in Parkinson's disease: A blinded evaluation. *Arch. Neurol.*, *68*, 12, 1550–1556.

Chang, H. Y., Lee, Y. Y., Wu, R. M., Yang, Y. R., & Luh, J. J. (2019). Effects of rhythmic auditory cueing on stepping in place in patients with Parkinson's disease. *Medicine (Baltimore).*, *98*, 45, e17874.

Chivers Seymour, K., Pickering, R., Rochester, L., Roberts, H. C., Ballinger, C., Hulbert, S., Kunkel, D., Marian, I. R., Fitton, C., McIntosh, E., Goodwin, V. A., Nieuwboer, A., Lamb, S. E., & Ashburn, A. (2019). Multicentre, randomised controlled trial of PDSAFE, a physiotherapist-delivered fall prevention programme for people with Parkinson's. *J. Neurol. Neurosurg. Psychiatry*, *90*, 7, 774–782.

Chung, K. A., Lobb, B. M., Nutt, J. G., & Horak, F. B. (2010). Effects of a central cholinesterase inhibitor on reducing falls in Parkinson's disease. *Neurology*, *75*, 14, 1263–1269.

Clarke, C. E., Patel, S., Ives, N., Rick, C. E., Dowling, F., Woolley, R., Wheatley, K., Walker, M. F., & Sackley, C. M. (2016). Physiotherapy and occupational Therapy vs No Therapy in mild to moderate Parkinson disease. *JAMA Neurol.*, *73*, 3, 291–299.

ClinRisk Ltd, 2019. QFracture-2016 [WWW Document]. URL https://qfracture.org/ (accessed 6.30.20).

Compston, J., Cooper, A., Cooper, C., Gittoes, N., Gregson, C., Harvey, N., Hope, S., Kanis, J. A., McCloskey, E. V., Poole, K. E. S., Reid, D. M., Selby, P., Thompson, F., Thurston, A., & Vine, N. (2017). UK clinical guideline for the prevention and treatment of osteoporosis. *Arch. Osteoporos.*, *12*, 1, 43.

Compston, J. E., McClung, M. R., & Leslie, W. D. (2019). Osteoporosis. *Lancet*, *393*, 364–376.

Contin, M., Riva, R., Baruzzi, A., Albani, F., Macri', S., & Martinelli, P. (1996). Postural Stability in Parkinson's Disease: The Effects of Disease Severity and Acute Levodopa Dosing. *Park. Relat. Disord.*, *2*, 1, 29–33.

Creaby, M. W., & Cole, M. H. (2018). Gait characteristics and falls in Parkinson's disease: A systematic review and meta-analysis. *Park. Relat. Disord 57*, 1–8.

Critchley, R. J., Khan, S. K., Yarnall, A. J., Parker, M. J., & Deehan, D. J. (2015). Occurrence, management and outcomes of hip fractures in patients with Parkinson's disease. *Br. Med. Bull.*, *115*, 1, 135–142.

Cummings, S. R., Martin, J. S., McClung, M. R., Siris, E. S., Eastell, R., Reid, I. R., et al. (2009). Denosumab for Prevention of Fractures in Postmenopausal Women with Osteoporosis. *N. Engl. J. Med.*, *361*, 8, 756–765.

Curtis, E. M., Moon, R. J., Harvey, N. C., & Cooper, C. (2017). Reprint of: The impact of fragility fracture and approaches to osteoporosis risk assessment worldwide. *Int. J. Orthop. Trauma Nurs.*, *26*, 7–17.

Dance for PD 2000 [WWW Document], URL https://danceforparkinsons.org/ (accessed 3.7.20).

Deane, K. H. O., Flaherty, H., Daley, D. J., Pascoe, R., Penhale, B., Clarke, C. E., Sackley, C., & Storey, S. (2014). Priority setting partnership to identify the top 10 research priorities for the management of Parkinson's disease. *BMJ Open*, *4*, 12, e006434–e16434.

Delgado-Alvarado, M., Marano, M., Santurtún, A., Urtiaga-Gallano, A., Tordesillas-Gutierrez, D., & Infante, J. (2020). Non-pharmacological, nonsurgical treatments for freezing of gait in Parkinson's disease: A systematic review. *Mov. Disord.*, *35*, 2, 204–214.

Domingos, J. M., Godinho, C., Dean, J., Coelho, M., Pinto, A., Bloem, B. R., & Ferreira, J. J. (2015). Cognitive impairment in fall-related studies in Parkinson's disease. *J. Parkinsons. Dis.*, *5*, 3, 453–469.

Doruk, D., Gray, Z., Bravo, G. L., Pascual-Leone, A., & Fregni, F. (2014). Effects of tDCS on executive function in Parkinson's disease. *Neurosci. Lett.*, *582*, 27–31.

Duncan, R. P., Cavanaugh, J. T., Earhart, G. M., Ellis, T. D., Ford, M. P., Foreman, K. B., Leddy, A. L., Paul, S. S., Canning, C. G., Thackeray, A., & Dibble, L. E. (2015). External validation of a simple clinical tool used to predict falls in people with Parkinson's disease. *Parkinsonism Relat. Disord.*, *21*, 8, 960–963.

Ehlen, F., Schindlbeck, K., Nobis, L., Maier, A., & Klostermann, F. (2018). Relationships between activity and well-being in people with Parkinson's disease. *Brain Behav.*, *8*, 5, 1–8.

Ekker, M. S., Janssen, S., Seppi, K., Poewe, W., de Vries, N. M., Theelen, T., Nonnekes, J., & Bloem, B. R. (2017). Ocular and visual disorders in Parkinson's disease: Common but frequently overlooked. *Park. Relat. Disord.*, *40*, 1–10.

Enemark, M., Midttun, M., & Winge, K. (2017). Evaluating outcomes for older patients with parkinson's disease or dementia with lewy bodies who have been hospitalised for hip fracture surgery: potential impact of drug administration. *Drugs and Aging*, *34*, 5, 387–392.

Evatt, M. L., DeLong, M. R., Khazai, N., Rosen, A., Triche, S., & Tangpricha, V. (2008). Prevalence of vitamin D insufficiency in patients with Parkinson's disease and Alzheimer disease. *Arch. Neurol.*, *65*, 10, 1348–1352.

Fasano, A., Aquino, C. C., Krauss, J. K., Honey, C. R., & Bloem, B. R. (2015). Axial disability and deep brain stimulation in patients with Parkinson disease. *Nat. Rev. Neurol.*, *11*, 2, 98–110.

Feller, K. J., Peterka, R. J., & Horak, F. B. (2019). Sensory re-weighting for postural control in Parkinson's disease. *Front. Hum. Neurosci.*, *13*, 1–17.

Fietzek, U. M., Schroeteler, F. E., Ziegler, K., Zwosta, J., & Ceballos-Baumann, A. O. (2014). Randomised cross-over trial to investigate the efficacy of a two-week physiotherapy programme with repetitive exercises of cueing to reduce the severity of freezing of gait in patients with Parkinson's disease. *Clin. Rehabil.*, *28*, 9, 902–911.

Follett, K. A., Weaver, F. M., Stern, M., Hur, K., Harris, C. L., Luo, P., Marks, W. J., Rothlind, J., Sagher, O., Moy, C., Pahwa, R., Burchiel, K., Hogarth, P., Lai, E. C., Duda, J. E., Holloway, K., Samii, A., Horn, S., Bronstein, J. M., Stoner, G., Starr, P. A., Simpson, R., Baltuch, G., De Salles, A., Huang, G. D., & Reda, D. J. (2010). Pallidal versus subthalamic deep-brain stimulation for Parkinson's disease. *N. Engl. J. Med.*, *362*, 22, 2077–2091.

Frenklach, A., Louie, S., Koop, M. M., & Bronte-Stewart, H. M. (2009). Excessive postural sway and the risk of falls at different stages of Parkinson's disease. *Mov. Disord.*, *24*, 3, 377–385.

Gandolfi, M., Tinazzi, M., Magrinelli, F., Busselli, G., Dimitrova, E., Polo, N., Manganotti, P., Fasano, A., Smania, N., & Geroin, C. (2019). Four-week trunk-specific exercise programme decreases forward trunk flexion in Parkinson's disease: A single-blinded, randomised controlled trial. *Park. Relat. Disord.*, *64*, 268–274.

Gao, Q., Leung, A., Yang, Y., Wei, Q., Guan, M., Jia, C., & He, C. (2014). Effects of Tai Chi on balance and fall prevention in Parkinson's disease: A randomised controlled trial. *Clin. Rehabil.*, *28*, 8, 748–753.

Gazibara, T., Pekmezovic, T., Tepavcevic, D. K., Tomic, A., Stankovic, I., Kostic, V. S., & Svetel, M. (2014). Circumstances of falls and fall-related injuries among patients with Parkinson's disease in an outpatient setting. *Geriatr. Nurs. (Minneap).*, *35*, 5, 364–369.

Gervasoni, E., Cattaneo, D., Messina, P., Casati, E., Montesano, A., Bianchi, E., & Beghi, E. (2015). Clinical and stabilometric measures predicting falls in Parkinson disease/parkinsonisms. *Acta Neurol. Scand.*, *132*, 4, 235–241.

Giladi, N., Horak, F. B., & Hausdorff, J. M. (2013). Classification of gait disturbances: Distinguishing between continuous and episodic changes. *Mov. Disord.*, *28*, 11, 1469–1473.

Giladi, N., & Nieuwboer, A. (2008). Understanding and treating freezing of gait in Parkinsonism, proposed working definition, and setting the stage. *Mov. Disord.*, *23*, S423–S425.

Gillespie, W. J., Gillespie, L. D., & Parker, M. J. (2010). Hip protectors for preventing hip fractures in older people. In M. J. Parker (Ed.), *Cochrane Database of Systematic Reviews*, 10, Chichester, UK: John Wiley & Sons, Ltd.

Ha, A. D., Brown, C. H., York, M. K., & Jankovic, J. (2011). The prevalence of symptomatic orthostatic hypotension in patients with Parkinson's disease and atypical Parkinsonism. *Park. Relat. Disord.*, *17*, 8, 625–628.

Henderson, E. J., Lord, S. R., Brodie, M. A., Gaunt, D. M., Lawrence, A. D., Close, J. C. T., Whone, A. L., & Ben-Shlomo, Y. (2016). Rivastigmine for gait stability in patients with Parkinson's disease (ReSPonD): a randomised, double-blind, placebo-controlled, phase 2 trial. *Lancet Neurol.*, *15*, 3, 249–258.

Henderson, E. J., Lord, S. R., Close, J. C. T., Lawrence, A. D., Whone, A., & Ben-Shlomo, Y. (2013). The ReSPonD trial: rivastigmine to stabilise gait in Parkinson's disease a phase II, randomised, double blind, placebo controlled trial to evaluate the effect of rivastigmine on gait in patients with Parkinson's disease who have fallen. *BMC Neurol.*, *13*, 1, 1–10.

Henderson, E. J., Lyell, V., Bhimjiyani, A., Amin, J., Kobylecki, C., & Gregson, C. L. (2019). Management of fracture risk in Parkinson's: A revised algorithm and focused review of treatments. *Park. Relat. Disord.*, *64*, 181–187.

Hoehn, M. M., & Yahr, M.D. (1967) Parkinsonism onset, progression, and mortality. *Neurology.*, *17*, 427.

Horak, F. B., Nutt, J. G., & Nashner, L. M. (1992). Postural inflexibility in Parkinsonian subjects. *J. Neurol. Sci.*, *111*, 1, 46–58.

House, P. A., Weaver, F. M., Follett, K. A., Stern, M., Hur, K., & Harris, C. L. (2009). Bilateral Deep Brain Stimulation vs Best Medical Therapy for Patients With Advanced Parkinson Disease: A Randomised Controlled Trial. *Yearb. Neurol. Neurosurg.*, *301*, 1, 207–209.

IJmker, T., & Lamoth, C. J. C. (2012). Gait and cognition: the relationship between gait stability and variability with executive function in persons with and without dementia. *Gait Posture*, *35*, 1, 126–130.

Isaacson, S. H., & Skettini, J. (2014). Neurogenic orthostatic hypotension in Parkinson's disease: Evaluation, management, and emerging role of droxidopa. *Vasc. Health Risk Manag.*, *10*, 169–176.

Ivkovic, V., Fisher, S., & Paloski, W. H. (2016). Smartphone-based tactile cueing improves motor performance in Parkinson's disease. *Park. Relat. Disord.*, *22*, 42–47.

Jehu, D., & Nantel, J. (2018). Fallers with Parkinson's disease exhibit restrictive trunk control during walking. *Gait Posture*, *65*, 246–250.

Kanis, J., University of Sheffield, 2008. FRAX Fracture Risk Assessment Tool [WWW Document]. URL https://www.sheffield.ac.uk/FRAX/ (accessed 6.30.20).

Karachi, C., Cormier-Dequaire, F., Grabli, D., Lau, B., Belaid, H., Navarro, S., Vidailhet, M., Bardinet, E., Fernandez-Vidal, S., & Welter, M. -L. (2019). Clinical and anatomical predictors for freezing of gait and falls after subthalamic deep brain stimulation in Parkinson's disease patients. *Parkinsonism & related disorders, 62,* 91–97.

Karachi, C., Grabli, D., Bernard, F. A., Tande, D., Wattiez, N., Belaid, H., Bardinet, E., Prigent, A., Nothacker, H. -P., Hunot, S., Hartmann, A., Lehericy, S., Hirsch, E. C., & Francois, C. (2010). Cholinergic mesencephalic neurons are involved in gait and postural disorders in Parkinson disease. *J. Clin. Invest.*, *120*, 8, 2745–2754.

Karadsheh, M. S., Weaver, M., Rodriguez, K., Harris, M., Zurakowski, D., & Lucas, R. (2015). Mortality and Revision Surgery Are Increased in Patients With Parkinson's Disease and Fractures of the Femoral Neck. *Clin. Orthop. Relat. Res.*, *473*, 10, 3272–3279.

Kataoka, H., & Ueno, S. (2015). Low FAB score as a predictor of future falling in patients with Parkinson's disease: a 2.5-year prospective study. *J. Neurol.*, *262*, 9, 2049–2055.

Kemmler, W., Kohl, M., & von Stengel, S. (2017). Long-term effects of exercise in postmenopausal women. *Menopause*, *24*, 1, 45–51.

Kleinschmidt-DeMasters, B. K. (1989). Early progressive supranuclear palsy: pathology and clinical presentation. *Clin. Neuropathol.*, *8*, 2, 79–84.

Koay, L., Rose, J., & Abdelhafiz, A. H. (2018). Factors that lead to hospitalisation in patients with Parkinson's disease—A systematic review. *Int. J. Clin. Pract.*, *72*, 1, 1–5.

Koller, W., & Glatt, S. (1989). Falls and Parkinson's disease. *Clin.* Neuropharmacol. *12*, 2, 98–105.

Lamb, S. E., Jørstad-Stein, E. C., Hauer, K., & Becker, C. (2005). Development of a common outcome data set for fall injury prevention trials: The Prevention of Falls Network Europe consensus. *J. Am. Geriatr. Soc.*, *53*, 9, 1618–1622.

Lawson, R. A., Richardson, S. J., Yarnall, A. J., Burn, D. J., & Allan, L. M. (2020). Identifying delirium in Parkinson's disease: a pilot study. *Int. J. Geriatr. Psychiatry, 35*, 5, 547–552.

Lee, H. K., Ahn, S. J., Shin, Y. M., Kang, N., & Cauraugh, J. H. (2019). Correction to: Does transcranial direct current stimulation improve functional locomotion in people with Parkinson's disease? A systematic review and meta-analysis (J NeuroEng Rehabil (2019) 16 (84). *J. Neuroeng. Rehabil.*, *16*, 1, 1–13. doi: 10.1186/s12984-019-0562-4.

Li, F., Harmer, P., Fitzgerald, K., Eckstrom, E., Stock, R., Galver, J., Maddalozzo, G., & Batya, S. S. (2012). Tai chi and postural stability in patients with Parkinson's disease. *N. Engl. J. Med.*, *366*, 6, 511–519.

Li, Z., Yu, Z., Zhang, Jinbiao, Wang, J., Sun, C., Wang, P., Zhang, & Jiangshan (2015). Impact of rivastigmine on cognitive dysfunction and falling in Parkinson's disease patients. *Eur. Neurol.*, *74*, 1–2, 86–91.

Lindholm, B., Eek, F., Skogar, Ö., & Hansson, E. E. (2019). Dyskinesia and FAB score predict future falling in Parkinson's disease. *Acta Neurol. Scand.*, *139*, 6, 512–518.

Lindholm, B., Hagell, P., Hansson, O., & Nilsson, M. H. (2015). Prediction of falls and/or near falls in people with mild Parkinson's disease. *PLoS One*, *10*, 1, 1–11.

Lisk, R., Watters, H., & Yeong, K. (2017). Hip fracture outcomes in patients with Parkinson's disease. *Clin. Med.*, *17*, S3, P20.

Lord, S., Galna, B., Yarnall, A. J., Morris, R., Coleman, S., Burn, D., & Rochester, L. (2017). Natural history of falls in an incident cohort of Parkinson's disease: early evolution, risk and protective features. *J. Neurol.*, *264*, 11, 2268–2276.

Lord, S. R., Bindels, H., Ketheeswaran, M., Brodie, M. A., Lawrence, A. D., Close, J. C. T., Whone, A. L., Ben-Shlomo, Y., & Henderson, E. J. (2020). Freezing of Gait in People with Parkinson's disease: Nature, Occurrence, and Risk Factors. *J. Parkinsons. Dis.*, *10*, 631–640.

Low, P. A., Opfer-Gehrking, T. L., McPhee, B. R., Fealey, R. D., Benarroch, E. E., Willner, C. L., Suarez, G. A., Proper, C. J., Felten, J. A., Huck, C. A., & Corfits, J. L. (1995). Prospective Evaluation of Clinical Characteristics of Orthostatic Hypotension. *Mayo Clin. Proc.*, *70*, 7, 617–622.

Low, V., Ben-Shlomo, Y., Coward, E., Fletcher, S., Walker, R., & Clarke, C. E. (2015). Measuring the burden and mortality of hospitalisation in Parkinson's disease: A cross-sectional analysis of the English Hospital Episodes Statistics database 2009-2013. *Park. Relat. Disord.*, *21*, 5, 449–454.

Mactier, K., Lord, S., Godfrey, A., Burn, D., & Rochester, L. (2015). The relationship between real world ambulatory activity and falls in incident Parkinson's disease: Influence of classification scheme. *Park. Relat. Disord.*, *21*, 3, 236–242.

Mancini, M., Zampieri, C., Carlson-Kuhta, P., Chiari, L., & Horak, F. B. (2009). Anticipatory postural adjustments prior to step initiation are hypometric in untreated Parkinson's disease: an accelerometer-based approach. *Eur. J. Neurol.*, *16*, 9, 1028–1034.

Marjama-Lyons, J., Smith, L., Mylar, B., Nelson, J., Holliday, G., & Seracino, D. (2002). Tai Chi and reduced rate of falling in Parkinson's disease: a single-blinded pilot study. *Mov. Disord.*, *17*(Suppl 5), S70–S71.

Martin, T., Weatherall, M., Anderson, T. J., & Macaskill, M. R. (2015). A Randomised Controlled Feasibility Trial of a Specific Cueing Programme for Falls Management in Persons with Parkinson disease and Freezing of Gait. *J. Neurol. Phys. Ther.*, *39*, 3, 179–184.

Masud, T., Binkley, N., Boonen, S., & Hannan, M. T. (2011). Official Positions for FRAX® Clinical Regarding Falls and Frailty: Can Falls and Frailty be Used in FRAX®? From Joint Official Positions Development Conference of the International Society for Clinical Densitometry and International Osteoporosis Foundati. *J. Clin. Densitom.*, *14*, 3, 194–204.

Mathias, C. J., & Kimber, J. R. (1998). Treatment of postural hypotension. *J. Neurol. Neurosurg. Psychiatry*, *65*, 3, 285–289.

Matinolli, M., Korpelainen, J. T., Korpelainen, R., Sotaniemi, K. A., & Myllylä, V. V. (2009). Orthostatic hypotension, balance and falls in Parkinson's disease. *Mov. Disord.*, *24*, 5, 745–751.

McDonald, C., Newton, J. L., & Burn, D. J. (2016). Orthostatic hypotension and cognitive impairment in Parkinson's disease: Causation or association? *Mov. Disord.*, *31*, 7, 937–946.

Merola, A., Romagnolo, A., Rosso, M., Lopez-Castellanos, J. R., Wissel, B. D., Larkin, S., Bernardini, A., Zibetti, M., Maule, S., Lopiano, L., & Espay, A. J. (2016). Orthostatic hypotension in Parkinson's disease: Does it matter if asymptomatic? *Park. Relat. Disord.*, *33*, 65–71.

Mirelman, A., Rochester, L., Maidan, I., Del Din, S., Alcock, L., Nieuwhof, F., et al. (2016). Addition of a non-immersive virtual reality component to treadmill training to reduce fall risk in older adults (V-TIME): a randomised controlled trial. *Lancet* 388(10050) 1170–1182.

Miller, K. J., Suárez-Iglesias, D., Seijo-Martínez, M., & Ayán, C. (2019). Physiotherapy for freezing of gait in Parkinson's disease: A systematic review and meta-analysis. *Rev. Neurol.*, *70*, 5, 161–169.

Moro, E., Hamani, C., Poon, Y. Y., Al-Khairallah, T., Dostrovsky, J. O., Hutchison, W. D., & Lozano, A. M. (2010). Unilateral pedunculopontine stimulation improves falls in Parkinson's disease. *Brain*, *133*, 1, 215–224.

Morris, M. E., Iansek, R., Matyas, T. A., & Summers, J. J. (1996). Stride length regulation in Parkinson's disease: Normalisation strategies and underlying mechanisms. *Brain*, *119*, 2, 551–568.

Morris, M. E., Iansek, R., Matyas, T. A., & Summers, J. J. (1994). The pathogenesis of gait hypokinesia in Parkinson's disease. *Brain*, *117*, 5, 1169–1181.

Morris, M. E., Menz, H. B., McGinley, J. L., Watts, J. J., Huxham, F. E., Murphy, a. T., Danoudis, M. E., & Iansek, R. (2015). A Randomised Controlled Trial to Reduce Falls in People With Parkinson's Disease. *Neurorehabil. Neural Repair*, *29*, 8, 777–785.

Morris, M. E., Taylor, N. F., Watts, J. J., Evans, A., Horne, M., Kempster, P., Danoudis, M., McGinley, J., Martin, C., & Menz, H. B. (2017). A home programme of strength training, movement strategy training and education did not prevent falls in people with Parkinson's disease: a randomised trial. *J. Physiother.*, *63*, 2, 94–100.

Naismith, S. L., Shine, J. M., & Lewis, S. J. G. (2010). The specific contributions of set-shifting to freezing of gait in Parkinson's disease. *Mov. Disord.*, *25*, 8, 1000–1004.

National Institute for Health and Care Excellence, (2017). Biphosphonates for treating osteoporosis (Technology Appraisal Guidance 464). Available at: https://www.nice.org.uk/guidance/ta464 [Accessed 13 July 2020].

National Institute for Health and Care Excellence (2017). Parkinson's Disease in Adults (NICE Guideline 71). Available at: https://www.nice.org.uk/guidance/NG71 [Accessed 13 July, 2020].

National Institute for Health and Care Excellence (2018). Referral to physiotherapy, occupational therapy or speech and language therapy in Parkinson's disease (Quality Standard 164, Quality Statement 3). Available at: https://www.nice.org.uk/guidance/qs164/chapter/quality-statement-3-referral-to-physiotherapy-occupational-therapy-or-speech-and-language-therapy [Accessed 13 July 2020].

Newton, J. L., & Frith, J. (2018). The efficacy of nonpharmacologic intervention for orthostatic hypotension associated with aging. *Neurology, 91*, 7, e652–e656.

Nieuwboer, A. (2015). Cueing effects in Parkinson's disease: Benefits and drawbacks. *Ann. Phys. Rehabil. Med., 58*, e70–e71.

Nieuwboer, A. (2008). Cueing for freezing of gait in patients with Parkinson's disease: A rehabilitation perspective. *Mov. Disord., 23*, S2, S475–S481.

Nieuwboer, A., Baker, K., Willems, A. M., Jones, D., Spildooren, J., Lim, I., Kwakkel, G., Van Wegen, E., & Rochester, L. (2009). The short-term effects of different cueing modalities on turn speed in people with parkinson's disease. *Neurorehabil. Neural Repair, 23*, 8, 831–836.

Nilsson, M. H., Rehncrona, S., & Jarnlo, G. B. (2011). Fear of falling and falls in people with Parkinson's disease treated with deep brain stimulation in the subthalamic nuclei. *Acta Neurol. Scand., 123*, 6, 424–429.

Nutt, J. G., Bloem, B. R., Giladi, N., Hallett, M., Horak, F. B., & Nieuwboer, A. (2011a). Freezing of gait: Moving forward on a mysterious clinical phenomenon. *Lancet Neurol., 10*, 8, 734–744.

Nutt, J. G., Horak, F. B., & Bloem, B. R. (2011b). Milestones in gait, balance, and falling. *Mov. Disord., 26*, 6, 1166–1174.

Okun, M. S., Gallo, B. V., Mandybur, G., Jagid, J., Foote, K. D., Revilla, F. J., Alterman, R., Jankovic, J., Simpson, R., Junn, F., Verhagen, L., Arle, J. E., Ford, B., Goodman, R. R., Stewart, R. M., Horn, S., Baltuch, G. H., Kopell, B. H., Marshall, F., Peichel, D. L., Pahwa, R., Lyons, K. E., Tröster, A. I., Vitek, J. L., & Tagliati, M. (2012). Subthalamic deep brain stimulation with a constant-current device in Parkinson's disease: An open-label randomised controlled trial. *Lancet Neurol., 11*, 2, 140–149.

Owen, C. L., Ibrahim, K., Dennison, L., & Roberts, H. C. (2019). Falls Self-Management Interventions for People with Parkinson's Disease: A Systematic Review. *J. Parkinsons. Dis., 9*, 2, 283–299.

Parkinson, J. (1817). *An essay on the shaking palsy*. London: Sherwood, Neely and Jones.

Paul, S. S., Allen, N. E., Sherrington, C., Heller, G., Fung, V. S. C., Close, J. C. T., Lord, S. R., & Canning, C. G. (2014). Risk factors for frequent falls in people with Parkinson's disease. *J. Parkinsons. Dis., 4*, 4, 699–703.

Pickering, R. M., Grimbergen, Y. A. M., Rigney, U., Ashburn, A., Mazibrada, G., Wood, B., Gray, P., Kerr, G., & Bloem, B. R. (2007). A meta-analysis of six prospective studies of falling in Parkinson's disease. *Mov. Disord., 22*, 13, 1892–1900.

Pieruccini-Faria, F., Jones, J. A., & Almeida, Q. J. (2014). Motor planning in Parkinson's disease patients experiencing freezing of gait: The influence of cognitive load when approaching obstacles. *Brain Cogn., 87*, 76–85.

Pouwels, S., Bazelier, M. T., De Boer, A., Weber, W. E. J., Neef, C., Cooper, C., & De Vries, F. (2013). Risk of fracture in patients with Parkinson's disease. *Osteoporos. Int., 24*, 8, 2283–2290.

Ramirez-Zamora, A., & Ostrem, J. L. (2018). Globus pallidus interna or subthalamic nucleus deep brain stimulation for Parkinson disease: a review. *JAMA Neurol. 75*, 3, 367–372

Reid, I. R., Black, D. M., Eastell, R., Bucci-Rechtweg, C., Su, G., Hue, T. F., Mesenbrink, P., Lyles, K. W., & Boonen, S. (2013). HORIZON Pivotal Fracture Trial and HORIZON Recurrent Fracture Trial Steering Committees. Reduction in the Risk of Clinical Fractures After a Single Dose of Zoledronic Acid 5 Milligrams. *J. Clin. Endocrinol. Metab., 98*, 2, 557–563.

Rochester, L., Galna, B., Lord, S., & Burn, D. (2014). The nature of dual-task interference during gait in incident Parkinson's disease. *Neuroscience, 265*, 83–94.

Rochester, L., Hetherington, V., Jones, D., Nieuwboer, A., Willems, A. M., Kwakkel, G., & Van Wegen, E. (2004). Attending to the task: Interference effects of functional tasks on walking in Parkinson's disease and the roles of cognition, depression, fatigue, and balance. *Arch. Phys. Med. Rehabil., 85*, 10, 1578–1585.

Rock Steady 2000[WWW Document] URL https://www.rocksteadyboxing.org/ (accessed 3.7.20).

Rosano, C., Brach, J., Studenski, S., Longstreth, W. T., & Newman, A. B. (2008). Gait variability is associated with subclinical brain vascular abnormalities in high-functioning older adults. *Neuroepidemiology*, *29*, 3–4, 193–200.

Royal Osteoporosis Society, n.d. Information and support [WWW document]. Retrieved June 30, 2020, from https://theros.org.uk/information-and-support/.

Savica, R., Wennberg, A. M. V., Hagen, C., Edwards, K., Roberts, R. O., Hollman, J. H., Knopman, D. S., Boeve, B. F., Machulda, M. M., Petersen, R. C., & Mielke, M. M. (2017). Comparison of Gait Parameters for Predicting Cognitive Decline: The Mayo Clinic Study of Aging. *J. Alzheimer's Dis.*, *55*, 2, 559–567.

Scientific Advisory Committee on Nutrition. (2016). Vitamin D and Health. *Scientific Advisory Committee on Nutrition*.

Scottish Intercollegiate Guidelines Network. Diagnosis and pharmacological management of Parkinson's disease [pdf]. 2010. National Clinical guideline.

Senard, J. M., Raï, S., Lapeyre-Mestre, M., Brefel, C., Rascol, O., Rascol, A., & Montastruc, J. L. (1997). Prevalence of orthostatic hypotension in Parkinson's disease. *J. Neurol. Neurosurg. Psychiatry*, *63*, 5, 584–589.

Sheehy, T. L., McDonough, M. H., & Zauber, S. E. (2017). Social Comparisons, Social Support, and Self-Perceptions in Group Exercise for People With Parkinson's disease. *J. Appl. Sport Psychol.*, *29*, 3, 285–303.

Shen, X., & Mak, M. K. Y. (2015). Technology-assisted balance and gait training reduces falls in patients with Parkinson's disease: A randomised controlled trial with 12-month follow-up. *Neurorehabil. Neural Repair*, *29*, 2, 103–111.

Sherrington, C., Canning, C., Dean, C., Allen, N., & Blackman, K. (2008). *Weight-bearing Exercise for Better Balance. (WEBB)*.

Siris, E. S., Selby, P. L., Saag, K. G., Borgström, F., Herings, R. M. C., & Silverman, S. L. (2009). Impact of Osteoporosis Treatment Adherence on Fracture Rates in North America and Europe. *Am. J. Med.*, *122*, S3–S13.

Slaug, B., Nilsson, M. H., & Iwarsson, S. (2013). Characteristics of the personal and environmental components of person-environment fit in very old age: A comparison between people with self-reported Parkinson's disease and matched controls. *Aging Clin. Exp. Res.*, *25*, 6, 667–675.

Smith, M. D., Ben-Shlomo, Y., & Henderson, E. (2019). How often are patients with progressive supranuclear palsy really falling? J. *Neurol.*, *266*, 8, 2073–2074.

Spildooren, J., Vinken, C., Van Baekel, L., & Nieuwboer, A. (2019). Turning problems and freezing of gait in Parkinson's disease: a systematic review and meta-analysis. *Disabil. Rehabil.*, *41*, 25, 2994–3004.

St George, R. J., Carlson-Kuhta, P., Burchiel, K. J., Hogarth, P., Frank, N., & Horak, F. B. (2012). The effects of subthalamic and pallidal deep brain stimulation on postural responses in patients with Parkinson disease. *J. Neurosurg.*, *116*, 6, 1347–1356.

Tai Chi Health Institute, 2018. History of Tai Chi [WWW Document]. URL https://taichiforhealth-institute.org/history-of-tai-chi-2/ (accessed 6.10.20).

Taylor, D., Hale, L., Schluter, P., Waters, D. L., Binns, E. E., McCracken, H., McPherson, K., & Wolf, S. L. (2012). Effectiveness of tai chi as a community-based falls prevention intervention: A randomised controlled trial. *J. Am. Geriatr. Soc.*, *60*, 5, 841–848.

Testa, D., Monza, D., Ferrarini, M., Soliveri, P., Girotti, F., & Filippini, G. (2001). Comparison of natural histories of progressive supranuclear palsy and multiple system atrophy. *Neurol. Sci.*, *22*, 3, 247–251.

Thaut, M. H., Rice, R. R., Braun Janzen, T., Hurt-Thaut, C. P., & McIntosh, G. C. (2019). Rhythmic auditory stimulation for reduction of falls in Parkinson's disease: a randomised controlled study. *Clin. Rehabil.*, *33*, 1, 34–43.

The Consensus Committee of the American Autonomic Society and the American Academy of Neurology. (1996). Consensus statement on the definition of orthostatic hypotension, pure autonomic failure, and multiple system atrophy. *Neurology*, *46*, 5, 1470–11470.

Thevathasan, W., Debu, B., Aziz, T., Bloem, B. R., Blahak, C., Butson, C., Czernecki, V., Foltynie, T., Fraix, V., Grabli, D., Joint, C., Lozano, A. M., Okun, M. S., Ostrem, J., Pavese, N., Schrader, C., Tai, C. H., Krauss, J. K., & Moro, E. (2018). Pedunculopontine nucleus deep brain stimulation in Parkinson's disease: A clinical review. *Mov. Disord.*, *33*, 1, 10–20.

Tomlinson, C. L., Patel, S., Meek, C., Clarke, C. E., Stowe, R., Shah, L., Sackley, C. M., Deane, K. H., Herd, C. P., Wheatley, K., & Ives, N. (2012). Physiotherapy versus placebo or no intervention in Parkinson's disease (Review). *Cochrane Libr.*, 9, 1–101.

Torsney, K. M., Noyce, A. J., Doherty, K. M., Bestwick, J. P., Dobson, R., & Lees, A. J. (2014). Bone health in Parkinson's disease: a systematic review and meta-analysis. *J Neurol Neurosurg Psychiatry*, *85*, 10, 1159–1166.

Van Den Bos, F., Speelman, A. D., Samson, M., Munneke, M., Bloem, B. R., & Verhaar, H. J. J. (2013). Parkinson's disease and osteoporosis. *Age Ageing*, *42*, 2, 156–162.

Van der Kolk, N. M., de Vries, N. M., Kessels, R. P. C., Joosten, H., Zwinderman, A. H., Post, B., & Bloem, B. R. (2019). Effectiveness of home-based and remotely supervised aerobic exercise in Parkinson's disease: a double-blind, randomised controlled trial. *Lancet Neurol.*, *18*, 11, 998–1008.

van der Marck, M. A., Klok, M. P. C. C., Okun, M. S., Giladi, N., Munneke, M., Bloem, B. R., Arney, K., Browner, N. M., Caunter, M., Cianci, H. J., Dunlop, B., Eggert, K., Fisher, B., Hass, C. J., Hunter, C., Jabre, M., Kraakevik, J., Lyons, K. E., Phibbs, F., Scott, B. L., Shih, L., Tan, E. K., Tan, L., Varanese, S., Voss, T., Ashburn, A., Ballinger, C., Bhatti, M. T., Hausdorff, J., Lindvall, S., Morris, M. E., Nieuwboer, A., Schwalb, J. M., Studenski, S., & Wood, B. H. (2014). Consensus-based clinical practice recommendations for the examination and management of falls in patients with Parkinson's disease. *Park. Relat. Disord.*, *20*, 4, 360–369.

van Wegen, E., de Goede, C., Lim, I., Rietberg, M., Nieuwboer, A., Willems, A., Jones, D., Rochester, L., Hetherington, V., Berendse, H., Zijlmans, J., Wolters, E., & Kwakkel, G. (2006). The effect of rhythmic somatosensory cueing on gait in patients with Parkinson's disease. *J. Neurol. Sci.*, *248*, 1–2, 210–214.

Vanacore, N., Bonifati, V., Fabbrini, G., Colosimo, C., De Michele, G., Marconi, R., Nicholl, D., Locuratolo, N., Talarico, G., Romano, S., Stocchi, F., Bonuccelli, U., De Mari, M., Vieregge, P., & Meco, G. (2001). Epidemiology of multiple system atrophy. *Neurol. Sci.*, *22*, 1, 97–99.

Vaugoyeau, M., & Azulay, J. P. (2010). Role of sensory information in the control of postural orientation in Parkinson's disease. *J. Neurol. Sci.*, *289*, 1–2, 66–68.

Velseboer, D. C., de Haan, R. J., Wieling, W., Goldstein, D. S., & de Bie, R. M. A. (2011). Prevalence of orthostatic hypotension in Parkinson's disease: A systematic review and meta-analysis. *Park. Relat. Disord.*, *17*, 10, 724–729.

Vercruysse, S., Gilat, M., Shine, J. M., Heremans, E., Lewis, S., & Nieuwboer, A. (2014). Freezing beyond gait in Parkinson's disease: A review of current neurobehavioural evidence. *Neurosci. Biobehav. Rev.*, *43*, 213–227.

Volpe, D., Giantin, M. G., Maestri, R., & Frazzitta, G. (2014). Comparing the effects of hydrotherapy and land-based therapy on balance in patients with Parkinson's disease: A randomised controlled pilot study. *Clin. Rehabil.*, *28*, 12, 1210–1217.

Walker, R. W., Chaplin, A., Hancock, R. L., Rutherford, R., & Gray, W. K. (2013). Hip fractures in people with idiopathic Parkinson's disease: Incidence and outcomes. *Mov. Disord.*, *28*, 3, 334–340.

Walker, R. W., Palmer, J., Stancliffe, J., Wood, B. H., Hand, A., & Gray, W. K. (2014). Experience of care home residents with Parkinson's disease: Reason for admission and service use. *Geriatr. Gerontol. Int.*, *14*, 4, 947–953.

Weil, R. S., Schrag, A. E., Warren, J. D., Crutch, S. J., Lees, A. J., & Morris, H. R. (2016). Visual dysfunction in Parkinson's disease. *Brain*, *139*, 11, 2827–2843.

What exactly is PD Warrior? - PD Warrior [WWW Document]. URL https://pdwarrior.com/exactly-pd-warrior/ (accessed 3.7.20).

Wielinski, C. L., Erickson-Davis, C., Wichmann, R., Walde-Douglas, M., & Parashos, S. A. (2005). Falls and injuries resulting from falls among patients with Parkinson's disease and other Parkinsonian syndromes. *Mov. Disord.*, *20*, 4, 410–415.

Witt, I., Ganjavi, H., & Macdonald, P. (2019). Relationship between freezing of gait and anxiety in parkinson's disease patients: a systemic literature review. *Parkinsons. Dis.*, 2019.

Wong-Yu, I. S. K., & Mak, M. K. Y. (2019). Multisystem Balance Training Reduces Injurious Fall Risk in Parkinson's Disease. *Am. J. Phys. Med. Rehabil.*, *98*, 3, 239–244.

Yarnall, A. J., Rochester, L., Baker, M. R., David, R., Khoo, T. K., Duncan, G. W., Galna, B., & Burn, D. J. (2013). Short latency afferent inhibition: A biomarker for mild cognitive impairment in Parkinson's disease? *Mov. Disord.*, *28*, 9, 1285–1288.

Chapter 11

Exercise in Parkinson's

Bhanu Ramaswamy, Julie Jones and Katherine Baker

Chapter outline

Introduction

Most people want to stay physically active for as long as possible, whether or not they have Parkinson's, and research suggests that people who exercise at moderate intensity at least three times a week have less risk of developing the condition than those who do not exercise throughout their lives (LaHue et al., 2016). However, for people with Parkinson's, exercise is as vital as taking medication.

Pharmacological management remains the mainstay of intervention for many Parkinson's symptoms, but this neither targets underlying pathological processes nor limits the progression of the condition. Exercise has been shown to benefit motor and non-motor symptoms, and evidence suggests that exercise may also slow the progression of Parkinson's through varied neuroprotective mechanisms at the cellular level, resulting in lower mortality risk (Ellis & Rochester, 2018; Keus et al., 2014; LaHue et al., 2016). Although there are known negative side effects to taking medication, there are no known adverse effects to taking exercise.

All members of the multidisciplinary team (MDT) should understand the benefits of physical activity (PA) and exercise for people with Parkinson's, so that they can encourage individuals to improve their health while also reducing deconditioning effects. This may include signposting to local community exercise groups.

The terms *physical activity* and *exercise* are used interchangeably in health, sport, and leisure settings, although there are distinct differences. It is important for professionals to understand the difference so that they can discuss the importance of staying active in relation to Parkinson's and set appropriate goals. The following definitions are used in this chapter:

Physical activity (PA) refers to movement produced by skeletal muscle expending energy. PA is behaviour-driven and includes daily routines such as moving around the kitchen to prepare a meal, walking to and around the shops, or gardening. Introducing PA as a means of staying active, getting active, or keeping fit and healthy is a good starting point for people who are not already exercising but who want to remain active (Keus et al., 2014).

Exercise is structured PA and includes goals that target a specific aspect of health and builds on fitness components such as strength or balance. It is performance-driven activity aimed at maintaining or improving movement.

Exercise interventions delivered by health professionals are mainly designed to improve specific aspects of an individual's clinical performance. This includes targeting strength and flexibility to improve chair or bed transfers, gait-specific exercise to improve walking and reduce falls risk, and balance and strength programmes for safety when mobilising, particularly with regard to climbing and descending stairs, which is especially important for hospitalised individuals prior to discharge home.

Research informs our understanding of the mechanisms and benefits of exercise, providing the scientific basis for different exercise strategies used in the management of people with Parkinson's. For instance, a programme planned to benefit an individual with a bradykinetic-rigid presentation of Parkinson's will be different from one planned for a person with tremor-dominant Parkinson's. Some exercise styles target changes to muscles, soft tissue and joints, aiming to improve posture and balance, while others may focus on breathing, communication, and swallowing; or they may target non-motor symptoms (NMS), such as those involving sleep or mood.

Discussions with individuals about exercise should explore different ways and places to exercise (at home, in the gym, or outdoors), in company or alone. It is also important to stress that, along with physical improvements, exercise can have cognitive and emotional benefits.

This chapter describes the evidence for the benefits of PA and exercise. It explores recommended exercise prescriptions as well as barriers and motivators to exercise for individuals with Parkinson's, addressing this for the different stages of the condition:

1. At diagnosis: when it is important to encourage and enable uptake or increase of exercise from the outset
2. Maintenance stage: when general PA and exercise advice is required to keep the person fit and active for as long as possible
3. Complex and palliative stage: when exercise is aimed at the performance of functional activities

The chapter concludes with resources for professionals and signposting suggestions.

Evidence for the benefits of exercise

Exercise should be an integral component of Parkinson's management, of equal importance to medication rather than only complementary (Keus et al., 2014).

Specific areas addressed in recent research include training for gait, strength, aerobic capacity, balance, and combating Parkinson's-specific symptoms with power and amplitude (large movement) training (Radder et al., 2020).

The optimal type and dosage of exercise remain underdetermined from systematic reviews (SRs), as aims and objectives of trials vary and include physical improvement, improvement in mental health (including cognition), and the promotion of social inclusion. The different types of exercise and assorted outcome measures researched make it difficult to compare studies and draw robust conclusions.

We have therefore based this chapter's recommendations on the European Physiotherapy Guideline for Parkinson's Disease (Keus et al., 2014), relevant studies published since the guideline—including SRs, meta-analyses, and theoretical reviews—and an exercise framework resource developed for health professionals (Parkinson's UK, 2017).

Earlier chapters have detailed the key motor and NMS associated with Parkinson's and how manifestations of the symptoms differ between individuals. A personalised approach to managing symptoms also enables the exploration of the particular physical activities that interest the individual and what would keep them motivated to exercise as far through the course of Parkinson's as possible.

Impact of reduced activity and effects of exercise on symptoms

Most research focuses on the motor symptom effects of exercise (Keus et al., 2014; Radder et al.; 2020). Over time, bradykinesia can compromise joint range of movement and strength, and the combined effects of rigidity and tremor further limit flexibility. All changes alter the biomechanics of movement, leading to movement dysfunction and impaired balance. Collectively, these symptoms reduce PA levels, which may lead to muscle atrophy, joint stiffness, and reduced physical capacity. Progression of the condition manifests as greater complexity in symptom development as well as reduced physical capacity and mobility, which in turn underpin inactivity.

The cycle of deterioration is affected by a range of other pathologies and NMS, including apathy, fatigue, anxiety, pain and fear of falling. These contribute to further muscle weakness or shortening, balance dysfunction, reduced aerobic capacity and functional performance, social isolation and reduced participation in activity (Figure 11.1).

Several literature reviews into exercise benefits for motor symptoms (Bouça-Machado et al., 2019; Ellis & Rochester, 2018; Keus et al., 2014; Oliveira de Carvalho et al., 2018; Radder et al., 2020) indicate that regular exercise correlates with the improvement of motor symptoms. Specific improvements are cited in strength, balance, gait and function, each reducing the risk for falls. Improvements were also seen regardless of whether exercise was done individually or as part of a group.

These reviews showed that regular exercise (varied styles) additionally reduced fatigue, apathy, depression, insomnia and constipation. Exercise-related improvements have also been reported in global cognitive function, processing speed, sustained attention and mental flexibility in people with Parkinson's (da Silva et al., 2018; Paul et al., 2019).

Owing to the diversity of symptoms, an individualised, varied, and progressive approach to exercise prescription is required in order to maintain or achieve the full benefits for health and reduce premature mortality (Table 11.1).

Neurophysiological benefits of exercise

Aerobic exercise performed at the correct intensity is reported to attenuate Parkinson's symptoms through disease-modifying effects that delay underlying pathological processes and improve motor symptoms and NMS (Ahlskog, 2018; Ellis & Rochester, 2018; Hirsch et al., 2018; Oliveira de Carvalho et al., 2018). Most of our current knowledge comes from animal research, but the effects of exercise are being replicated in small-sample studies of people with Parkinson's and are showing similar effects (Ellis & Rochester, 2018; Hirsch et al., 2018; LaHue et al., 2016). The possible mechanisms discussed in these papers include exercise-associated inducements of structural adaptation within the brain, leading to widespread neuro-molecular changes including the following:

- Improved vascularisation and angiogenesis (the formation of new blood vessels)
- Increased levels of proteins associated with the promotion of dopaminergic neuron survival, such as brain- or glial-derived neurotropic factors (BDNFs or GDNFs)
- Transmission through improved synaptogenesis (formation or strengthening of neuronal junctions to pass electrical or chemical signals onward)

The consequences of these enhanced mechanisms are seen in reduced neuroinflammation, aiding overall brain health, and, more specifically for people with

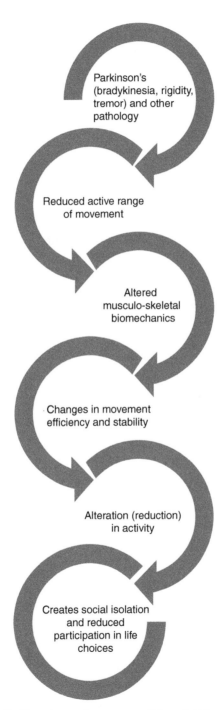

FIGURE 11.1   How Parkinson's symptoms can result in reduced movement and reduced activity

TABLE 11.1 Benefits of exercise in Parkinson's

Target of exercise	Effective exercise style
Improvement in motor symptoms	
Bradykinesia and rigidity	Large-amplitude and power movements
Tremor	Stretching or body-weighted activity through hands (e.g. cycling, which may have a possibly short-lived effect)
Postural instability	Resistance training and balance work (e.g., exercises to prevent falls)
Reduction in falls risk	Strength and balance exercises and exercises targeting functional activities
Improvement in non-motor symptoms	
Fatigue, apathy, depression, insomnia and constipation	Aerobic exercise and social styles of exercise (e.g. walking, dance, tai chi and yoga)
Neurophysiologic changes	
Synaptogenesis Angiogenesis Dopamine system changes • Reduced dopamine loss • Preserved or restored terminals • Increased neurotrophic factors • Improved increased dopamine turnover • Dopaminergic neurone survival	Aerobic exercise at a vigorous intensity and in large amounts

Parkinson's, improvements in how dopamine is preserved and used (Ellis & Rochester, 2018).

The direct impact and benefits of exercise on the underlying condition is therefore suggestive of a neuroprotective role, which either inhibits the degenerative effect (as from oxidative stress or mitochondrial dysfunction) on the nervous system or enhances regenerative effects. The terms often used to describe these two effects are *neuroprotection* and *neurorestoration*. In view of the time-limited benefits of medication, they present an exciting prospect.

Types of physical activity and exercise beneficial in Parkinson's

Regardless of the type exercise must be motivating for the individual, which means fun for some, social inclusion for others, or just the satisfaction of having done exercise that helps attain a specific (personal) goal; this is another reason why exercise recommendations should be individualised.

Selecting the most appropriate exercise for each individual also requires an understanding of the challenges involved in the way people move. Most physical tasks combine several fitness components; for example, rising from a seated position, which requires flexibility, strength and balance. Much exercise research is therefore based on the delivery of a multimodal exercise programme. The "one size fits all" approach is unlikely to be effective for the needs of a particular individual who requires a tailored approach (Ellis & Rochester, 2018).

It is recommended that people with Parkinson's should undertake five different types of exercise: strength, balance, aerobic/endurance, flexibility and function-based exercise (Keus et al., 2014). Symptom diversity means that research cannot conclusively define the optimal exercise type or dose; therefore recommendations have been informed by the results of research, anecdotal information from exercisers with Parkinson's, and input from professionals who prescribe exercise.

As an example, Table 11.2 shows three exercise types relevant to people with Parkinson's: muscle strength, balance and aerobic effects. Prescribers of exercise should understand that all exercise requires an element of cognitive input from the person with Parkinson's, which includes planning and coordinating the movement sequence and remembering how to use the equipment safely.

Compared with research trials that often study one exercise type or style, in practice individual exercises are combined to achieve the physical ability to perform a task (muscular strength, power, and endurance-related attributes), to carry it out safely (balance attributes) and in a state of good health (cardiovascular and metabolic attributes) in an environment to motivate the person to keep exercising.

A large number of studies into the types of exercise available for people with Parkinson's have been undertaken. Many are small in scale, but all are available to the reader via a simple database search. Table 11.3 summarises the types of activity that have research evidence in Parkinson's as well as popular exercise styles and classes that people with Parkinson's can take up. It is not a comprehensive list; online forums for people with Parkinson's include comments from individuals sharing experiences of the positive benefits of exercise as diverse as acrobatics, gymnastics and body popping!

Cycling. Studies included static or dynamic and tandem cycling (where the rider with Parkinson's was forced by the rider without Parkinson's to increase the pedaling rate). Individuals who freeze when walking tend not to freeze when cycling. Cycling gave short-term improvements in tremor, gait speed, and the ability to plan and organise.

Walking, but not running, resulted in improvements in motor symptoms, balance, quality of life (QoL), and (not surprisingly) walking itself. This was whether on a treadmill, which also improved cognitive function when conducted for longer periods, or using styles such as Nordic Walking.

Dance is popular and can be fast paced (Zumba Gold) or slower. It can be more creative (balletic) or partnered (ballroom or square dancing); it addresses

TABLE 11.2 Specific exercise styles: insights from research

Muscle strength, power, and endurance

Exercises that make the muscle work harder than usual are required to build tissue and improve endurance. Exercises against resistance are such an example.

Evidence from research

- Strength and power training is well tolerated in people with mild to moderate Parkinson's.
- It improves both physical function and quality of life. Specific benefits include increased strength, reduced cardiovascular stress while lifting and carrying a given weight, and increased muscular endurance during work or play.

Balance

Exercises to improve the control of the body over its base of support helps to achieve postural equilibrium and orientation.

Evidence from research

- Specific balance exercise has been shown to improve the performance of balance tasks, such as improved stability for steady standing tasks (static balance), dynamic balance anticipating perturbation, or responding to changes in surfaces underfoot.
- It remains unclear if balance exercises reduce falls or improve quality of life.

Aerobic exercise

Aerobic exercise is activity using large muscle groups that can be maintained continuously and is rhythmic in nature (Riebe et al., 2018). The exercise should stimulate a faster heart and breathing rate to sustain the demand. This exercise component is also called cardiovascular or cardiorespiratory endurance.

Evidence from research

- Aerobic exercise, especially through endurance training, is associated with positive cardiovascular effects, including lowering of the resting heart rate and blood pressure, better responses to increases in submaximal activity, improvements in muscle oxygen delivery systems and toxin extraction capacities and the reduction of atherogenic risk factors.
- Reduced metabolic risk by enhancing glycaemic control and lipid profile.

Adapted from (Bouça-Machado et al., 2019; Ellis & Rochester, 2018; Keus et al., 2014; Oliveira de Carvalho et al., 2018; Radder et al., 2020)

balance, endurance, speed and aerobic exercise. All dance forms improved motor and NMS and QoL. As a social form of exercise, dance is considered a leisure (for pleasure) activity rather than sport.

Exergaming: Evidence for exercise-based computer games (exergaming) as a rehabilitation tool for people with Parkinson's is growing. A SR of commercial games (Nintendo Wii Fit™ and Microsoft Kinect™) designed for home use (Garcia-Agundez et al., 2019) showed that slower, less complex games were safe for participants. People enjoyed the games, their gameplay performance improved, and the literature concluded that exergaming could be useful for rehabilitating motor skills in people with Parkinson's. This is resulting in the development of tailored games that are safe and practical for people with Parkinson's to use in rehabilitation and home settings.

TABLE 11.3 Examples of activity and dose taken up by people with Parkinson's

Exercise type	Recommended dose	Researched examples
Balance	One to three times a week	Specific balance class Tai chi Gaming consoles
Endurance—cardiorespiratory and muscular	150 minutes total per week at moderate intensity (e.g. 30 minutes five times a week); OR 75 minutes vigorous intensity	Aerobic classes Jog/run Swimming Cycling Nordic walking
Flexibility—including amplitude training	Two to three times a week	Yoga Pilates Stretching/posture classes
Function-based, specific to Parkinson's	Daily	Chair stands Rolling in bed Stair practice PD Warrior PWR!
Strength	Twice a week	Weight/resistance training Boxing training Circuit class

Parkinson's-specific programmes are multimodal programmes that target power and amplitude of movement to recalibrate bradykinetic (slow) and hypokinetic (small) movement. These use complex and exaggerated physical movements such as arm- swing or high stepping as well as strength and flexibility to improve control, the fluidity of movement responses, coordination and speed. They also include activities that challenge cognition (e.g., counting, naming, and listing tasks while doing the physical exercise) to encourage the ability to carry out more than one task at a time (dual- or multitasking) for as long as possible. For those who experience on/off problems or freezing, addressing falls risk with movement strategies can improve safety. Examples of such programmes include the following:

- LSVT-BIG (Lee Silverman Voice Therapy for movement): Amplitude-oriented training (large movements in set activities) was effective in reducing motor impairments for people with mild Parkinson's (McDonnell et al., 2017).
- HiBalance programme: Improved stability (Joseph et al., 2018).
- Boxing: Improved fitness and function (from the Rock Steady Boxing programme) (Larson et al., 2021) (Combs et al., 2013).
- PD Warrior (McConaghy, 2015) and Parkinson's Wellness and Recovery (PWR!). Although large communities of people follow the programme, there are no published evaluations.

Exercise Environment

Traditionally, exercise intervention has been delivered on a 1:1 basis or in a group format.

However, exercise programmes are increasingly available online through downloadable printed exercise sheets, video classes (live or recorded) and online programmes. Technology offers many advantages, allowing exercise to be undertaken at a convenient time and enabling novice exercisers to develop self-efficacy with exercise prior to considering participation in a wider group. Technology may also provide opportunities for exercise when accessibility to groups is challenging, such as for those in remote and rural areas or during times of holidays, poor weather or pandemic-related lockdown.

The use of technology may also offer opportunities for exercise participation to be monitored through fitness apps on smartphones and watches. These can be motivational and promote behaviour change, encouraging self-management (Dobkin, 2017). The area of artificial intelligence is also growing, evolving to help individuals progress their goals once they have achieved a programmed objective.

However, the provision of online exercise programmes offers less opportunity for socialisation and the development of a sense of community, which is clearly a valued component of group exercise for people with Parkinson's and their caregivers (Hunter et al., 2019).

Areas to Target for Exercise

It is important for therapists to be aware of which key body areas to focus on. The body areas in Figure 11.2 are involved in everyday tasks with which many people with Parkinson's report having difficulty. These include rolling or getting out of bed, washing and dressing (may be slow, off balance, poor flexibility), preparing meals, shopping, gardening and performing leisure activities. As with all the exercise examples in the table, a tailored approach is required so that the safest option can be selected for those who are less steady or are exercising in a seated position.

Regular reviews of the exercise prescription should be carried out and changes made to take account of aging, comorbidities and the progression of Parkinson's.

Barriers and motivators to exercise

Although some people with Parkinson's use exercise as a regular part of their routine for managing their condition, many do not have an exercise habit and find it challenging to start or maintain an exercise programme. There are many reasons why exercise does not happen regularly enough (Keus et al., 2014) (Schootmeijer et al., 2020), most of which can be addressed with help from health and exercise professionals (Table 11.4).

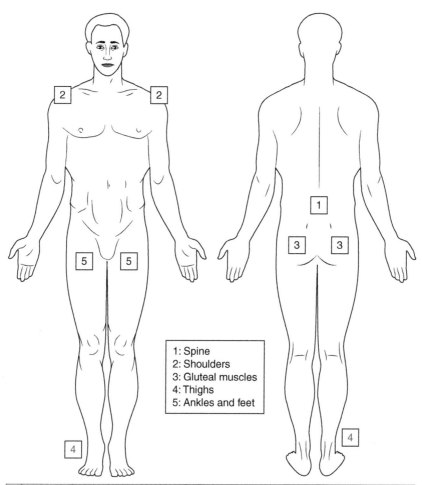

	Area	Rationale	Exercise recommendations
1.	**Spine**	Stiffness in the spine is a regularly reported symptom.	• Exercises for lower back stiffness include rotational spinal twists, side bends and lower spine stretches to regain flexibility (e.g., pelvic tilting with Pilates and stretches from yoga poses; both of which then progress to work up the whole spine). • If stiffness reduces the range of movement, consider exercises of the large-amplitude type, exaggerating the movement to return the movement to near-normal range. • If stiffness affects function, target the actual function. For example, tasks such as turning to look over one's shoulder (especially important for drivers), rolling over in bed, sitting up from lying, and reaching for objects to the side or on the ground.

FIGURE 11.2   Key body areas and examples of exercises to focus on

FIGURE 11.2   *(Cont.)*

	Area	Rationale	Exercise recommendations
2.	**Shoulders**	Many individuals are diagnosed with a frozen shoulder years before they are diagnosed with Parkinson's, most probably due to unrecognised tonal changes.	• Stiffness restricting movement at the shoulders and trunk can contribute to early loss of arm swing; therefore, exercises to loosen the shoulder girdle area are required. Examples include shoulder rolls and wide arm stretches, pulling the shoulder blades into retraction. • Arm extension can be a compensation for a forward stoop where the shoulder girdle, chest and hip/lower back areas are not kept active. Large movements through the range are recommended. For example: going from a squat into full toe raise, arms elevated. • Shoulder rolls are particularly useful for the shrugging action of putting on a coat, lifting the arms to hang out washing and reaching up into cupboards.
3.	**Gluteal or bottom muscles**	These provide stability around the hips and pelvis and are essential for tasks such as getting out of a chair, staying upright and stable when walking, as well as maintaining balance when moving around.	• Select functional exercises such as straight sit to stand and step climbing or a specific exercise set, such as a backward lunge with body upright.
4.	**Thighs**	Thigh muscle strength is vital for functional tasks such as sit to stand, stair climbing and walking. Strong muscles provide stability around the knee, providing steadiness when moving in upright positions.	• Gluteal workouts, as described earlier, done in the upright position will also work the thighs. • For seated exercises, the use of ankle weights for knee straightening is a good starting point.
5.	**Ankles and feet**	Keeping ankle joints strong and feet flexible is essential, as they help to maintain balance when the foot is on the ground, adapting to the terrain and keeping the body steady over the foot. Flexibility and stability of the numerous joints and timely recruitment of the muscles of the ankles and feet ensure foot clearance.	• Exercises to strengthen the anterior shin muscles for dorsiflexion are recommended. • Propulsive forces are required for forward walking; therefore controlled heel raises should be included.

TABLE 11.4 The main barriers to exercise, with possible management strategies

Barriers	Possible management strategies
Personal physical barriers	
1. Existing health problems including pain 2. Lack of energy 3. Parkinson's symptoms, including freezing episodes, or on/off phenomenon	**1 and 2:** Seek support from a health professional to guide how to manage the combination of problems experienced. May need referral to a professional qualified in motivational interviewing (MI) or cognitive behavioural therapies (CBT) or a clinical neuropsychologist **3:** Timing exercise when medication is at optimal level. Seek a physiotherapist to guide on the most effective exercise for current needs.
Personal mental barriers	
1. Fear of injury or pain 2. Perceived lack of time 3. Lack of will power 4. Lack of company 5. Cognitive changes, therefore difficult or daunting using equipment 6. Negative experience or attitude to exercise	**1:** May improve when medication for Parkinson's is optimal and analgesia taken in preparation for exercise. A physiotherapist can advise on the most effective exercise for current needs or a professional with MI or CBT qualifications may be of help. **2:** Use a diary to monitor issues with barriers. Establishing a daily routine can help identify when time for exercise might be available **3, 4, 5 and 6:** May require another person to be an external motivator and support, (friend, family or a professional such as a personal trainer). Monitor ability (e.g., with a fitness app).
Practical barriers	
1. Lack of time 2. Lack of local service 3. Lack of resources such as financial constraints 4. Adverse weather (too hot, cold or icy) 5. Difficult to get transport to exercise space	**1:** Consider a more vigorous approach, so that the person can spend less time on exercise; consider short-session exercise "snacks" (10 minutes). **2 and 3:** Consider online exercise resources (video, YouTube, exergaming (e.g., Wii or Kinnect). The exercise professional may run his or her own online classes. Many classes are free of charge and require no equipment. **4 and 5:** Have varied options such as plan A, B, and C for weather, mood, or when the body not as responsive; this may be a lift in a car to get to the exercise class.
Skill-related barriers	
1. Not in the habit 2. Does not know where to start 3. Unused to gym-based exercise equipment 4. Has cognitive impairment 5. Realises that the trainer lacks knowledge about Parkinson's	**1.** Start regular short walks in company to walk around the block or local park. Some might try a weekly class, but not all individuals enjoy groups. **2.** Seek professional input to explore the exercise framework suggestions. **3.** Look at alternatives for home exercise, exercising locally with friends, taking up an outdoor sport, or going with a personal trainer to learn the use of gym-type equipment. **4.** Seek support from another to help explain, set up, or exercise alongside the person (a professional, family member, or friend). Attend a class that can manage changes to cognition and alter or slow the exercise for the individual's needs.

Adults in the general population cite many barriers to exercise including these:

- Issues relating to their health
- Lack of interest
- Weakness
- Fear of falls and injury
- Pain
- Adverse weather
- Limited access to exercise resources

In addition to these, individuals with Parkinson's report low outcome expectations, lack of time, and fear of falling as most associated with reduced or absent exercise behaviour (Ellis et al., 2013). In studies of motivation, people with Parkinson's have also been shown to be more apathetic than controls, putting in the least effort for the lowest reward (Chong et al., 2015).

Motivation to take up exercise for the first time or to target exercise that is specific to individual need should start at the point of diagnosis, with recommendations to be active included from the outset by the neurologist or geriatrician and the Parkinson's disease nurse specialist. For more detailed conversations about activity and exercise, a referral can be made to a physiotherapist or exercise professional, preferably one with skills in motivational interviewing (McGrane et al., 2015; Miller & Rose, 2009). This is a directive and person-centred counseling approach that can enable behaviour change through the exploration and resolution of ambivalence—in this case, with regard to exercise.

Understanding what can motivate an individual is important. The motivators that encourage people to exercise and the barriers to being active and engaging in exercise are personal. They are dependent on individual circumstances, preferences, and opportunities and should be addressed on an individual basis.

Having another person present who can provide motivation is often helpful. In the first instance, this may be the physician at the point of diagnosis, advocating exercise, but it could also be the therapist setting the exercises or the carer or friend encouraging them. Peer recommendation, such as from the local Parkinson's group, is also an important factor (Chong et al., 2015; Ramaswamy et al., 2018).

Improving outcomes for both motor symptoms and NMS is another significant motivator. Individuals with Parkinson's who participate in exercise often report benefits that exceed the initial fitness outcomes. For example, over time, they might realise that their sleep quality has improved, they are less anxious, or their mood has improved. These subjective outcomes are not always recorded in research but are noted as anecdotes when individuals are chatting at the end of an exercise session. Exercise, particularly in groups, also offers additional social benefits such as feelings of belonging, a shared experience, camaraderie and being part of a community. This results in an enhanced sense of "taking control" among the individuals with Parkinson's as well as their caregivers (Claesson et al., 2019; Hunter et al., 2019).

These and other studies into motivation emphasise the importance of facilitating exercise programmes that are enjoyable, safe and address balance and fear of falling. In addition, programmes should aim to include social engagement and social support, both in rehabilitation and in-home settings (Claesson et al., 2019; Garcia-Agundez et al., 2019; Hunter et al., 2019). It is recommended that exercise should be scheduled shortly after medication administration when dopamine levels are highest, as these have an effect on motivation as well as on mobility.

The main barriers to exercise and suggestions for countering them are tabulated in Table 11.4.

Prescribing exercise

An exercise programme should comprise several components combined to suit the individual's needs, and all of them should be taken into consideration. The **exercise prescription** follows the FITT principles—frequency, intensity, type, and time (duration) of exercise. These are underpinned by the **training principles:** specificity, overload, progression, variance and reversibility.

Current guidelines and activity level recommendations exist for the adult population (UK Chief Medical Officers, 2019); they are appropriate for people with Parkinson's. This section of the chapter discusses only principles with Parkinson's-specific aspects that add to or differ from information provided for the general adult population. The UK Parkinson's Exercise Framework (Parkinson's UK, 2017) has been developed with these principles in mind (Table 11.7).

FITT principles

Frequency

It is recommended that people with Parkinson's, especially those new to exercise, work toward being able to achieve the following:

- Moderate or vigorous aerobic exercise, 30 minutes, five times a week
- Progressive resistance exercise, two to three times a week
- Parkinson's-specific exercise two to four times a week up to daily, depending on the goal

The exercise programme prescribed by a therapist will usually have functional elements focusing on managing motor symptoms. These may include the practice of sit to stand (10 repetitions, three times a day) to enable getting out of a chair more easily, or they may address standing posture, suggesting standing against a kitchen door for the time it takes for the kettle to boil, to reduce neck and low back pain. Such exercises often address issues directly related to how the individual manages activities of daily living.

Intensity

Intensity is described using the same terminology as that set out in the UK Chief Medical Officers' 2019 guidance: sedentary, light, moderate, vigorous or very vigorous.

Recent research has focused on the intensity of exercise training for people with Parkinson's because higher intensity (vigorous and very vigorous) programmes have shown possible disease-modifying effects. The more challenging balance programmes also show better results for falls-risk reduction compared with those that are less challenging.

The optimal exercise level required to influence Parkinson's at a neurophysiological? level has not yet been determined, but current research suggests that aerobic exercise delivered at 60% to 80% of maximal heart rate achieves the best outcomes. (Schenkman et al., 2018) Assessing intensity is complex, as exercise can be physically and/or cognitively demanding. Most individuals will not have access to equipment for measuring intensity, so they should be advised to use measures such as the following:

- The Borg Scale of Rate of Perceived Exertion (RPE), aiming for RPE of around 13/20 for 30 minutes per session, building up to five sessions a week
- Self-rating the exercise as easy, just right, and too hard
- Understanding that the effort they apply means that they should not be able to speak in full sentences while exercising

Like any other skill, it takes time to learn to exercise at higher intensities. A large proportion of people with Parkinson's are classified as sedentary, even from diagnosis, so enrolling in a high-intensity programme might initially be too daunting, putting them off exercise completely. There may also be a risk of injury if they begin with higher-intensity exercises. For such individuals a graded approach, working toward a higher intensity, is advisable.

Type and time (duration)

Earlier in this chapter we discussed type of exercise. In setting duration of a programme, multiple factors require consideration, including comorbidities, exercise history, physical ability, and access to exercise facilities or equipment.

Ultimately, the goal should be to work toward being comfortable and confident to exercise for a minimum of 30 minutes per session. However, in working with exercise novices, "exercise snacking" (small bouts of exercise that do not require a warm-up), may be desirable to build self-efficacy (belief in their ability to do the exercise) and confidence with exercise.

Training principles

Specificity means that the exercise should be relevant or related to the task the individual needs to improve.

For example, gym-based studies have established that people with Parkinson's demonstrate the same capacity for muscle hypertrophy as healthy controls, yet improved leg strength gained using a resistance machine may not result in improved walking or balance.

Similarly, using the treadmill has not consistently resulted in improvements in walking off the treadmill, although one study using both a treadmill and a virtual reality programme over 6 months of training has shown a reduced incidence of falls (Mirelman et al., 2016).

For those with cognitive and motor learning difficulties, a lack of familiarity with gym-based equipment can impair the training effect. For them, functional or task-specific training, combined with specific types of exercise—for instance, strength training—is more likely to result in improved functional ability.

Overload, progression, variance, and reversibility

Studies into the principles of overload (where the body is worked at a greater intensity than normal to improve fitness), progression, variance and reversibility do not currently provide consistent evidence of their benefits.

As most trials are only run for short periods, little is known about the principle of progression specifically in Parkinson's. Recommendations on how to progress the exercise would therefore be the same as for any adults undertaking exercise.

Discussions between health and exercise professionals on Parkinson's research sites (Table 11.6) provide pragmatic insight into the following issues regarding all exercise principles and their consideration alongside individual lifestyles and symptoms:

- Parkinson's motor symptoms can put individuals at higher risk of injury when exercising "cold," therefore care should be taken not to introduce the principle of overload or progression too early in a programme. Those less fit and new to exercise seem to show a better result (specific to the type of exercise being trained) to overload when the exercise programme is correctly prescribed compared with the regular exercisers. This is helpful in terms of motivation for those only beginning to engage in PA and exercise.
- Most people prefer to have some variation in an exercise programme. However, for people with Parkinson's experiencing cognitive changes, too much variation can affect adherence to the programme or result in suboptimal performance.

Timing of Exercise

As stated earlier, timing of exercise is important and careful consideration should be given to NMS such as fatigue, and many individuals report the best time for exercise is late morning or midafternoon. Creating a routine for exercise also helps develop a mindset of preparation for activity.

Timing of exercise can also refer to the point along the journey when a person will take up particular types of exercise. For example, earlier in the condition, power is affected more than general strength or endurance due to bradykinesia (reducing speed of movement) and muscles being prone to fatigue more easily. As there is often an element of reversible disuse in the early stages of the condition, a programme based on principles of progressive overload, gradually increasing stress placed upon the body during exercise training to build strength, is recommended.

As Parkinson's progresses, the expected outcomes of exercise change, with application of the FITT principles developing from assurance of improvement to a goal of maintaining fitness levels and finally to the expectation that the exercise will minimise or reduce the rate at which mobility and fitness deteriorate.

Promoting exercise

Guidelines can help in the translation of research findings into practice, and practice can be further enhanced by asking about the physical activity and exercise the person already undertakes (Keus et al., 2014). Taking into account the length of diagnosis and the individual's interest in being active and fit, PA and exercise should be set, monitored, and modified as their condition progresses. Examples of when and how this could be achieved and adapted are found in the Parkinson's Exercise Framework (see Table 11.6).

To assist professionals in thinking about exercise prescription, Table 11.5 offers ideas on the 'why, when and how to promote exercise'.

Summary

Many people with Parkinson's are less active and less motivated than age-matched peers. Early targeted exercise intervention reduces symptoms and speed of progression (Paul et al., 2019). The benefits of exercise include improvements in motor symptoms and NMS. People with Parkinson's often report that their ability to manage functional tasks, their energy levels, and their self-confidence improved as a direct consequence of engaging in exercise (Sheehy et al., 2017). Those who exercise are better able to participate in everyday activities and to maintain good cognitive functioning.

The role of the multidisciplinary team (MDT) is to promote regular exercise, using consultations to embed the exercise notion within an individual's lifestyle. It is important to emphasise the importance of taking up exercise, or encouragement to continue effective activity, from the outset. In this way, compliance with exercise even in the later stages of the condition will be easier. Professionals can utilise the evidence for exercise to support and educate individuals who might struggle with the concept of engaging in PA and exercise.

TABLE 11.5 Why, when, and how to promote exercise

Why (Objectives)	When	How to promote exercise
To promote general physical activity	Discussed at any point during progression of the condition	For those who are habitually more sedentary or who believe that their current level of activity is sufficient to keep them fit, try to gain an understanding of their attitude towards PA and exercise. Introduce them to local support group networks providing the opportunity to meet others; introduce the idea of the NEAT approach (non–exercise-activity thermogenesis)—a lifestyle where one undertakes to be as active as possible in all tasks (e.g., walking to the shops or an "exercise-snacking" approach). Keep a list of the exercises offered locally (charity, leisure centre or local authority activities). Such groups may be able to link each individual with an exercise buddy.
To promote an understanding of the importance of exercise	Newly diagnosed	The focus should be on encouraging the individual's investment in exercise and building it into a lifestyle choice. Discussions regarding specific sports, such as golf, can include the importance of muscle power and endurance in maintaining a good golf swing and walking around the golf course. Introducing exercise components for tennis players, bowlers, and those who just want to keep up their pace while playing with grandchildren are similar examples. The exercise prescriber should educate the person with Parkinson's to expect periods where improvements are very noticeable and periods when progress does not occur. To optimise performance, encourage the individual to vary the exercise. For example, from time to time, instead of always using a resistance band for the exercise programme, use free weights (including body weights or dumbbells).
To stress the importance of remaining active	Maintenance stage	The individual should be supported to maintain the effort with which they exercise while also ensuring that both body and mind are engaged so as to preserve memory, attention and learning and to aid in the management of non-motor symptoms such as sleep and mood.

(Continued)

TABLE 11.5 Why, when, and how to promote exercise (*Cont.*)

Why (Objectives)	When	How to promote exercise
To maintain independence in the face of progression of Parkinson's	Later stages	The focus of exercise becomes more functional as the performance of daily activities becomes affected. People may struggle to climb stairs or rise from a chair without using their arms. Targeting walking steadily, especially while the person is lifting and carrying objects, may be necessary, with specific exercises for building strength sufficient to withstand perturbations that could put the individual at risk of falling under such dual-task conditions. In asking carers and family members to help with exercise programmes, it is important to remember that this may be an additional stress for them.

TABLE 11.6 Resources

Resource	Details and websites
Parkinson's UK	Exercise resource page https://www.parkinsons.org.uk/information-and-support/exercise
	Exercise blogs Includes two blogs by Dr. Beckie Port, Parkinson's UK Research Communications Manager, as part of Parkinson's UK "Exercise and Parkinson's" drive 1. Is exercise good for Parkinson's? https://medium.com/parkinsons-uk/the-science-of-exercise-part-1-58c1054b50c6 2. Exercise in Parkinson's: what's best? https://medium.com/parkinsons-uk/the-science-of-parkinsons-exercise-part-2-2d680afa1a01
	Exercise professionals hub Hub support professionals delivering exercise to people with Parkinson's https://www.parkinsons.org.uk/professionals/exercise-hub
Michael J. Fox Foundation for Parkinson's Research	**Blog** https://www.michaeljfox.org/news/exercise-and-parkinsons-frequently-asked-questions
Parkinson's Foundation	**Blog** https://www.parkinson.org/Understanding-Parkinsons/Treatment/Exercise

TABLE 11.6 Resources (*Cont.*)

Resource	Details and websites
Sites that review outcome measures and assessment tools	Therapists can look up validated and reliable tools for clinical and research purposes **Shirley Ryan ability lab "rehabilitation measures" database:** https://www.sralab.org/rehabilitation-measures **Physiopedia outcome measures:** https://www.physio-pedia.com/Category:Outcome_Measures

Exercise can improve sense of empowerment and self-efficacy and provide an environment within which shared experience and learning are promoted, leading to the development of a social network of support for the individual.

Personal Perspectives

Both vignettes below are examples of how people with Parkinson's can be champions for exercise, depending on the roles they pursue.

The first story is from Mike, a person with Parkinson's with an interest in exercise. He knows that it does him good, but he does not read much further into its effects. Mike has acted as a peer contact for local people with Parkinson's who wanted to know about exercise.

Mike's story

Being a little bit fitter helps us with many of the difficulties of life. This is true of aging and of having conditions that seem to mimic aging, like Parkinson's. As someone with Parkinson's but with no specialist knowledge, I see my comrades benefiting in many ways from exercising with advice from physiotherapists, especially when they are encouraged to "challenge your balance!" There is the simple benefit of training ankles and hips to be ready for slips and jerks and to avoid bad falls. There's the fun of doing it together, practising the "hip hula"! There's the good company that gets you out of the house and doing something positive for your overall well-being.

Mike

The second story is from Bob, a person with Parkinson's who has read extensively about what might help his symptoms and kept up to date with the research. Bob then approached the local Parkinson's UK committee to start a boxing training class in 2014, which still runs to this day.

Bob's story

In 2011, Stephanie Combs and colleagues published a paper describing the benefits of boxing training for six people with Parkinson's. The research determined that despite the progressive nature of Parkinson's, the people in the study, even those with moderate to severe Parkinson's, showed both short- and long-term improvements in balance, walking, activities of daily living and quality of life after boxing training, plus that boxing training programme were feasible and safe for people with Parkinson's.

The findings of this research are confirmed by my own experience, as I decided in 2014 to "up my game" and embark on boxing training myself.

In combination with fitness activities, boxing training incorporates whole-body movements, with upper-extremity punching motions and lower-extremity footwork in multiple directions, all performed at speed. It provides both anaerobic and aerobic exercise in one session. Each session comprises a full-body workout that ensures I am getting fitter and fitter. I am especially keen on using the wall-mounted Speed Ball and have become quite proficient at it. I received one for my 70th birthday recently and am really enjoying using it in my home gym.

I have read somewhere that a 60-minute boxing training session results in energy expenditure similar to that of running about 9 km (5.6 miles) in 60 minutes on a treadmill. I could not run that far on a treadmill. Therefore, if this is true, the boxing training gives me that level of cardiorespiratory benefit, which is not immediately obvious but non-etheless real. And there is nothing quite like pounding a heavy punch bag as hard and as fast as you can! When I finish a session, I am physically tired but mentally very stimulated.

The combination of punches that I have to deliver to the various punch bags in the gym have benefitted my hand-eye coordination and improved my strength, flexibility, and balance. But the big surprise for me was the "brain training," which is also part of the package. By repeatedly moving my legs in predetermined patterns and by punching various combinations repeatedly, I am effectively training my brain and body to do this more automatically. This, in turn, has helped me handle concurrent multiple tasks, cognitive as well as physical. As the coach increases the combinations of punches I have to throw, it becomes more difficult to activate my legs and feet in conjunction with the punching. Nevertheless, I can see an improvement over time, although it requires intense concentration! At today's training session, I lost concentration and the heaviest bag I was using swung right back at me; I instinctively moved to my left and released a sequence of punches without thinking about it – an automatic movement proven!

I must make clear that boxing training, however wonderful it is for me, is not a cure, although I believe it helps to slow down the progress of the condition. I still have off days and off periods, but overall I am much stronger and fitter and more mobile and flexible than when I started, and this has helped me as I go about my daily life.

Bob

Top tips for exercise in Parkinson's

1. Exercise should be an integral component of Parkinson's management.

2. Discussions about exercise should explore different ways and places to exercise.

3. Because of the diversity of symptoms, an individualised, varied and progressive approach to exercise prescription is required.

4. Regardless of the type of exercise, each individual must be motivated to do it.

5. Parkinson's motor symptoms can put individuals at higher risk of injury when exercising "cold," so care should be taken not to introduce the principle of overload or progression too early in a programme.

6. Exercise should preferably be conducted when medication is optimised. For most people with Parkinson's, this will be approximately 30 minutes following the ingestion of medication.

7. A daily routine of PA and exercise should be advocated, making sure that individuals are aware of the benefits for Parkinson's symptoms and management.

8. Technology, such as apps and online exercise sessions, offers the advantage of enabling the individual to exercise at a convenient time; it can help novice exercisers to develop self-efficacy with exercise prior to considering participation in a wider group.

9. One can follow the European Physiotherapy Guideline for Parkinson's Disease and the Parkinson's UK Exercise Framework when an exercise programme is to be recommended.

10. It is best to be specific in offering exercise advice and to follow the FITT principles: frequency, intensity, type and duration.

11. If the health professional does not have sufficient knowledge and expertise in exercise, the individual can be referred to a specialist in exercise prescription. Parkinson's UK local advisors can help signpost the individual to a Parkinson's exercise specialist.

12. The exercise programme should be reviewed and adapted by the exercise professional regularly to suit the individual's physical and mental abilities as well as his or her needs.

References

Ahlskog, J. E. (2018). Aerobic exercise: evidence for a direct brain effect to slow Parkinson's disease progression. *Mayo Clinic Proceedings*, *93*(3), 360–372.

Bouça-Machado, R., Rosário, A., Caldeira, D., Castro Caldas, A., Guerreiro, D., Venturelli, M., et al. (2019). Physical activity, exercise and physiotherapy in Parkinson's disease: defining the concepts. *Movement Disorders Clinical Practice*, *7*(1), 7–15.

Chong, T. T. J., Bonnelle, V., Manohar, S., Veromann, K. -R., Muhammed, K., Tofaris, G. K., et al. (2015). Dopamine enhances willingness to exert effort for reward in Parkinson's disease. *Cortex*, *69*, 40–46.

Claesson, I. M., Ståhle, A., & Johansson, S. (2019). Being limited by Parkinson's disease and struggling to keep up exercising; is the group the glue? *Disability and Rehabilitation*, *42*(9), 1270–1274.

Combs, S. A., Diehl, M. D., Chrzastowski, C., Didrick, N., McCoin, B., Mox, N., et al. (2013). Community-based group exercise for persons with Parkinson's disease: a randomised controlled trial. *NeuroRehabilitation, 32*(1), 117–124.

da Silva, F. C., Iop, R. d. R., de Oliveira, L. C., Boll, A. M., de Alvarenga, J. G. S., Gutierres Filho, P. J. B., et al. (2018). Effects of physical exercise programmes on cognitive function in Parkinson's disease patients: a systematic review of randomised controlled trials of the last 10 years. *PLoS ONE, 13*(2), e0193113.

Dobkin, B. H. (2017). A rehabilitation-internet-of-things in the home to augment motor skills and exercise training. *Neurorehabilitation and Neural Repair, 31*(3), 217–227.

Ellis, T., Boudreau, J. K., DeAngelis, T. R., Brown, L. E., Cavanaugh, J. T., Earhart, G. M., et al. (2013). Barriers to exercise in people with Parkinson's disease. *Physical Therapy, 93*(5), 628–636.

Ellis, T., & Rochester, L. (2018). Mobilising Parkinson's disease: the future of exercise. *Journal of Parkinson's Disease, 8*(s1), S95–S100.

Garcia-Agundez A, Folkerts AK, Konrad R, Caserman P, Tregel T, Goosses M, Göbel S, Kalbe E. Recent advances in rehabilitation for Parkinson's Disease with Exergames: A Systematic Review. J Neuroeng Rehabil. 2019 Jan 29;16(1):17. doi: 10.1186/s12984-019-0492-1. PMID: 30696453; PMCID: PMC6352377.

Hirsch, M.A., van Wegen, E.E.H., Newman, M.A. et al. Exercise-induced increase in brain-derived neurotrophic factor in human Parkinson's disease: a systematic review and meta-analysis. Transl Neurodegener 7, 7 (2018). https://doi.org/10.1186/s40035-018-0112-1.

Hirsch, M. A., van Wegen, E. E. H., Newman, M. A., & Heyn, P. C. (2018). Exercise-induced increase in brain-derived neurotrophic factor in human Parkinson's disease: a systematic review and meta-analysis. *Translational Neurodegeneration, 7*(1).

Hunter, H., Lovegrove, C., Haas, B., Freeman, J., & Gunn, H. (2019). Experiences of people with Parkinson's disease and their views on physical activity interventions. *JBI Database of Systematic Reviews and Implementation Reports, 17*(4), 548–613.

Joseph, C., Leavy, B., Mattsson, S., Falk, L., & Franzén, E. (2018). Implementation of the HiBalance training programme for Parkinson's disease in clinical settings: a feasibility study. *Brain and Behaviour, 8*(8), e01021.

Keus, S.H. J., Munneke, M., Graziano, M., et al. (2014). European physiotherapy guideline for Parkinson's disease. KNGF/ParkinsonNet. Available at www.parkinsonnet.info.guidelines/parkinsons.

LaHue, S. C., Comella, C. L., & Tanner, C. M. (2016). The best medicine? The influence of physical activity and inactivity on Parkinson's disease. *Movement Disorders, 31*(10), 1444–1454.

Danielle Larson, Chen Yeh, Miriam Rafferty & Danny Bega (2021) High satisfaction and improved quality of life with Rock Steady Boxing in Parkinson's disease: results of a large-scale survey, Disability and Rehabilitation, DOI: 10.1080/09638288.2021.1963854.

McConaghy, M. (2015). *The new Parkinson's treatment; exercise is medicine. Australia:* Port Campbell Press.

McDonnell, M. N., Rischbieth, B., Schammer, T. T., Seaforth, C., Shaw, A. J., & Phillips, A. C. (2017). Lee Silverman Voice Therapy (LSVT)-BIG to improve motor function in people with Parkinson's disease: a systematic review and meta-analysis. *Clinical Rehabilitation, 32*(5), 607–618.

McGrane, N., Galvin, R., Cusack, T., & Stokes, E. (2015). Addition of motivational interventions to exercise and traditional physiotherapy: a review and meta-analysis. *Physiotherapy, 101*(1), 1–12.

Miller, W. R., & Rose, G. S. (2009). Toward a theory of motivational interviewing. The. *American Psychologist*, *64*(6), 527–537.

Mirelman, A., Rochester, L., Maidan, I., Del Din, S., Alcock, L., Nieuwhof, F., et al. (2016). Addition of a non-immersive virtual reality component to treadmill training to reduce fall risk in older adults (V-TIME): a randomised controlled trial. *The Lancet*, *388*(10050), 1170–1182.

Oliveira de Carvalho, A., Filho, A. S. S., Murillo-Rodriguez, E., Rocha, N. B., Carta, M. G., & Machado, S. (2018). Physical exercise for Parkinson's disease: clinical and experimental evidence. *Clinical Practice & Epidemiology in Mental Health*, *14*(1), 89–98.

Parkinson's UK (2017). Parkinson's exercise framework for professionals. Retrieved December 6, 2020, from https://www.parkinsons.org.uk/information-and-support/parkinsons-exercise-framework.

Paul, K. C., Chuang, Y. H., Shih, I. F., Keener, A., Bordelon, Y., Bronstein, J. M., et al. (2019). The association between lifestyle factors and Parkinson's disease progression and mortality. *Movement Disorders*, *34*(1), 58–66.

Radder, D. L. M., Lígia Silva de Lima, A., Domingos, J., Keus, S. H. J., van Nimwegen, M., Bloem, B. R., et al. (2020). Physiotherapy in Parkinson's disease: a meta-analysis of present treatment modalities. *Neurorehabilitation and Neural Repair*, *34*(10), 871–880.

Ramaswamy, B., Jones, J., & Carroll, C. (2018). Exercise for people with Parkinson's: a practical approach. *Practical Neurology*, *18*(5), 399–406.

Riebe, D., Ehrman, J. K., Liguori, G., Magal, M., & American College of Sports Medicine (2018). *ACSM's guidelines for exercise testing and prescription* (10th ed.). Philadelphia, Baltimore, New York: Wolters Kluwer.

Schenkman M, Moore CG, Kohrt WM, Hall DA, Delitto A, Comella CL, Josbeno DA, Christiansen CL, Berman BD, Kluger BM, Melanson EL, Jain S, Robichaud JA, Poon C, Corcos DM. Effect of High-Intensity Treadmill Exercise on Motor Symptoms in Patients With De Novo Parkinson Disease: A Phase 2 Randomised Clinical Trial. JAMA Neurol. 2018 Feb 1;75(2):219–226. doi: 10.1001/jamaneurol.2017.3517. PMID: 29228079; PMCID: PMC5838616.

Schootmeijer et al (2020). Barriers and motivators to engage in exercise for persons with Parkinson's Disease. Journal of Parkinson's Disease (10): 1293–1299.

Sheehy, T. L., McDonough, M. H., & Zauber, S. E. (2017). Social comparisons, social support, and self-perceptions in group exercise for people with Parkinson's disease. *Journal of Applied Sport Psychology*, *29*(3), 285–303.

UK Chief Medical Officers (2019). Physical Activity Guidelines. Retrieved December 6, 2020, from https://www.gov.uk/government/publications/physical-activity-guidelines-uk-chief-medical-officers-report.

Chapter 12

Care of the Hospitalised Person With Parkinson's

Rob Skelly, Lisa Brown and Sally Jones

Chapter outline

Introduction

People with Parkinson's are more likely than others to be admitted to hospital. Most admissions are non-elective, and those admitted are often in the complex or palliative stage of Parkinson's. On average, these individuals have a longer length of stay and a higher mortality rate; they are more likely to be discharged to a residential or care home than are other aged-matched patients. Cost of care is also higher, averaging £3338 ($5353) per non-elective Parkinson's admission in England (2009-2013) (Low et al., 2015). Complicated drug schedules, a high incidence of delirium and dysphagia, communication difficulties, and motor fluctuations all make caring for inpatients with Parkinson's challenging. This chapter describes how people with Parkinson's differ from the general population in relation to hospital admission; it includes descriptions of the complications and outcomes of hospital admission and discusses issues that arise in caring for Parkinson's inpatients, in particular medication management, dysphagia and delirium. Also covered is the role of the multidisciplinary team and an exploration of how care can best be organised. How emergency admissions can be avoided is also covered, and recommendations for the care of elective surgical patients with Parkinson's are offered.

Epidemiology of hospitalisation in people with Parkinson's

Which people with Parkinson's are admitted to hospital?

People with Parkinson's are 1.4 to 3.0 times more likely to be admitted to hospital than age-matched individuals in the general population (Guttman et al., 2004; Low et al., 2015). In England, around 45,000 people with Parkinson's are admitted to hospital each year; many are admitted more than once and 72% of these admissions are non-elective. Parkinson's itself was coded as the primary reason for admission in 10% of cases and a secondary cause in 90%. Admissions occur mainly in the older population, with 45% of admissions occurring in those 75 to 85 years of age and nearly 20% in those over 85 years of age (Low et al., 2015). In a Spanish study, the mean age of hospitalised Parkinson's patients was 78 years (Gil-Prieto et al., 2016). Admissions are more common among men (women, 40%, vs. men, 60%), reflecting the known, higher frequency of Parkinson's among males (Low et al., 2015). Not surprisingly, admitted patients are likely to have more advanced disease. In our own experience of non-elective admissions, only 3% of patients were Hoehn-Yahr stage 1 or 2, whereas 52% were stage 3, 25% stage 4, and 20% stage 5. Most (84%) of these patients were admitted from their own homes, 9% from residential care homes and 7% from nursing homes (Skelly et al., 2014).

Causes of admission

Common causes for admission include pneumonia, urinary tract infection and hip fracture. Parkinson's patients are more likely to have these diagnoses than are other patients. Pneumonia as a cause of admission is 1.6 to 1.9 times as frequent in people with Parkinson's than in the age- and sex-matched general

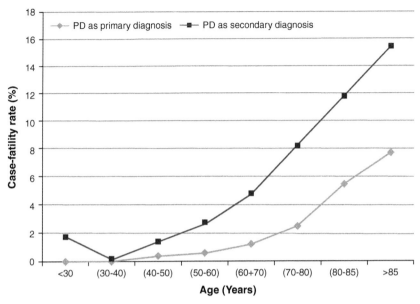

FIGURE 12.1   Case fatality rates in people with Parkinson's admitted to hospital in Spain (1997-2012). *Reproduced from Gil-Prieto et al., (2016).*

inpatient population; urinary tract infection is 2.3 to 2.6 times as common and hip fractures are 2.2 to 2.6 times as common (Guttman et al., 2004; Low et al., 2015; Lubomski et al., 2015).

In a systematic review and meta-analysis of hospital-based studies, infections accounted for 22% of admissions, worsening motor function for 19%, falls and fractures for 18%, cardiovascular comorbidities for 13% and neuropsychiatric complications for 8% (Okunoye et al., 2020).

Mortality

Mortality among Parkinson's inpatients is higher than that in age-matched patients without Parkinson's. Mortality rates are 3.7% in Australia, 6.5% in England and 10% in Spain. The differences may reflect the proportion of emergency admissions in each study: 34% in Australia and 86% in Spain. Mortality increases with age (Fig. 12.1) and is higher among men in all age groups.

Length of stay and destination upon discharge

In England the mean length of stay (LOS) was 7 days longer for Parkinson's patients than for those of a similar age without Parkinson's (16 vs. 9 days), and those with Parkinson's were twice as likely to have a very long LOS (>3 months) (Low et al., 2015). LOS increases with age and may be longer in men. At the end of the hospital stay people with Parkinson's were less likely to be discharged to their usual place of residence and more likely to be discharged to a care home. Rate of transfer to care homes is approximately 5.8%, but it can be as high as 32% if a percutaneous endoscopic gastrostomy (PEG) feeding tube has been inserted during admission (Brown et al., 2020).

Prescription and administration of dopaminergic medication

Parkinson's Foundation Centres of Excellence and UK Parkinson's specialists report lack of confidence that Parkinson's medication is given on time at their institutions and also report poor staff knowledge (Chou et al., 2011; Skelly et al., 2015). Medication errors may be the result of prescription errors or administration problems. Prescription errors are common and include failure to prescribe, wrong drug, incorrect preparation (e.g., dispersible, controlled release), incorrect dose, incorrect frequency and incorrect timings.

Frequency of medication errors

We found at least one prescription error in more than 50% of hospitalised Parkinson's patients, but the number of doses affected by prescription error was only 5%, suggesting that initial prescribing errors are generally identified and remedied (Skelly et al., 2014). Hou et al. (2012) reported that 21% of inpatients with Parkinson's were prescribed a contraindicated medication and 8.3% of dopaminergic medications were omitted; of these, 7.7% were delayed more than 30 minutes. The proportion of medication given on time improved after the first 2 days and was higher if there had been a neurology consultation. In a study from the United Kingdom, 9% of inpatients with Parkinson's were given a contraindicated antidopaminergic medication (for example, haloperidol, prochlorperazine or metoclopramide), and 39% of Parkinson's medications were delayed or omitted (Skelly et al., 2017a).

If levodopa (L-dopa) medication is delayed, people with Parkinson's may become stiff and immobile, get anxious, struggle to swallow and communicate, have painful dystonia and experience other pain syndromes. Errors of medication administration can also be associated with a decline in motor function (see Fig. 12.2) (Gerlach et al., 2013).

Those with long disease duration or motor fluctuations are most likely to have such symptoms, whereas those with early-stage disease who are receiving L-dopa three times daily may tolerate some delays. It should be appreciated that sicker patients (confused, unconscious, unable to swallow) are more likely to miss medication, which might further worsen their situation. We could not confirm that delays in medication increased LOS, but a study from the Basque region of Spain showed that the omission of dopaminergic medication was

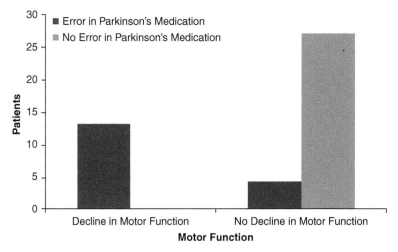

FIGURE 12.2 Relationship between medication errors and motor decline during hospital admission in a study of Dutch Parkinson's patients. *Data from Gerlach et al. (2013).*

associated with increased mortality (OR 1.9) and prolonged LOS by 4 days (Lertxundi et al., 2017; Skelly et al., 2017a).

Causes of errors in the administration of medications

Reasons for failing to administer medication include patient refusal, patient off ward, drug out of stock, patient not permitted to take anything by mouth (NBM), patient unable to take medication because of drowsiness or a swallowing problem. Of all omitted medications, around 25% are omitted because they were out of stock. Dopamine agonists and monoamine oxidase inhibitors are more likely than L-dopa preparations to be out of stock (8% vs. 2% of prescribed doses).

L-dopa/carbidopa/entacapone is more likely to be out of stock than co-beneldopa or co-careldopa (4% vs. 2%) (Skelly et al., 2017b). Clinicians must work with pharmacists to make sure that nurses know where stores of critical medication are kept. Parkinson's specialists must suggest substitution policies so that available L-dopa preparations are used rather than omitting medication (Lertxundi et al., 2015). Although medication problems are prevalent in most hospitals, it is possible to make significant improvements, as shown in the case study later in this chapter.

Reconciliation of medications

Pharmacists have a crucial role in improving medication safety for people with Parkinson's. In the general inpatient population, pharmacists typically detect prescription errors in some 40% to 50% of admissions. Shared computer systems can help: allowing secondary care pharmacists access to general practitioner (GP) summary care records facilitates reconciliation and is likely to improve the medication experience for people with Parkinson's, although evidence for this is currently lacking.

Self-administration of medication

Motor function may be better when patients are in control of their own medication (Gerlach et al., 2013). Patients should be assessed to see if they can safely self-medicate. Although this bypasses institutional failures to provide medication on time, it has already been noted that hospitalised people with Parkinson's are elderly (mean age 78 years) and that the incidence of delirium may be as high as 56.6% (Lawson et al., 2020); thus self-administration is often not possible. Furthermore, concordance with medication schedules in the community may be even lower than in the hospital. A study using electronic medicine bottles that record the date and time of cap opening showed that a median of 97% of prescribed doses were taken, but a median of only 24% of doses were taken at the correct time (Grosset et al., 2009).

Non-oral dopaminergic therapy

Concerns about swallowing may lead to nil by mouth (NBM) orders. Risks of aspiration must be balanced against risks of malnutrition and motor decline. Our own hospital guideline recommends that NBM status be reviewed early, as swallowing may have improved following treatment of the acute illness that led to the admission. Staff should ask if swallowing is any different from normal and whether there is already a plan in place to reduce aspiration risk; they should also consider if an individual's swallow is safe enough to permit oral medication. If medication cannot be given by mouth, non-oral options must be considered (Fig. 12.3). The choice is between L-dopa by nasogastric tube, a rotigotine patch and subcutaneous apomorphine. There are advantages and drawbacks to each option, but a randomised controlled trial to compare treatment strategies has not been conducted.

Rotigotine patches

Rotigotine is a non-ergot dopamine agonist delivered via transcutaneous patch. Bioavailability can vary depending on where the patch is applied: patches on shoulders may have higher bioavailability than those on thighs. It takes about 3 hours for rotigotine to reach detectable levels in the plasma and 2 to 3 days to reach steady state concentration. It is metabolised in the liver and excreted mainly as inactive metabolites in the urine and faeces. It takes 5 to 7 hours to wear off after the patch has been removed. The use of rotigotine in place of L-dopa is a compromise: it is slow to reach therapeutic levels and has to be used at a lower

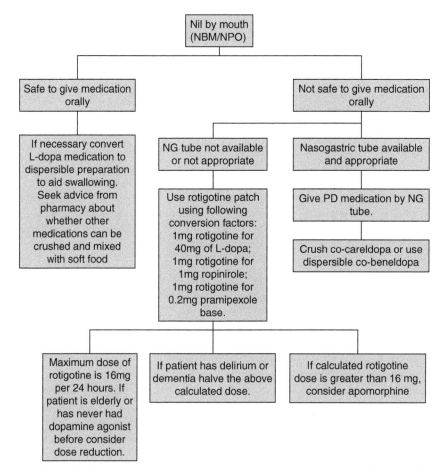

FIGURE 12.3 Flowchart for Parkinson's medication management when an individual is unable to take oral medication. Conversion factors given in this table are based on those provided by Brennan & Genever (2010) and are given as an aid to management but prescribers should consult their pharmacist and the drug's summary of product characteristics before prescribing.

dose to reduce side effects; it may therefore be less effective. Whenever a usual Parkinson's medication has had to be altered because a patient is NBM the Parkinson's team should be informed and they should arrange to review the patient as soon as possible and further adjust the medication as appropriate.

Nasogastric medication

Co-beneldopa dispersible tablets and co-careldopa tablets (crushed and dispersed) can be given by nasogastric (NG) tube. Controlled-release medication should be converted to dispersible tablets, and a dose reduction may be needed; we usually reduce the dose by 50% because controlled-release preparations have approximately 60% bioavailability compared to immediate release (and

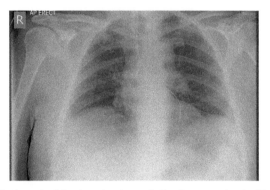

FIGURE 12.4   Radiograph of the chest showing a misplaced nasogastric tube. The tube has passed down the left main bronchus to terminate in the posterior segment of the lower lobe of the left lung. The tube does not cross the diaphragm in the midline. Courtesy of Radiology Department, University Hospitals of Derby and Burton, NHS Foundation Trust.

some rounding is necessary). Controlled release dopamine agonists should not be given by NG tube. Standard release dopamine agoinsts should be given instead and the daily dose divided into (typically) three doses per day. Pharmacy advice should be sought. NG tubes may be uncomfortable and can easily be dislodged. The position of the tube must be confirmed by testing the acidity of the aspirate before each medication is given. If no aspirate is obtained, a chest radiograph must be obtained, and such x-rays need expert interpretation. There are potentially serious consequences (e.g., pneumonitis) of giving medication via a misplaced tube (Fig. 12.4). NG medication is the preferred solution to NBM status because it enables a medication regimen very similar to the patient's usual one but, for various reasons, the NG route may often be unavailable.

Subcutaneous apomorphine

Apomorphine is a morphine derivative with dopamine agonist properties. Its onset of action is typically within 15 minutes; its plasma half-life is 40 minutes. Some experts use apomorphine in preference to rotigotine when oral L-dopa for NG delivery is not available. For example, a test dose of 2 mg apomorphine is given subcutaneously; if, after an hour, there is no nausea or hypotension, a dose of 3 mg is given. Further doses of 3 mg can be given four times daily. If the 3-mg dose is well tolerated but ineffective, a 4-mg dose can be tried after 2 hours (Sharma & Bolla, 2015). Apomorphine is not specifically licenced to replace non-oral Parkinson's medication. Prescribers should consult the summary of product characteristics or pharmaceutical company full prescribing information before prescribing. The dosage information given is an illustration of dosing used in one hospital and does not constitute prescribing advice. Domperidone reduces nausea but is only available orally and is not available in the US. Ondansetron should not be used with apomorphine. Maximal apomorphine daily dosing on this regime is 16 mg, equivalent to about 160 mg of L-dopa. Advantages of apomorphine include its rapid onset of action and reliable route of administration. Disadvantages are the potential for nausea and QTc prolongation, short duration of action and lack of staff experience with this medication.

Optimal calculator

Applications (apps) such as the Optimal Calculator (www.parkinsonscalculator. com), designed for use by non-specialists, can take the pain out of calculating a new dose. The user decides whether or not an NG tube is to be used. The user then inputs the patient's Parkinson's medication and the calculator advises what should be put through the NG tube or what dose of rotigotine patch to use. Parkinson's specialists should help train pharmacists to advise front-line staff on appropriate options for non-oral dopaminergic therapy.

Parkinson's hyperpyrexia syndrome

If dopaminergic medication is stopped suddenly, patients may develop a condition resembling the neuroleptic malignant syndrome: Parkinson's hyperpyrexia syndrome. This can follow after the sudden discontinuation or marked dose reduction of dopaminergic medication and is characterised by high fever in the absence of sepsis, severe stiffness, myoclonus, autonomic instability and impaired consciousness. The level of creatine kinase is raised, as is the neutrophil count. It may be complicated by venous thromboembolism, aspiration pneumonia, and acute kidney injury and is fatal in up to 20% of cases. Treatment involves restarting dopaminergic therapy, antipyretics, fluids, venous thromboembolism prophylaxis, a broad-spectrum antibiotic if sepsis cannot be excluded, and dantrolene if the individual is failing to improve on first line treatment. Sudden cessation of dopamine agonists can lead to dopamine agonist withdrawal syndrome, consisting of drug craving, agitation, sweating, depression, panic attacks, pain and postural hypotension.

Case study: a quality improvement project that worked!

Background

In 2015, a large National Health Service trust in England audited the administration of Parkinson's medications in their organisation. Interrogation of their electronic prescribing system showed that in the preceding 12 months, over 14,000 doses had been delayed and 3500 missed altogether. A quality improvement (QI) team was formed to tackle the problem via a QI project.

Three primary drivers were agreed on: education, patient identification and medication administration. Different interventions were put in place for each of these primary drivers, with "plan, do, study, act" cycles for each as required, starting in one ward area and then scaling up and spreading each intervention across the trust as a whole.

	Ward	Name	Drug Description	Scheduled	Administered	Period
	H₂₁		ROPINIROLE XL 8 mg Tablets	03/02 06:00	03/02 06:10	00:10
	H₂₁		CO-CARELDOPA 25/100 Tablets	03/02 08:00	03/02 07:52	00:00
	H₂₁		CO-CARELDOPA 25/100 Tablets	03/02 13:30	03/02 12:56	00:00
	H₂₁		CO-CARELDOPA 25/100 Tablets	03/02 19:00	03/02 18:20	00:00

Results 1-4

FIGURE 12.5   Electronic dashboard filtered by ward.

Education

The QI team felt that all staff should be aware of the time-critical nature of Parkinson's medications, of the consequences of missed medications, and of what to do if a person with Parkinson's were NBM. Interventions developed to achieve this included delivering many teaching sessions tailored to specific staff groups, the inclusion of a brief session on Parkinson's management at institutional induction, and the development of both an app and a website with guidance for non-specialists on aspects of Parkinson's care, including what to do if a person with Parkinson's was NBM. A short educational film that included powerful patient stories was also developed. This was shown to all wards, at induction to the institution, and at all the teaching sessions. This film is available for general viewing under a Creative Commons licence and can be accessed at https://vimeo.com/148216230

Patient identification

The QI team felt that there should be early identification of people with Parkinson's, that medication reconciliation should become a priority in this patient group, and that there should be active reminders of patients requiring time-critical medications at every nursing handover. Therefore, in addition to the interventions already mentioned, information technologists on the team developed a dashboard linked to the electronic prescribing system. The live part of this dashboard (Fig. 12.5) enables teams to filter patients by ward and obtain a live list of people under their care as well as when their medications are due. Throughout the day, the ward sister, doctor, or pharmacist would then be able to see if medication were delayed and, if so, why, enabling problem solving in real time. The dashboard included a function where teams could look at their retrospective data, track progress and compare themselves against other areas within the hospital.

Administration of medication

It was agreed that Parkinson's medication should always be available, not just during normal office hours; that systems should be in place to ensure that patients who were NBM received medication promptly via an alternative route; and that

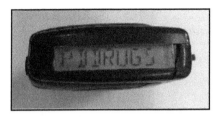

FIGURE 12.6   Parkinson's drug administration bleep.

patients should be able to receive their drugs at specified times even if outside the time of standard drug rounds. A change was made to ensure that Parkinson's medication was routinely stocked within the drug cupboards on medical admissions units and elderly care wards, with an electronic system informing other ward areas where these drugs were stocked. Commonly used Parkinson's drugs were also added to emergency drug cupboards within the emergency departments. Flowcharts with NBM guidance were added to the junior doctors' app and intranet. A bleep was also provided to each ward, which was linked to the electronic prescribing system for the ward and would automatically go off 10 minutes before a Parkinson's drug on that ward was due to be administered (Fig. 12.6).

Results

On the initial target ward, the proportion of Parkinson's drugs given on time improved from 48% before the QI project to 88% afterward (Fig. 12.7). Similarly, when interventions were rolled out across the three hospital sites, the trust-wide percentage of Parkinson's drugs given on time improved from 48% to 80%.

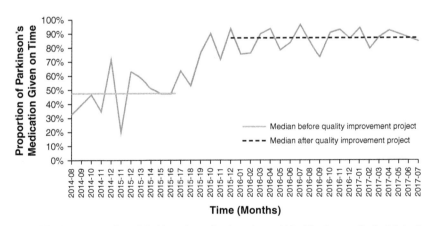

FIGURE 12.7   Proportion of Parkinson's medication given within 30 minutes of scheduled administration time. Improvement in the timely administration of Parkinson's drugs on the initial target ward is shown. The three-year historical median was 48% and new median 88%, which was sustained over 18 months.

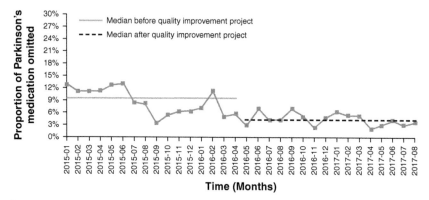

FIGURE 12.8   Proportion of Parkinson's medications omitted across the institution. This fell from a 3-year historical median of 10% to a new median of 4%.

The number of omitted Parkinson's medications also fell across the institution from a median of 10% to 4% (Fig. 12.8). Staff reported greater confidence in treating people with Parkinson's, and patient feedback was also positive.

Dysphagia

Most people with Parkinson's will develop swallowing impairment at some point, and those admitted to hospital are highly likely to have swallowing difficulties. Predictors of dysphagia include Hoehn-Yahr stage 4 or 5, dementia, unexplained weight loss, and drooling. Consequences of dysphagia include reduced quality of life, aspiration pneumonia, malnutrition and depression. Not all individuals with dysphagia are aware the problem. Half of those without a subjective sense of swallowing difficulty are found to have such difficulties on formal testing (Suttrup & Warnecke, 2016). All Parkinson's patients admitted to hospital should therefore have a swallow assessment by a speech and language therapist (SLT) as soon as possible. Many admitted patients are already known to the SLT department and, if there has been no change in swallowing symptoms, advice already in place in the community can be followed. Impaired swallowing does not always respond to L-dopa therapy because cognitive deficits, peripheral nerve damage, and neuromuscular pathology may contribute to swallowing problems. Non-etheless, where dysphagia is a wearing-off symptom or subject to 'on/off' fluctuations, optimisation of L-dopa therapy may improve swallowing.

Tube feeding

Sometimes dysphagia worsens during an acute illness, such as an infection. An acute change in swallowing associated with intercurrent illness may be reversible; therefore temporary use of an NG tube to facilitate medication administration and support nutrition should be considered. In the presence of chronic severe dysphagia, temporary use of an NG tube may help inform the decision to place a percutaneous endoscopic gastrostomy (PEG). Decisions about PEG feeding for chronic dysphagia in Parkinson's are not easy. Although discussions should have taken place in the outpatient clinic, this does not always happen. Indeed, in a UK audit of PEG feeding in Parkinsonian conditions, 82% of PEGs were placed during an emergency admission and only 22% of patients had made future care planning decisions (Brown et al., 2020). Tube feeding is discussed further in Chapter 7.

Delirium

Delirium occurs in up to 56% of Parkinson's inpatients (Lawson et al., 2020). The criteria listed in the *Diagnostic and Statistical Manual of Mental Disorders*, 5th Edition (American Psychiatric Association, 2013), for delirium include:

- Impaired attention and awareness
- Acute onset
- Disordered thinking not explained by an underlying neurocognitive condition
- Evidence of an underlying medical cause

Some features of delirium overlap with those of Parkinson's dementia: tremor, confusion, hallucinations, drowsiness and fluctuations in level of confusion. Delirium is associated with motor decline, increased mortality, prolonged LOS and institutionalisation. People with Parkinson's, in particular those who are older, may be at increased risk of developing delirium (Lawson et al., 2019). For practical purposes a search for an underlying medical cause should be undertaken in all Parkinson's inpatients presenting with confusion. Infections, metabolic disturbance, hypoxia, constipation, urinary retention, subdural haemorrhage, adverse effects of drugs and alcohol withdrawal all must be considered. If no medical cause for delirium can be identified, the possibility of Parkinson's psychosis should be considered.

The underlying cause should be treated and multicomponent interventions such as the following implemented:

- Maintain good hydration
- Treat constipation
- Minimise noise
- Use clocks and calendars for orientation
- Make sure that spectacles and hearing aids are available and in working order

Drugs with a significant anticholinergic burden—oxybutynin, tolterodine, amitriptyline—should be discontinued. Opiates may have to be reduced.

Long-standing anticholinergic medication given for tremor (e.g., trihexyphenidyl, procyclidine) may have to be withdrawn gradually. Pharmacists should help identify offending medications; tools to assess anticholinergic drug burden can be used.

If a patient presents with delirium shortly after an increase in his or her Parkinson's medication, the change should be reversed. There is a lack of evidence to guide other changes to Parkinson's medication. Temporarily using a simpler regimen with co-beneldopa or co-careldopa only should be considered (Aminoff et al., 2011). Rivastigmine may be continued if already on stable dosing but should not be commenced in the setting of delirium (van Eijk et al., 2010). Haloperidol should be avoided. Electronic prescribing systems can help to prevent inadvertent prescription of drugs contraindicated in Parkinson's, including haloperidol, prochlorperazine and metoclopramide. If a sedative is required, lorazepam can be considered. Quetiapine can be used by specialists but may cause prolongation of the QT interval, drowsiness and postural hypotension; it is also linked to an increased risk of stroke.

Surgical patients

Surgical patients with Parkinson's stay longer in hospital, have more falls and remain longer in intensive care units than those without Parkinson's (Mueller et al., 2009). Orthopedic patients with Parkinson's are at high risk of delirium and decubitus ulcers and may recover more slowly (Jonsson et al., 1995). In a US study including 234 elective surgical admissions with Parkinson's, the following complications were more common among Parkinson's patients than others: aspiration pneumonia (OR 3.8), postoperative delirium (OR 2.5), hypotension (OR 2.5), and urinary tract infection (OR 2.0) (Pepper & Goldstein, 1999). Proactive care of older people undergoing elective surgery involves comprehensive geriatric assessment and can reduce LOS among such patients (Partridge et al., 2018). Attention is paid to nutrition, cognition, functional status, home environment, exercise capacity and comorbidities. Such an approach is likely to be beneficial for people with Parkinson's and could be delivered by the Parkinson's MDT. As a rule, Parkinson's patients should be placed first on the operating list to reduce the risk of disrupting their medication schedules. Morning Parkinson's medication should be given as usual. If the patient has a deep brain stimulator (DBS), the surgeon should be informed. Diathermy is best avoided but, if needed, bipolar diathermy should be used (Brennan & Genever, 2010). If the gastrointestinal route of administration will be unavailable postoperatively, the Parkinson's specialist should advise on the use of rotigotine or apomorphine. For elective surgery, should the oral route be unavailable, the Parkinson's team should help plan peri-operative and post-operative changes in medication.

Multidisciplinary care for people with Parkinson's admitted to hospital

Care from the multidisciplinary team

The MDT has a crucial role to play in the assessment and management of frail, elderly inpatients with Parkinson's. Although medical factors are important, a holistic assessment should include assessment of cognition, mood, function (e.g., self-care abilities), home environment and social support. Inpatient comprehensive geriatric assessment reduces mortality and improves the chance of living at home 6 to 12 months after assessment (Ellis et al., 2011). For inpatients, the importance of the role of the SLT in regard to swallowing has been highlighted. The physiotherapist and occupational therapist (OT) are also crucial to ensuring the best outcome and avoiding longer LOSs. People with Parkinson's should mobilise as soon as possible, and therapists should be aware of the timing of the medication schedule so that intervention can be delivered at the optimal time.

The MDT must understand cues and strategies to enable the management of problems such as FOG and transfers (see Tables 6.1 and 7.6). They should consider the environment and try to reduce distractions and obstacles. Having a laser pen available to provide visual cueing is a good idea. An understanding of the effect of non-motor symptoms such as anxiety and apathy on performance is important, as individuals with these problems need a tailored approach. Practical tips for the ward MDT are shown at the end of the chapter.

In our hospital, the specialist therapists from the Parkinson's MDT offer an in-reach service to support the therapists and care staff on the wards. The specialist therapists may support therapy sessions for individuals with more complex problems, advocate for timely medication where this is important, and offer management advice and support to therapists and other ward professionals. In addition, patients often find familiar faces reassuring.

Lack of similarity between the home and hospital environments is a potential barrier to successful rehabilitation. An acute-care therapy pathway that includes early home-based therapy, photographs of the home and enhanced liaison with community services has shown promise, but further evidence is needed (Lovegrove & Marsden, 2019).

Nursing care

The ward nurse has a key role in coordinating the care of a Parkinson's inpatient. He or she can improve the patient experience and reduce LOS by ensuring prompt investigations, assessments and the involvement of other MDT members. Ensuring accurate medication administration, recording postural blood pressures and keeping fluid and food charts are all important. Unavailable Parkinson's medications should be ordered urgently. Nursing staff should

TABLE 12.1 Actions to improve inpatient care for people with Parkinson's

Hospital guideline for the management of people with Parkinson's

Electronic prescription and drug administration system

Clear guidance on medication administration if person is to take nothing by mouth

Avoidance of anticholinergic and antidopaminergic drugs

Electronic alert system to notify Parkinson's team of patient admission

Dysphagia assessment protocol

Multicomponent interventions to reduce incidence of delirium

In-reach service from members of the Parkinson's team

Front-door Parkinson's review

Falls risk and bone health assessment and action plan

Comprehensive geriatric assessment

Staff education programme

Low threshold for referral to Parkinson's specialist teams

Patient and carer information sheets on delirium, postural hypotension, and nasogastric tubes, discharge planning, future care planning, and mental capacity

provide timely feedback to the medical team and commence discharge planning from the point of admission. The patient's experience can be enhanced when the ward nurse liaises with the caregiver, gathering information about the exact medication regimen and care needs while updating the caregiver on progress and discharge plans. Nursing staff should monitor and optimise eating, drinking, and swallowing; bladder and bowel function; mobility and falls risk; communication; sleep; and mental well-being. Involving family in care can be helpful, and open visiting should be considered. On the other hand, caregiver strain can be an issue; nursing staff have a key role in identifying this and advocating for increased social care and support on discharge.

Organisation of care

Individuals with Parkinson's do not always report a good experience of care in hospital (Barber et al., 2001). Strategies to improve care must be multifaceted. Suggested actions to improve care are shown in Table 12.1.

Specialist involvement

Hospitalisations where Parkinson's is the primary cause for admission might be best managed on a neurology or Parkinson's ward, but these account for only 5% to 10% of Parkinson's admissions and have not increased significantly over

15 years. On the other hand, hospitalisations where Parkinson's is a comorbidity account for the majority of admissions and are increasing by 15% per year (Gil-Prieto et al., 2016). In the United Kingdom, many of these people will be cared for on "medicine for the elderly" wards. Others will be cared for on a wide variety of general medical wards. This is significant, as it means that clinicians from many specialties will be caring for inpatients with Parkinson's. These disparate professionals may have little expertise in Parkinson's, so it is crucial that they are properly supported with clear guidelines, effective training, and easy access to expert advice. Early notification of the Parkinson's team has been recommended (Aminoff et al., 2011). This can be done by the admitting team or automated. The electronic case records of people with Parkinson's can be tagged to alert the Parkinson's team when the patient is admitted. The Parkinson's nurse, neurologist or geriatrician can advise on medication issues while specialist therapists support staff with early mobilization and prompt discharge. Early specialist consultation may reduce LOS and improve outcomes (Mehta et al., 2008). Cohorting Parkinson's patients with general medical problems may be effective: a specialist Parkinson's disease unit on an elderly care ward reduced length of stay; it also improved medication management and patients' experience of care (Skelly et al., 2014).

Guidelines

It is important for hospitals to have guidelines for frontline staff on how to give Parkinson's medication if the oral route becomes unavailable. An example guideline is shown in Figure 12.9. This guideline gives general advice about care during the first 24 hours of in hospital. Parkinson's UK (2021) also includes example hospital guidelines on its website (https://www.parkinsons.org.uk).

Staff education

Staff with no specialist knowledge of Parkinson's will care for most hospitalised people with Parkinson's. It is important that they have effective and accessible training. Simple on-ward training programmes can be effective in improving staff knowledge (Skelly et al., 2014). Brief training videos showing people with "on/off" fluctuations can be especially useful in demonstrating the effects of omitted medication. Videos or whiteboard animations with local influential clinicians have salience. Training materials from charitable organisations are also helpful.

Admission avoidance

It is important for both the person with Parkinson's and health services to avoid unnecessary admission to hospital. Outpatient neurologist-supervised care is associated with a reduced rate of admission for psychosis, traumatic injury and

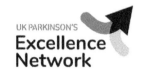

British Geriatrics Society
Improving healthcare
for older people

Inpatient Parkinson's Disease Management:
The first 24 hours

	ACTIVITY	COMMENTS
ED / Medical Admissions	Gather information re: usual PD medication regime - Check with patient / relatives / GP summary / clinic letter / discharge summary	
	Check when last dose given and when next dose due (including patches)	
	Ensure all PD medication prescribed at correct DOSE and TIME - Medications ALWAYS available via on-call pharmacist - ZERO TOLERANCE FOR 'DRUG UNAVAILABLE'	
	Assess swallow early if concerns: - If NBM MUST consider alternative route (NGT or patch) and medical team to prescribe ASAP - Use www.pdmedcalc.co.uk (or local algorithm)	
	Check not prescribed: - Haloperidol, metoclopramide, Prochlorperazine (dopamine blockers)	
First 24 Hours	Sit out early as appropriate: - Bed rest increases rigidity and risk of chest infections	
	Involve physio early	
	Request urgent Movement Disorders review if: - Unsafe swallow - Acute delirium with hallucinations - Severe dyskinesia - Complex medication regime: ➤ Apomorphine, Duodopa, >2 classes of PD meds, >5x / day - Deep brain stimulator (NB MRI / diathermy)	
	Caution with End of Life Care Pathway unless reviewed by a Movement Disorders specialist	

Designed and developed by Dr Sara Evans, Royal United Hospitals Bath, in cojunction with the British Geriatrics
Society, Movement Disorders Section   Version 1 (RUH, 2016)

FIGURE 12.9 British Geriatrics Society, Movement Disorders Section (BGSMDS) guideline for management of inpatients with Parkinson's: the first 24 hours. Used by permission of Dr. Sara Evans and BGSMDS.

urinary tract infection. More frequent review (at least five times in 4 years) is better than infrequent review (Willis et al., 2012). A Parkinson's advanced symptoms unit providing rapid-access multidisciplinary assessment has reduced all of the following: admissions to hospital by 7%, admission to care homes by 50%, hip fracture by 50%, and LOS by 38% (Archibald, 2018). Those most at risk for admission because of recurrent falls or troublesome hallucinations were prioritised and seen in the advanced symptoms unit within an average of 10 days from referral.

An intervention that included an educational intervention for care home staff and advance (future) care planning in institutionalised patients with dementia resulted in a 55% reduction in emergency admissions without increasing mortality (Garden et al., 2016). Although this intervention was not specifically for people with Parkinson's it is likely that similar benefits would be seen.

Inclusion of a palliative medicine specialist in the Parkinson's MDT might improve advance (future) care planning and sharing of skills (Skelly, 2016). Better compliance with medication is associated with better motor function and lower rates of hospitalisation (Muzerengi et al., 2016). Physiotherapy-led interventions can reduce falls in people with Parkinson's, and the prescription of bisphosphonates for the secondary prevention of fragility fractures reduces hospitalisations for fractures.

Personal perspective: David's story

I worked in the pharmaceutical industry for over 30 years and have had Parkinson's for 13 years, always managing my medication myself.

Unfortunately, in July 2019, I had a fall and broke my hip, which resulted in my being admitted to hospital for surgery. I found that I was not allowed to self-administer my medication, and my usual timing of medication was not correctly recorded (although I had written it down several times). The nursing staff insisted that they had to follow the medication timings as stated on the hospital computer system, and most of the time it was a different nurse dispensing the medication on each occasion; on some occasions, medication was completely omitted or doubled up! I was very aware of the importance of getting my medication on time. When my medication is working well, I can do most things for myself—dress myself, walk independently, catch the bus, and cook meals. If I forget to take my medication, I am totally the opposite, experiencing difficult freezing and struggling to walk. I have to depend on people to get around, and I certainly wouldn't catch a bus as I would be frightened of the consequences.

This distressing hospital scenario continued for over 3 weeks, and if I wanted to go to the toilet, two members of staff had to assist me. They were not always immediately available, so I had to wait. Eventually I was transferred to a rehabilitation unit, but unfortunately I had the same problems there. However, having regular physiotherapy there enabled me to get home, and I thought that I would finally be able to get back to "normal." However, I found that my discharge medication blister pack was missing one of the vital Parkinson's medications. As a result, my wife had to go to the GP for an emergency prescription! It took 2 weeks, once I was home, for me to begin to feel that things were returning to normal.

It is essential to get one's Parkinson's medications on time.

Top tips for the ward's multidisciplinary team

1. Be aware that acute illness may be associated with a reversible decline in motor function, delirium and fatigue.
2. Early mobilisation and therapeutic intervention are key to reducing deconditioning related to acute illness.
3. Review previous inpatient and outpatient interventions to find out what has or has not worked in the past.
4. Review the current home situation and caregiver support, previous discharges, safety concerns and capacity issues.
5. Consider the timing of therapy sessions (i.e., when medication is optimal but also for advice on the management of "off"-related symptoms).
6. Use cues and strategies.
7. Carry a laser pen in your pocket to provide a visual cue for freezing.
8. Try to minimise the distractions (TV, people, noise, etc.) in the area in which you are working with the individual.
9. Be aware of non-motor symptoms that can affect therapy (e.g., depression, anxiety, postural hypotension).
10. Consider which activities the patient must to be able to perform for a safe home discharge and create a prioritised problem list to guide inpatient therapy.
11. Request a review by the Parkinson's nurse specialist or doctor if there has been a change in the control of Parkinson's symptoms.
12. Make sure that Parkinson's follow-up for patients who will be discharged is in place.

References

American Psychiatric Association (2013). *Diagnostic and Statistical Manual of Mental Disorders.* Fifth ed. Arlington, VA.

Aminoff, M. J., Christine, C. W., Friedman, J. H., Chou, K. L., Lyons, K. E., Pahwa, R., et al. (2011). Management of the hospitalised patient with Parkinson's disease: Current state of the field and need for guidelines. *Parkinsonism Relat Disord, 17*(3), 139–145.

Archibald, N. (2018). Parkinson's Advanced Symptoms Unit (PASU) Business Case 2017/18 [online]: South Tees Hospitals NHS Foundation Trust. Available at: https://multiplesclerosisacademy.org/wp-content/uploads/sites/2/2019/07/PASU-business-case-2017.18.pdf/.

Barber, M., Stewart, D., Grosset, D., & McPhee, G. (2001). Patient and carer perception of the management of Parkinson's disease after surgery [2]. *Age and Ageing, 30*(2), 171–172.

Brennan, K. A., & Genever, R. W. (2010). Managing Parkinson's disease during surgery. *BMJ, 341*, c5718.

Brown, L., Oswal, M., Samra, A. -D., Martin, H., Burch, N., Colby, J., et al. (2020). Mortality and institutionalisation after percutaneous endoscopic gastrostomy in Parkinson's disease and related conditions. *Mov Disord Clin Pract.*

Chou, K. L., Zamudio, J., Schmidt, P., Price, C. C., Parashos, S. A., Bloem, B. R., et al. (2011). Hospitalisation in Parkinson disease: a survey of National Parkinson Foundation Centres. *Parkinsonism Relat Disord, 17*(6), 440–445.

Ellis, G., Whitehead, M. A., Robinson, D., O'Neill, D., & Langhorne, P. (2011). Comprehensive geriatric assessment for older adults admitted to hospital: meta-analysis of randomised controlled trials. *BMJ, 343*, d6553.

Garden, G., Green, S., Pieniak, S., & Gladman, J. (2016). The Bromhead Care Home Service: the impact of a service for care home residents with dementia on hospital admission and dying in preferred place of care. *Clin Med (Lond)*, *16*(2), 114–118.

Gerlach, O. H., Broen, M. P., & Weber, W. E. (2013). Motor outcomes during hospitalisation in Parkinson's disease patients: a prospective study. *Parkinsonism Relat Disord*, *19*(8), 737–741.

Gil-Prieto, R., Pascual-Garcia, R., San-Roman-Montero, J., Martinez-Martin, P., Castrodeza-Sanz, J., & Gil-de-Miguel, A. (2016). Measuring the Burden of Hospitalisation in Patients with Parkinson s Disease in Spain. *PLoS ONE*, *11*(3), e0151563.

Grosset, D., Antonini, A., Canesi, M., Pezzoli, G., Lees, A., Shaw, K., et al. (2009). Adherence to antiparkinson medication in a multicenter European study. *Mov Disord*, *24*(6), 826–832.

Guttman, M., Slaughter, P. M., Theriault, M. E., DeBoer, D. P., & Naylor, C. D. (2004). Parkinsonism in Ontario: comorbidity associated with hospitalisation in a large cohort. *Movement Disorders*, *19*(1), 49–53.

Hou, J. G., Wu, L. J., Moore, S., Ward, C., York, M., Atassi, F., et al. (2012). Assessment of appropriate medication administration for hospitalised patients with Parkinson's disease. *Parkinsonism Relat Disord*, *18*(4), 377–381.

Jonsson, B., Sernbo, I., & Johnell, O. (1995). Rehabilitation of hip fracture patients with Parkinson's Disease. *Scand J Rehabil Med*, *27*(4), 227–230.

Lawson, R. A., McDonald, C., & Burn, D. J. (2019). Defining delirium in idiopathic Parkinson's disease: A systematic review. *Parkinsonism Relat Disord*, *64*, 29–39.

Lawson, R. A., Richardson, S. J., Yarnall, A. J., Burn, D. J., & Allan, L. M. (2020). Identifying delirium in Parkinson's disease: a pilot study. *Int J Geriatr Psychiatry*.

Lertxundi, U., Isla, A., Solinís, M. A., Domingo-Echaburu, S., Hernandez, R., & García-Monco, J. C. (2015). A proposal to prevent omissions and delays of anti-Parkinsonian drug administration in hospitals. *Neurohospitalist*, *5*, 53e54.

Lertxundi, U., Isla, A., Solinis, M. A., Echaburu, S. D., Hernandez, R., Peral-Aguirregoitia, J., et al. (2017). Medication errors in Parkinson's disease inpatients in the Basque Country. *Parkinsonism Relat Disord*, *36*, 57–62.

Lovegrove, C. J., & Marsden, J. (2019). Service evaluation of an acute Parkinson's therapy pathway between hospital and home. *International Journal of Therapy and Rehabilitation*, *27*(7), 1–6.

Low, V., Ben-Shlomo, Y., Coward, E., Fletcher, S., Walker, R., & Clarke, C. E. (2015). Measuring the burden and mortality of hospitalisation in Parkinson's disease: A cross-sectional analysis of the English Hospital Episodes Statistics database 2009-2013. *Parkinsonism Relat Disord*, *21*(5), 449–454.

Lubomski, M., Rushworth, R. L., & Tisch, S. (2015). Hospitalisation and comorbidities in Parkinson's disease: a large Australian retrospective study. *J Neurol Neurosurg Psychiatry*, *86*(3), 324–330.

Mehta, S., Vankleunen, J. P., Booth, R. E., Lotke, P. A., & Lonner, J. H. (2008). Total knee arthroplasty in patients with Parkinson's disease: impact of early postoperative neurologic intervention. *Am J Orthop (Belle Mead NJ)*, *37*(10), 513–516.

Mueller, M. C., Juptner, U., Wuellner, U., Wirz, S., Turler, A., Hirner, A., et al. (2009). Parkinson's disease influences the perioperative risk profile in surgery. *Langenbeck's Archives of Surgery*, *394*(3), 511–515.

Muzerengi, S., Herd, C., Rick, C., & Clarke, C. E. (2016). A systematic review of interventions to reduce hospitalisation in Parkinson's disease. *Parkinsonism Relat Disord*, *24*, 3–7.

Okunoye, O., Kojima, G., Marston, L., Walters, K., & Schrag, A. (2020). Factors associated with hospitalisation among people with Parkinson's disease – A systematic review and meta-analysis. *Parkinsonism & Related Disorders* doi: 10.1016/j.parkreldis.2020.02.018.

Parkinson's UK (2021). Guidelines. Retrieved 27 September 2021 from https://www.parkinsons. org.uk/professionals/guidelines

Partridge, J., Sbai, M., & Dhesi, J. (2018). Proactive care of older people undergoing surgery. *Aging Clin Exp Res*, *30*(3), 253–257.

Pepper, P. V., & Goldstein, M. K. (1999). Postoperative complications in Parkinson's disease. *J Am Geriatr Soc*, *47*(8), 967–972.

Sharma, J. C., & Bolla, B. (2015). *Guidance for the Management of the acutely ill Parkinson's Disease patient.* United Lincolnshire Hospitals NHS Trust.

Skelly, R., Brown, L., Fakis, A., Kimber, L., Downes, C., Lindop, F., et al. (2014). Does a specialist unit improve outcomes for hospitalised patients with Parkinson's disease? *Parkinsonism & Related Disorders*, *20*, 1242–1247.

Skelly, R., Brown, L., Fakis, A., & Walker, R. (2015). Hospitalisation in Parkinson's disease: A survey of UK neurologists, geriatricians and Parkinson's disease nurse specialists. *Parkinsonism Relat Disordr*, *21*, 277–281.

Skelly, R., Brown, L., & Fogarty (2017a). Delayed administration of dopaminergic drugs is not associated with prolonged length of stay of hospitalised patients with Parkinson's disease. *Parkinsonism Relat Disord*, *35*, 25–29.

Skelly, R., Brown, L., Gosrani, S., & Fogarty, A. (2017b). Omission of Dopaminergic Drugs in Hospitalised Parkinson's Patients: A Study of Drug Availability. *Age & Ageing*, *46*(suppl_2), ii19–ii119.

Skelly, R. H. (2016). Specialist palliative medicine in Parkinson's disease - improving quality and achieving patients' preferences for end of life care. *Age and Ageing*, *45*(eLetters Supp.).

Suttrup, I., & Warnecke, T. (2016). Dysphagia in Parkinson's Disease. *Dysphagia*, *31*(1), 24–32.

van Eijk, M. M., Roes, K. C., Honing, M. L., Kuiper, M. A., Karakus, A., van der Jagt, M., et al. (2010). Effect of rivastigmine as an adjunct to usual care with haloperidol on duration of delirium and mortality in critically ill patients: a multicentre, double-blind, placebo-controlled randomised trial. *Lancet*, *376*(9755), 1829–1837.

Willis, A. W., Schootman, M., Tran, R., Kung, N., Evanoff, B. A., Perlmutter, J. S., et al. (2012). Neurologist-associated reduction in PD-related hospitalisations and health care expenditures. *Neurology*, *79*(17), 1774–1780.

Chapter 13

Atypical Parkinsonian Syndromes

Jade Donnelly, Luke Massey, Sarah McCracken and Boyd Ghosh

Chapter outline

Introduction

Atypical Parkinsonian syndromes (APS) are comprised of the conditions progressive supranuclear palsy (PSP), corticobasal syndrome (CBS) and multiple system atrophy (MSA). Although these conditions differ from Parkinson's and from each other, they share some similarities and it can be quite difficult to differentiate between them, particularly in the early stages. Owing to their similarities, they are often seen in the same clinics. These are rare neurological conditions with no curative treatment and an average duration from onset to death of 6 years. Individuals rapidly develop severe problems, leading to full dependence on caregivers. The conditions affect vision, thinking, speech, swallow, movement, bladder and bowel function. Relentless progression of these conditions often requires significant involvement by the multidisciplinary team (MDT) in order to support the individual and caregiver through a rapidly changing series of problems. This chapter discusses the three conditions, using case studies for each of the APSs to highlight cardinal features. Also discussed is the role of the MDT in managing these individuals. In particular, it will be seen that many of the team members' roles overlap, and therefore good communication is of vital importance for effective and efficient care.

Progressive supranuclear palsy

PSP is a life-limiting condition caused by the accumulation of an abnormal form of the protein tau in brain cells. It typically presents between the ages of 40 and 80, with a mean age at diagnosis of 63 years. It is more common in men than women and is associated with a median survival of about 6 years (Litvan et al., 1996). Recent diagnostic criteria have been established for the various subtypes of PSP, as outlined in Table 13.1, and the PSP Association has published a list of useful red flags (PSP Association, 2019b) to prompt diagnosis. These are outlined in Table 13.2. Although initial stages can be separated into subtypes, all subtypes will generally evolve into the same phenotype of Richardson syndrome (Hoglinger et al., 2017). Individuals present with instability, often falling frequently in the early stages. This should be a red flag to therapists as it is unusual in early Parkinson's. Individuals also present with slowing or paralysis of fast eye movements (saccades), which is the key diagnostic sign. Individuals may have subcortical dementia with slowing of thought processes, difficulty retrieving information, motor recklessness and impulsivity. In addition, the individual's swallowing and speech deteriorate over the course of the condition. As is the case for all the atypical Parkinsonian syndromes, there is no medication to cure or slow the condition's progression. Intervention, both therapy and medication, is aimed at controlling symptoms.

Case study

Henry is 67 years old; over the past 2 years he and his wife have noticed that he is less stable on his feet, often tripping up kerbs and losing his balance when stepping backward—for example, when opening the fridge. He has had a few bad falls that required sutures. Henry's wife has noticed that he is much quieter in social situations and offers less input in group conversations. He has developed a sweet tooth and now tends to overfill his mouth, which has led to episodes of choking. Despite being aware that his balance is poor and having been warned by his wife not to, Henry still attempts to answer the doorbell. This often results in falls or near misses.

On examination, Henry was unable to look down and had slow saccades horizontally. He had marked postural instability demonstrated by a positive pull test. In attempting to sit, he fell down into his chair in an uncontrolled manner. He had axial rigidity, most noticeable in his neck, but also had rigidity in his limbs. He was impulsive, often starting a task or activity before the clinician had

TABLE 13.1 Diagnostic criteria in progressive supranuclear palsy

	PSP-RS	PSP-PGF	PSP-P	Others
Definite	Defined by pathology			
Probable	Vertical gaze palsy or slowing of vertical saccades			
	Unprovoked falls <3 years or fall on pull test <3 years	Progressive gait freezing within 3 years; not responsive to dopa	Akinesia and rigidity, either axial or limb; either dopa responsive or not	PSP-F: Vertical gaze palsy or slow vertical saccades with frontal cognition deficits (three of reduced fluency, apathy, bradyphrenia, dysexecutive, impulsivity)
Possible	> Two steps back on pull test <3 years	Progressive gait freezing <3 years; not responsive to dopa		PSP-CBS: Vertical gaze palsy or slow saccades with one cortical sign (sensory loss, apraxia, alien limb) and 1 MD sign (rigidity, akinesia, myoclonus)
Suggestive	Macro SWJ or eyelid opening apraxia, WITH either a fall on the pull test or more than two steps back on pull test.		Bradykinesia, either axial or limb; dopa responsive or not WITH one of SWJ or EOA or falls <3 years or fall on pull test <3years or speech disorder or frontal cognition or dopa resistance or hypokinetic dysarthria or dysphagia or photophobia	PSP-PI: Unprovoked falls <3 years or fall on pull test <3years PSP-CBS: One cortical sign (sensory loss, apraxia, alien limb) and one MD sign (rigidity, akinesia, myoclonus)

Abbreviations: PSP-RS, PSP Richardson syndrome; PSP-PGF, PSP progressive gait failure; PSP-P, PSP Parkinsonism; PSP-F, PSP with frontal lobe, cognitive or behavioural signs; PSP-CBS, PSP corticobasal syndrome; PSP-PI, PSP with postural instability; SWJ, square-wave jerks; EOA, eyelid opening apraxia; sensory loss, cortical sensory loss; MD, movement disorder; rigidity, cogwheel rigidity; speech disorder, non-fluent aphasia or apraxia of speech
The frontal phenotype comprises at least three of the following: apathy, bradyphrenia, dysexecutive syndrome, reduced phonemic verbal fluency, impulsivity, perseveration and disinhibition. Mandatory inclusion: Age greater than 40 at first symptom, gradually progressive and sporadic. Mandatory exclusions: Signs suggestive of another disease such as Motor neuron disease, mulitple system atrophy, Alzheimer's disease, prion disease and encephalitis; Imaging suggestive of another disease e.g. normal pressure hydrocephalus; lab findings suggestive of another disease (e.g. neurosyphilis, Wilson disease, Niemann Pick disease).
Adapted from Höglinger et al. (2017).

TABLE 13.2 Red flags for a diagnosis of progressive supranuclear palsy

1	Falls	Often backwards and without warning
2	Postural instability	Axial rigidity
3	Slowness of movement	Bradykinesia
4	Motor recklessness	Impulsivity
5	Eye problems	Restricted eye movement. May describe finding it difficult to walk downstairs due to problems with downward gaze, reduced blink, double vision
6	Speech	Slurring of speech, soft voice
7	Swallowing difficulties	Liquids and solids, excessive saliva
8	Cognitive changes	Change in personality, irritability, apathy
9	Emotional lability	Easily brought to tears or laughter
10	No presenting tremor	

Adapted from https://pspassociation.org.uk/information-and-support/for-professionals/red-flags-for-gps/

requested it. In a verbal fluency test, he generated only eight words, demonstrating problems with retrieval. He scored 34 out of a possible 100 on the PSP rating scale, a validated measure to monitor progression. This score would usually be expected to increase by about 11 points per year (Ghosh et al., 2013) which can be useful to inform prognosis.

Henry's presentation has many of the hallmarks of PSP, as described earlier (see Table 13.1), although individuals may not present with all of the features described.

The important aspects of this case are Henry's poor balance and his impulsivity. His compromised balance has led to several falls and hospital admissions, including some injuries requiring sutures. To manage his problems, health professionals—including physiotherapists, occupational therapists (OTs), speech and language therapists (SLTs), Parkinson's disease nurse specialists (PDNSs) and orthotic specialists—must work together.

In the early stages of the condition, vertical eye movements are often slower; as the condition progresses, there is complete loss of vertical eye movement. If there is a limitation of vertical gaze, the vestibulo-ocular reflex (VOR) or "doll's-head manoeuvre" can be carried out, although neck rigidity may prevent it. This would show the full range of eye movements in the vertical direction, confirming that the paresis stems from a supranuclear deficit rather than a structural limitation of eye movement, which can sometimes be found in the elderly.

Henry tripped when stepping up kerbs owing to his inability to look down. In the early stages, therapy may include optimising eye movements and tracking between targets combined with balance challenges. As the condition progresses or if eye movements are already very restricted, there is little to be gained; thus therapy is more likely to cause frustration. Careful consideration must be given to safety and balance. Marking the edges of furniture with tape may help. Individuals frequently experience light sensitivity, so closing blinds and recommending wraparound sunglasses can be helpful. If individuals experience double vision, the use of an eye patch can be helpful. The therapist should advise that if an eye patch is used, the eyes are to be covered alternately.

Owing to the reduced downgaze, reading and eating can become difficult; some individuals find it increasingly difficult to find the plate, making mealtimes challenging. It can be helpful to raise the plate on a block; prism eyeglasses that direct the vision downward can also be useful. Prism glasses are available free of charge from the PSP association. It should be noted that they should not be used during walking.

Postural instability

Postural instability is a major aspect of the condition, with falls, as seen in the case study, being a common presentation. The pull test or retropulsive pull test is carried out to assess postural stability. The clinician stands behind the individual and pulls on his or her shoulders so as to displace them. This may initially be done with a very gentle pull to gauge the effect and then repeated with more force. The individual may take one or several steps to recover but, classically, those with PSP make no stepping reaction; their reaction is described as "falling like a tree."

To target postural instability in the early stages, therapy should focus on balance, gait, and turning, taking into account the gaze palsy, rigidity, and backward lean. To help limit problems with axial rigidity later in the condition, early intervention should include promoting axial rotation and range-of-movement exercises for the neck. Such exercises may include knee rolling, rolling over in bed, and specific range-of-movement exercises for the neck. Therapy should also focus on the individual's ability to move from sitting to standing, with an emphasis on hip flexion (hip hinge) to move weight anteriorly both on "sit to stand" and "stand to sit." It is important to teach caregivers to provide prompting for this activity in order to reenforce the kinaesthetic learning.

For those individuals whose centre of mass (COM) falls behind them when standing and who then frequently fall backwards, consideration should be given to the use of heel wedges. These are small orthoses that can be placed inside the shoe to bring the COM forward and may help with alignment in standing. Alternatively, a shoe with a small wedge may help.

Walking aids should be considered, although standard wheeled walkers can often be pulled over. An alternative is the U-step, a specially designed, sturdy walking aid with a reverse braking system and wheel-resistance mechanism that prevents the frame from rolling away from the individual; it is also difficult to tip over. However, as the condition progresses, walking aids may be more of a hindrance than a help as, because of cognitive deficits, they are often not used.

In the early stages, the emphasis will be on falls prevention. This includes balance exercises, that focus on weight transfers and core strength, focusing on abdominals, gluteals, and lateral hip muscles. Intervention for transfers, with the focus on taking a side step rather than a backwards step in order to turn, and a power stance (one foot forward and one back) when opening doors, can also help to limit falls.

Individuals with PSP will fall, despite all efforts, and an important role of the therapist is to teach individuals and their caregivers the techniques for getting up off the floor. This will include teaching backward chaining, which breaks the task into small steps. The OT should consider provision of lifting equipment such as the Raizer chair lift, a battery-operated mobile lifting chair or the pneumatic Mangar camel chair lift, which inflates beneath the individual.

Part of the role of therapists in the management of APS is to preempt potential problems. Owing to the progressive nature of the condition, early referral for a wheelchair is recommended. How quickly one chooses to do this may depend on the psychological impact of the referral on the individual. Current waiting list times in the health service locally may also be a factor. Initially, a standard wheelchair may be appropriate, but as the condition progresses, the individual may benefit from one with tilt-in-space options as well as lateral support. Because of the visual problems and bradyphrenia experienced by people with PSP, an electric wheelchair or scooter would not be indicated for most, but each case should be assessed individually. Adaptations in the individual's home may also have to be considered. These can include walk-in wet rooms, ceiling track hoist systems and downstairs living. Because individuals with PSP tend to be impulsive, stair lifts can be dangerous; therefore a careful, individualised assessment should be made. The PSP Association (2020) has produced useful guidance for therapists.

Impulsivity

The other important aspect of the case study is impulsivity, which is a frontal deficit. Henry does not wait for his wife to answer the door but impulsively stands up to do it himself. This demonstrates motor recklessness and impulsive behaviour, not only in not waiting for his wife but also by not considering his own safety. Management can be challenging and requires an MDT approach, particularly the physiotherapist, OT and SLT. The MDT should reinforce that this is a symptom of the condition rather than a sign of obstructiveness, as it can be a source of frustration for caregivers.

Impulsivity, combined with deteriorating balance as the condition progresses, is challenging and can often lead to hospital admission and caregiver breakdown. The progression of mobility, cognition and ocular changes over time in PSP is illustrated in Figure 13.1 (Ghosh et al., 2013). Sensors can detect when an individual has stood up from a chair or got out of bed, providing an alert to the caregiver, but sensors are only as effective as those who are responding to the alarm. Because of their impulsivity and the inability to recognise risk,

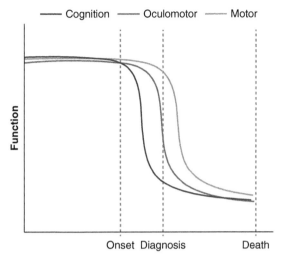

Cognition —— Oculomotor —— Motor

Function

Onset Diagnosis   Death

FIGURE 13.1 Decline of various functions in progressive supranuclear palsy. *Based on data from Ghosh et al., (2013).*

individuals with PSP rarely sit down when the alarm sounds. The OT or community physiotherapist can assess whether such devices are appropriate in an individual's situation, whether this is at home or in a care home.

As demonstrated in the case study, individuals can also exhibit impulsivity when eating. They may overfill their mouths, putting themselves at risk of choking. To limit this, the OT can offer advice regarding appropriate cutlery (for instance, smaller implements) or eating and drinking aids. The SLT can offer prompts and exercises to promote a safer swallowing technique and limit the risk of choking. One-way-valve straws and specialist cups may be considered. As the condition progresses, increasing bradykinesia can lead to loss of dexterity, and the individual may need assistance with feeding. Although this signifies a certain loss of independence, the risk of choking from impulsive mouth filling is reduced.

Henry is impulsive when he is eating, but this is not the case for all individuals. As the condition progresses, each mealtime can take more than an hour. In these situations, the food often grows cold and plate warmers may be recommended. This might also prompt conversations about feeding tubes if they have not been discussed already.

Speech and swallowing

SLT involvement throughout the course of the condition is vital. In the early stages this may focus on communication, considering both low- and high-technology options, with the former usually more effective as PSP progresses. Voice legacy and voice banking, recording the individual's voice for posterity or for future use in electronic communication, respectively, should be considered.

Dysphagia management is another key feature for SLT management. Early management includes education for both the individual and the caregiver regarding dietary modifications, such as using thicker liquids, including milkshakes or prescribed thickeners. Later management includes altering food textures and the consideration of feeding tubes as part of the MDT discussion, particularly with the dietitian. The mytube videos produced by the MND society are a useful resource that may be of interest to individuals considering feeding tubes: https://mytube.mymnd.org.uk/

Corticobasal syndrome

Corticobasal syndrome (CBS) comprises a collection of conditions including Alzheimer's disease and corticobasal degeneration (CBD, a tau protein condition similar to PSP), which all present in a similar way. Although different pathologies can cause the same phenotype, the following discussion concentrates largely on the condition caused by CBD pathology. Individuals typically present between the ages of 60 and 80. There are different subtypes, with recent diagnostic criteria outlined in Table 13.3 (Armstrong et al., 2013). The PSP Association (2019a) has published a list of red flags for CBS (Table 13.4), which may help to prompt diagnosis. Presenting symptoms for CBS include:

- A dystonic upper limb
- Difficulty executing motor programmes (apraxia)
- Gait disorder
- Visuospatial dysfunction, with difficulty piecing together visual information to make a whole visual representation
- Corticosensory loss, where sensory information such as a drawing a shape on the palm of the hand cannot be integrated into a perceived shape such as a number
- Language disorder with non-fluent aphasia
- Dementia with subcortical problems, as found in PSP (Graham et al., 2003; Mahapatra et al., 2004).

Mean survival is 7.9 years, during which individuals progress rapidly toward dependence, with difficulties in mobility, swallowing, speech and cognition.

Case study

Carol is 74 years old and has recently noticed that her right hand is clumsier and feels stiff; it does not always do what she wants it to do. She has to struggle to put her earrings on and is finding that manipulating the remote control for the TV is more challenging. Previously, she was a keen seamstress, but now she finds that the process of rethreading the needle of her sewing machine confusing. She has recently given up driving, as she was finding it increasingly difficult to work out the spaces between obstacles. She has had difficulty finding

TABLE 13.3 Diagnostic criteria for corticobasal degeneration

Probable CBD	Possible CBD	FBSS*	NAV of PPA*	PSPS*
Age ≥50, less than two relatives with CBD and asymmetric presentation of two of a, b, and c AND two of d, e or f.	Asymmetric presentation of one of a, b, and c AND two of d, e or f.	Two of: Executive dysfunction; Behavioural or personality change; Visuospatial deficits	Effortful agrammatic speech with one of the following: Impaired sentence but preserved word comprehension; Groping, distorted speech production (apraxia of speech)	Three of the following: Axial or symmetric limb rigidity or akinesia or postural instability or falls or urinary incontinence Behavioural changes or slowing or paralysis of vertical saccades
a. Limb rigidity or akinesia b. Limb dystonia c. Limb myoclonus				
d. Orobuccal or limb apraxia e. Corticosensory deficit f. Alien-limb phenomenon				

Abbreviations: FBSS, frontal behavioural-spatial syndrome; NAV of PPA, non-fluent or agrammatic variant of primary progressive aphasia; PSPS, PSP syndrome.
*Presentation must be insidious with a minimal duration of 1 year. Permitted phenotypes for probable CBD include probable CBD OR FBSS or NAV WITH one CBD feature (a to f). Permitted phenotypes for possible CBD are possible CBD OR FBSS, NAV OR PSPS WITH one CBD feature (b to f). Exclusion criteria include evidence of other conditions (e.g., MSA, amyotrophic lateral sclerosis, Lewy body disease, structural lesion, genetic cause or alternative primary progressive aphasia.
Adapted from Armstrong et al. (2013).

TABLE 13.4 Red flags for a diagnosis of corticobasal degeneration

1	**Highly asymmetric progressive presentation**	One side affected much earlier and worse than the other
2	**Apraxia**	Clumsy, awkward hands
3	**Dystonia**	Odd posture of hand, foot, arm or leg
4	**Myoclonus**	Quick involuntary jerks
5	**Alien limb**	Reaching or grasping automatically
6	**Speech**	Slurring or distortion of speech, halting, stuttering
7	**Cognitive and behavioural changes**	Change in personality, irritability, apathy, low mood, difficulties with organisation and planning
8	**Poor response to levodopa**	

Adapted from https://pspassociation.org.uk/information-and-support/for-professionals/red-flags-for-gps/

the icons on her computer screen and has had more trouble reading. She has had appointments with the optician on several occasions but, despite new glasses, her eyesight remains poor.

On examination, Carol struggles to interpret Navon figures, which are, for example, where a large letter *H* is drawn out of lots of the small letter *t*'s. This is a sign of visuospatial difficulty. She has dystonia in her right upper limb—a stiffness throughout the whole range of movement of the arm as opposed to spasticity. When asked to copy meaningless gestures with her hand, she was able to do so with her left hand but not her right. Similarly, miming meaningful gestures, such as brushing her teeth, was more difficult with her right hand than her left, suggesting limb apraxia. She also had orobuccal apraxia, as she was unable to mime yawning or to blow a kiss to her husband in clinic.

Many features of PSP are commonly seen in CBS. Figure 13.2 highlights those that are common to both disorders and those that are more specific to PSP or CBS. Much of the advice that we offer to people with PSP is equally relevant for those with CBS. However, in this scenario, two main difficulties are specific for individuals with CBS. These are the difficulties that Carol has with dexterity and visuospatial function.

Dexterity

In the early stages of CBS, individuals may complain of unilateral stiffness and clumsiness in an arm or leg, sometimes progressing to severe dystonia such that the hand clenches into a fist. This can lead to problems with tissue breakdown and hand hygiene, as cleaning and drying the hand may become difficult. If the hand is clenched too tightly, the fingernails may dig into the palm.

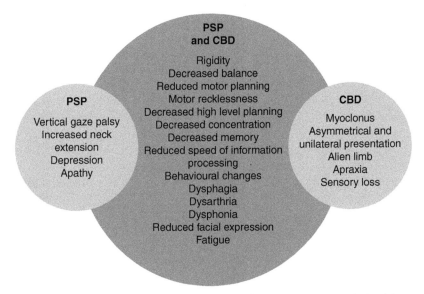

FIGURE 13.2 Common impairments in progressive supranuclear palsy and corticobasal degeneration. *Reproduced with permission from the PSP Association (2020).*

Several members of the MDT have a role to play in this scenario. Early referral to a physiotherapist and OT to encourage use and stretching of the limb is important. A mirror may be helpful for visual feedback when working with the upper limb. As the condition progresses, assessment for splinting, either off-the-shelf or custom made, or referral to specialist hand therapy services may be appropriate. In severe cases, injection of botulinum toxin into the flexor muscles of the hand can be carried out to weaken them. Intensive therapy, including splinting, should be carried out after this to stretch the fingers. Hard splints that gradually increase in size (serial casting) may then help to obtain more range of movement without tonic flexion of the hand.

Visuospatial dysfunction

Individuals with CBS may develop visuospatial dysfunction, leading to difficulty in integrating visual information. They may have difficulty making sense of the world around them. In Carol's case, this explains why she had difficulty parking her car and finding icons on the computer screen. Along with the apraxia, it is also the reason why she is experiencing difficulties threading the needle on her sewing machine.

Many members of the MDT are needed to treat this type of problem. Carol had already given up driving, but all individuals with CBS who are still driving must be assessed and advised regarding their ability to drive.

The OT may provide equipment for use around the house that can improve day-to-day function, such as kettle tippers or electric can openers. Adjusting settings, font sizes and color on screens may help with computer work. As problems progress, an ophthalmologist may certify the individual as partially sighted, opening up the possibility of more help such as a blue badge for car parking and contact with the Royal National Institute for the Blind for talking books or aids such as a white stick.

In the early stages, to optimise mobility, the physiotherapist should focus on coordination and bilateral tasks with the use of visual targets. As the condition progresses, the focus will shift to compensatory strategies, balancing safety with function. Because of the unilateral nature of the upper limb problems, different walking aids may be needed. The Evolution four-wheel walker with monobrake and arm trough and the U-Step are worth considering. Both these aids have a single hand-braking mechanism.

Multiple system atrophy

MSA is a rare condition, with a prevalence of 3.4 to 4.4 per 100,000 (Bjornsdottir et al., 2013; Schrag et al., 1999). Mean age of presentation is around 60 years, and MSA is slightly more common in women than in men. The mean time between onset and death is 5.7 years (Bjornsdottir et al., 2013). MSA is caused by the accumulation of alpha-synuclein protein in the brain, in contrast to PSP and CBS, which are caused by the accumulation of tau protein.

As its name would suggest, MSA is a condition of many systems, and individuals may present with any of the following features:

- Parkinsonism, with bradykinesia and rigidity
- A cerebellar syndrome with ataxia
- Autonomic dysfunction, with bowel, bladder or blood pressure problems
- Respiratory symptoms including stridor and obstructive sleep apnoea
- Bulbar issues, with speech and swallowing difficulties

Unlike PSP and CBS, cognition is not usually significantly affected in MSA. Established diagnostic criteria are outlined in Table 13.5, with supportive and non-supportive features for the diagnosis listed in Table 13.6 (Gilman et al., 2008).

Case study

David is 49 years old. He lives with his wife and two children and works as an accountant. For the last 2 years he has often felt "very wobbly" on his feet, frequently staggering and bumping into things; his work colleagues were concerned that he had a drinking problem. He often feels lightheaded when he gets up first thing in the morning and after big meals. His wife has noticed that he has very noisy breathing at night, and David often reports feeling tired during the day and that he is sleeping poorly at night. He developed erectile dysfunction about 3 years ago. He feels that he is constantly waking at night to pass urine and he is constipated. His speech is becoming faint and slightly squeaky. He is

TABLE 13.5 Diagnostic criteria for multiple system atrophy

Probable MSA	Possible MSA
Autonomic failure involving urinary incontinence (inability to control the release of urine from the bladder) and erectile dysfunction in males *or* an orthostatic decrease in blood pressure within 3 minutes of standing by at least 30 mm Hg systolic or 15 mm Hg diastolic *and*	At least one feature suggesting autonomic dysfunction (otherwise unexplained urinary urgency, frequency or incomplete bladder emptying; erectile dysfunction in males or significant orthostatic blood pressure drop that does not meet the requirement for probable MSA) *and*
Parkinsonism (bradykinesia with rigidity, tremor, or postural instability) that is poorly responsive to levodopa *or* a cerebellar syndrome (gait ataxia with cerebellar dysarthria, limb ataxia, or cerebellar oculomotor dysfunction)	Parkinsonism (bradykinesia with rigidity, tremor or postural instability) *or* a cerebellar syndrome (gait ataxia with cerebellar dysarthria, limb ataxia, or cerebellar oculomotor dysfunction) *and* at least one of the following:
	For possible MSAp or MSAc Babinski sign with hyperreflexia Stridor **For possible MSAp** Rapidly progressive Parkinsonism Poor response to levodopa Postural instability within 3 years of motor onset Cerebellar signs Dysphagia within 5 years of motor onset Atrophy on MRI of putamen, middle cerebellar peduncle, pons or cerebellum Hypometabolism on FDG-PET in putamen, brainstem or cerebellum **For possible MSAc** Parkinsonism Atrophy on MRI of putamen, middle cerebellar peduncle or pons Hypometabolism on FDG-PET in putamen Presynaptic nigrostriatal dopaminergic denervation on SPECT or PET

Abbreviations: FDG-PET, fluorodeoxyglucose positron emission tomography; MRI, magnetic resonance imaging; MSAc, cerebellar variant of MSA; MSAp, Parkinsonian variant of MSA; SPECT, single photon emission computed tomography
Adapted from Gilman et al. (2008).

less inclined to use the telephone as he is becoming conscious of people struggling to understand him.

On examination, David has finger-nose ataxia and heel-shin ataxia (incoordination). He also has dysdiadochokinesis: difficulty with smoothly tapping the palm and back of one hand on the palm of the other. He has an unsteady, ataxic gait. He has increased tone and brisk reflexes in his legs and upgoing plantar

TABLE 13.6 Supportive and non-supportive features for the diagnosis of multiple system atrophy

Supportive	Non-supportive
Orofacial dystonia	Classic pill-rolling tremor
Disproportionate antecollis	Clinically significant neuropathy
Camptocormia (severe anterior flexion of the spine) and/or Pisa syndrome (severe lateral flexion of the spine)	Hallucinations not induced by drugs
Contractures of hands or feet	Onset after the age of 75 years
Inspiratory sighs	Family history of ataxia or Parkinsonism
Severe dysphonia	Dementia
Severe dysarthria	White matter lesions suggesting multiple sclerosis
New or increased snoring	
Cold hands or feet	
Pathological laughter or crying	
Jerky, myoclonic postural/action tremor	

Adapted from Gilman et al. (2008).

reflexes. When doing finger and thumb taps on each hand, his movements are slow and decreasing in amplitude, suggestive of a Parkinsonian bradykinesia.

MSA may be either predominantly Parkinsonian, with slowness of movement, termed MSAp, or cerebellar, with ataxia termed MSAc. Autonomic dysfunction and upper motor neuron signs may also be present. David's presentation is not uncommon for MSAc, where the cerebellar features of ataxia predominate over the features of Parkinsonism. Frequently, individuals experience symptoms for several years preceding a diagnosis of MSA. This case study focuses on the autonomic and respiratory features of the condition. Many aspects of the care suggested earlier for individuals with PSP and CBS are also relevant for MSA, although there are some differences. The use of prism glasses for those with PSP was discussed earlier, but prism glasses can correct for either looking up or looking down. Those with MSA often find that owing to antecollis (forward head flexion), prism glasses that correct for the head-down position are effective for activities such as watching television and seeing other people's faces. Antecollis can be painful; a collar may be helpful as the condition progresses.

Autonomic symptoms

The autonomic symptoms of the condition are summarised in Table 13.7. They include bladder and bowel dysfunction, respiratory problems, erectile dysfunction and orthostatic hypotension.

TABLE 13.7 Autonomic features and symptoms of multiple system atrophy

Autonomic feature	Symptoms
Bladder dysfunction	Urgency, frequency, nocturia, urinary retention
Sexual dysfunction	Reduced or absent erections in males
Respiratory dysfunction	Inspiratory sighs, stridor, snoring, apnoea, oxygen de-saturation
Postural hypotension	Dizziness, blurred vision, "coat-hanger" pain, altered consciousness, falls
Cold extremities	Cold feet and hands
Sweating disturbance	Sweating after meals, increased or de-creased sweating
Bowel dysfunction	Constipation, diarrhoea, or both

Orthostatic hypotension (OH) occurs when there is a fall in blood pressure when the person quickly moves from lying to standing or sitting. This can result in significant symptoms in individuals with MSA, leading to fainting. OH is discussed at length in Chapter 10 but not further here.

Urinary problems

Urinary problems—including urgency, frequency, nocturia (nighttime frequency) and retention—are common. Often these symptoms precede the diagnosis of MSA. Many individuals may already have been seen in a urology service and have undergone interventions. If they have not already been seen, it is important to make a referral, as urinary flow studies and bladder scans may be required to determine the cause of the problem.

Nocturia may occur because the bladder is more irritable and does not fill much before it needs to empty or because the bladder fills more quickly.

An irritable bladder is a common occurrence in the general population as well as in people with MSA; it often causes urinary urgency during the day as well as night. Measures to relax the bladder muscle are helpful. Conservative measures include reducing or stopping caffeine. Medications include anticholinergics, such as solifenacin or oxybutynin, although caution should be exercised, as this class of drugs can cause cognitive dysfunction, blurred vision, constipation and dry mouth. Mirabegron and botulinum toxin treatment to the bladder can also be used.

Increased frequency may also be due to incomplete emptying of the bladder or increased urine production by the kidneys. Incomplete emptying, caused by a dysfunctional autonomic nervous system in MSA, would result in a significant residual of urine in the bladder after voiding. This can be ascertained by carrying out a post-voiding bladder ultrasound scan to determine the volume of urine remaining. Such an examination is often carried out by the continence service when they are investigating causes of urinary frequency. Treatment includes intermittent self-catheterisation, a fixed urinary catheter, or a suprapubic catheter. If hand dexterity becomes an issue, a caregiver may have to assist with intermittent catheterisation; therefore an indwelling or suprapubic catheter may be more appropriate.

Increased urine production by the kidneys can occur in MSA when autonomic dysfunction leads to the pooling of fluid in the legs during the day. When individuals like David lie flat at night, this fluid reenters the circulation, increasing the perfusion of the kidneys and causing more urine production. There are some options to help deal with this. Raising the head of the bed by 30 degrees can help to avoid overperfusion of the kidneys, thus slowing down urine production and reducing nocturia. A medication such as desmopressin may be helpful to limit urine production, but in that case blood monitoring would be necessary, as the use of desmopressin can lead to hyponatremia due to fluid retention in the circulation.

Constipation

Constipation, a common concern, is due to the slowing of bowel movements due to autonomic dysfunction. Initially the PDNS or dietitian can give advice regarding diet and fluid intake. The physiotherapist may encourage the individual to mobilise as much as possible to assist bowel motility. Along with the OT, the physiotherapist may also advise on posture for toileting and adaptations that can help in the process. If individuals find it difficult to sit and balance, they will be less able to effectively empty their bowels. To make this easier, the OT or physiotherapist can consider a raised toilet seat with both a back rest and arm supports as well as a footstool. If this is insufficient, referral to a local continence service may be indicated.

Medication may be useful and can be divided into four main types:

- Bulking agents, such as ispaghula husk (Fybogel), which increase the weight of the stool and stimulates bowel movements
- Softeners, such as docusate, which retain water and soften the stool
- Osmotic laxatives, such as lactulose, which draw water from the rest of the body to the bowel to soften the stool
- Stimulants, such as bisacodyl, which stimulate the bowel to move

It is also worthwhile considering what other medications, such as opiates, the individual is taking and whether these could affect bowel function. Some individuals may also require suppositories, enemas or bowel irrigation. It is important to note that periods of prolonged straining on the toilet followed by standing up can cause a fall in blood pressure, OH and faintness. In extreme cases it can cause loss of consciousness. The MSA Trust's guidelines on bowel management may be useful.

Erectile dysfunction

Erectile dysfunction, as experienced in David's case, is an early feature of the condition and is the inability to achieve or sustain an erection sufficient for penetration. In MSA, autonomic dysfunction may also lead to problems with ejaculation. The general practitioner or neurologist can prescribe an oral medication, such as sildenafil (Viagra), to enable increased blood flow to the penis and a stronger erection. However, it is important to remember that these medications can reduce overall blood pressure, possibly leading to syncope. Vacuum pumps can also be considered. There is little research into female sexual dysfunction. For more information, please refer to the MSA Trust's fact sheet on relationships, sex and MSA.

Sleep disorders

In the case study, David was found to have a sleep disorder, as highlighted by his feelings of fatigue and his wife's report of noisy breathing. Sleep disorders are common in MSA, affecting 40% of those with the condition. These features often precede other physical symptoms such as walking difficulties and autonomic dysfunction. Sleep symptoms include reduced and fragmented sleep, excessive daytime sleepiness, Rapid-eye-movement sleep behaviour disorder (RBD), obstructive sleep apnoea (OSA) and stridor.

In RBD, individuals act out their dreams because they have lost the body's normal paralysis during the dream phase of sleep. For example, a person so affected may be dreaming of being in a fight and start attacking his wife lying next to him, which is obviously unsettling. A small dose of clonazepam may be helpful, allowing the person to stay in a deeper sleep phase for longer. However, it may cause more sedation, which can lead to more falls.

OSA is a phenomenon wherein breathing at night is intermittently obstructed by collapse of the airway. The predominant cause in the general population is obesity. In MSA, however, this is thought to be caused by narrowing of the upper airway due to hypokinesia, dystonia, and weakness of bulbar muscles. This narrowing is worsened during sleep when muscle tone is reduced. In addition, central deficits, caused by neurodegeneration of the respiratory centres in the brainstem, cause a disordered response to respiration, leading to further sleep apnoea (Gaig & Iranzo, 2012). Constant arousals due to hypoxia lead to a lack of restful sleep and increased tiredness during the day. A lack of adequate ventilation during the night can lead to hypercapnia (abnormal levels of carbon dioxide in the bloodstream) and early-morning headache. Management includes referral to respiratory services, and continuous positive airways pressure (CPAP) is often recommended. CPAP provides air to the individual (through a flow generator and mask) at a higher-than-normal pressure, which makes it easier to overcome the resistance of narrowed airways and greatly facilitates ventilation, thus enabling the individual to avoid multiple awakenings during the night.

Stridor is a characteristic wheezing sound that occurs on inhaling due to narrowing of the airway. In MSA, both glottal narrowing and selective paralysis of the vocal cord abductors contribute to stridor. It can occur during the day or at night, but nighttime stridor is more common and is associated with shortened survival. Deep-breathing exercises, such as diaphragmatic breathing techniques, can be practised with a physiotherapist or SLT. As in the management of OSA, individuals may be referred to respiratory services and also to the ear/nose/throat team. Positive-pressure non-invasive ventilation may also be considered in the management of mild to moderate stridor, as well as surgical options such as tracheostomy or arytenoidectomy. There is some evidence of improved survival with the use of tracheostomy and, to a more limited extent, with CPAP (Cortelli et al., 2019). As a rule, CPAP seems to be effective for nighttime stridor. Daytime stridor suggests that stridor is occurring more often and without the reduction in resting tone that usually occurs at night. This indicates that daytime stridor may be more problematic. Thus, to maintain maximal independence, the surgical option of a tracheostomy may be more effective and appropriate. Treatment decisions for stridor must be considered carefully with the individual, as well as the respiratory, neurological and ear/nose/throat teams.

General management of atypical Parkinsonian syndromes

Challenges in diagnosis

Although this chapter has shown that PSP, CBD, and MSA are clearly different entities, they all present with similar problems and are often seen in the same clinic. Initially they can appear very similar to Parkinson's. Table 13.8 outlines some similarities and differences between these syndromes. However, the initial similarities can lead to significant delays in diagnosis, which, in the case of PSP, for example, can be 2 to 3 years after onset of the condition. This uncertainty in diagnosis can have significant psychological consequences for both the individual and family. Many individuals may be diagnosed with Parkinson's prior to their diagnosis of APS. Their comparison of their own disease trajectory against that of their peers with Parkinson's, which deteriorates more slowly, may be upsetting. Psychological support after the diagnosis, if possible, can be beneficial, and clinicians should offer referral soon after the diagnosis is made.

After 3 to 4 years, individuals with these conditions are often severely affected by their symptoms. In fact, the severity of their symptoms will be similar to or may be even worse than that of those entering palliative care with cancer diagnoses (Higginson et al., 2012). Not surprisingly, quality of life (QoL) for both the individual with one of these conditions and their caregiver deteriorates as the condition progresses. In a recent service evaluation project at our specialist regional clinic for these conditions, we found that both those affected and their caregivers had very poor QoL as measured by the condition-specific

TABLE 13.8 Differences between various syndromes

	IPD	PSP	CBD	MSA
Tremor	Resting	X	X	✓
Bradykinesia	✓	✓	✓	✓
Rigidity	✓	✓	✓	✓
Unstable	✓	✓✓	✓	✓
Symmetric	X	✓	X	X/✓
Cognitive	X	✓	✓	X
Response to levodopa	✓	X	X	X/✓
Dystonia	X	X	✓	X
Disease duration	++	+	+	+
Magnetic resonance imaging findings	X	Midbrain	X	#

Abbreviations: CBD, corticobasal degeneration; IPD, idiopathic Parkinson's disease; MSA, multiple system atrophy; PSP, progressive supranuclear palsy
X signifies that this symptom or sign is not present; more ✓s indicate an increasing severity of symptoms or signs. In the MRI section: the term *midbrain* refers to atrophy of the midbrain and a midbrain-to-pontine ratio of <0.52 (Massey et al., 2013); the term # refers to MRI changes in MSA which involve atrophy of the putamen, pons, cerebellum and middle cerebellar peduncle. These changes may be seen as putaminal atrophy, or a hyperintense putaminal rim and the "hot cross bun" sign due to atrophy of the pons (Kim et al., 2017). MRI findings do not enable a definitive diagnosis as these can be found in other conditions or may not be found at all; they only provide support to the clinical impression.

and caregiver-specific scales—PSP QoL, MSA QoL, and carer QoL (Pillas et al., 2016; Schrag et al., 2007; Schrag et al., 2006).

Calvert et al. (2013) used the EQ-5D, a QOL questionnaire, to compare people with PSP and MSA to those with other conditions. They found that PSP and MSA have the worst QoL of all the conditions that were considered, including motor neuron disease. Similar research has shown that caregivers for individuals with PSP have worse caregiver burdens and more depression than those caring for individuals with Parkinson's and have a similar level to caregivers of individuals with Alzheimer's disease (Schmotz et al., 2017).

Hospital admissions

These conditions are expensive to treat, with costs estimated at £44,700 ($61,400) per person per year for PSP and £33,060 ($45,420) for MSA, both greater than for Alzheimer's disease at £22,670 ($31,140) (McCrone et al., 2011). Inpatient admissions account for 40% of the PSP costs and 25% of MSA costs. Recent research carried out by our group (in preparation) shows that a significant number of people with PSP are admitted to hospital each year. For example, in 2019, there were 2165 admissions out of a total estimated patient population of only

2799. In our experience, owing to the nature of the condition, many individuals have multiple admissions. Although it is difficult to know exactly what proportion of these are emergency or elective admissions, it is clear that reducing the number of admissions per person would benefit QoL for both individuals and their caregivers as well as having a financial benefit to the provider by reducing healthcare costs.

Medication

There is no cure for these conditions. Medication for specific symptoms has been highlighted earlier. In addition, dopamine and amantadine are generally trialed at some point during the course of these conditions. Our practice involves a trial of co-beneldopa or co-careldopa to 50/200 mg three times daily, if tolerated, after diagnosis. About one-third of individuals with APS conditions may have a mild response to this level of dopamine, with a slight decrease in the number of falls or apathy somewhat reduced. However, a large response should prompt a reconsideration of the diagnosis. We have also found amantadine to be useful, particularly later in the course of the condition, for its energising effect, sometimes enabling individuals to communicate with single words where previously they were mute.

Drooling or excessive salivation (sialorrhea) can be problematic in all three conditions. Initially, atropine eye drops could be considered. Three to four drops can be placed around the gums and under the tongue, with the aid of a cotton bud, up to three times a day. Later, a hyoscine patch, with care about its effect on cognition, or glycopyrronium, could be considered. Botulinum toxin injections to the salivary glands may be helpful if these medications fail.

Multidisciplinary intervention

As well as medication for symptoms, the other mainstay of treatment is utilising the MDT for support. Therapy should have realistic goals, such as promoting QoL and engagement in meaningful activities, while being honest with the individual and caregiver about what can be offered and achieved, particularly regarding time frames.

All individuals with APS are likely to require a wheelchair, but there are subtle differences in the conditions. Unlike PSP and CBS, MSA rarely produces such profound cognitive and visual impairment; therefore an electric wheelchair is often advocated early in the condition, especially if OH is problematic. This can provide the individual with improved independence and QoL.

Bed mobility can be challenging in all APS conditions. Appropriate assessment for equipment needs, which may include a profiling bed or WendyLett sheets, should be carried out. Sleep systems and specialist seating assessments will have to be considered in the later stages of these conditions.

Hydrotherapy, or aquatic therapy, can be considered for all APS conditions. Swimming or any exercise in a pool may be particularly beneficial for MSA because of the counteractive effect of hydrostatic pressure on OH; however, the effects of excessive heat should be considered and managed appropriately.

Although there is currently very little if any literature to support therapy and MDT work in these conditions, early access to the MDT and a named contact to coordinate care is recommended (MSA Trust, 2015; PSP Association, 2011, 2018). The NHS England Rightcare Toolkit for progressive neurological conditions highlights the priorities that should be considered when a service for people with MSA, PSP, and/or CBS is being provided (NHS Rightcare, 2019). These guidelines and numerous published expert opinions suggest that all three of these conditions benefit from MDT work.

However, it is not clear that this is being offered routinely to these individuals. A national audit carried out by our service reviewed service provision for those with APS. Only half of hospital trusts contacted replied, with the predominance from specialist centres. An estimated 1 in 6 individuals were not seen in a specialist setting. These individuals are less likely to have access to a key worker to coordinate their care or regular input from a MDT. Although this finding implies that many were seen in specialist centres and appeared to have access to a coordinator, the predominance of replies from these centres will have skewed these results. This suggests that if information for all individuals were known, a significant number would be from non-specialist centres and therefore would not be receiving coordinated and MDT care as suggested.

Advanced care planning

Early referral to palliative care, discussions around advanced care planning, and individuals being put on the GP's "at risk" register should be part of routine practice. Early discussions, including individuals and caregivers as well as all members of the MDT, to consider lasting powers of attorney for both health and finances should also be encouraged.

There are various models of clinic that could be used to facilitate specialist input while also providing access to the MDT. As an example, a community palliative MDT is described in the following box. Other models of MDTs are discussed in Chapter 3, on MDTs.

A community palliative multidisciplinary team for atypical Parkinsonian syndromes led by a Parkinson's disease nurse specialist

Having worked as a Parkinson's disease nurse specialist (PDNS) for 15 years, I can see trends and patterns as atypical Parkinsonian syndromes (APSs) progress, particularly when compared to people with idiopathic Parkinson's. End-of-life care for these individuals can be complex and changes in their condition can be sudden and unpredictable; therefore they need access to a range of specialist clinicians in a timely manner.

Our community multidisciplinary team (MDT) includes a neurology specialist, physiotherapists, OTs and an SLT. We work together in people's homes and care homes, supporting these individuals and helping them to make complex decisions. I lead the service, prescribing, adjusting, and stopping medications as well as advising on anticipatory palliative medications. I can even verify death. Our team can facilitate treatment by helping individuals to make advance care plans and advance decisions to refuse treatment (ADRTs). We work collaboratively to carry out complex mental capacity assessments.

As an example of our work, our team has been working with 84-year-old Robert, who is in the palliative stage of progressive supranuclear palsy (PSP). The members of the MDT know him well. Over the past 4 years I have spent time with Robert's family and advised them regarding applying for a power of attorney for health and finance. He has written a will and completed an ADRT and Recommended Summary Plan for Emergency Care and Treatment (ReSPECT) form (a person-centred form, reflecting the individual's wishes regarding future clinical intervention), stating that he wishes no enteral feeding or resuscitation. Robert has moved into 24-hour care. I am the key contact for him, but he continues to see other members of the MDT. Robert is now on a palliative trajectory toward the last days of his life. The SLT is helping him with swallowing, feeding, and communication, and the physiotherapist and I are making joint visits.

APSs pose challenges, as the presenting symptoms cannot always be treated medically. Levodopa does not always help in PSP, corticobasal degeneration, or multiple system atrophy. Bulbar symptoms can advance rapidly in PSP and autonomic complications are difficult to control in multiple system atrophy. It is important to treat the person, not the condition, and to work collaboratively to deliver the best possible palliative care.

Sarah McCracken, PDNS

Conclusion

Currently there is no cure for APSs. They are demanding conditions that make heavy demands on resources. Although there is little established evidence for the benefits of an MDT in these conditions, our experience shows that effective communication and close work among members of the MDT are essential in their management.

Practitioners treating these individuals in the community or aiming to set up a specialist clinic should seek advice from the MSA Trust and the PSP Association (PSPA), or their US equivalent CurePSP. They have useful fact sheets and guidance, which have been referenced throughout this chapter. The PSPA has also developed an interactive tool to support professionals in their work. These organisations are responsive to the needs of clinicians and can provide assistance regarding tailoring services for individuals.

Individuals may be treated for Parkinson's before a formal diagnosis is made. Therapists and the PDNS should be alert for red flags, highlighting concerns if individuals do not fit the normal pattern for Parkinson's. Those with knowledge of the conditions can play a key role in continuing healthcare funding applications, ensuring that individuals receive the appropriate levels of care and funding.

Although these conditions have no cure and individuals deteriorate rapidly, there is an enormous amount that can be done by the clinician and the MDT to maintain the individual's QoL and independence for as long as possible. As Dame Cicely Saunders, founder of the hospice movement, said "You matter because you are you, and you matter to the end of your life. We will do all we can, not only to help you die peacefully but also to live until you die."

Top tips for atypical Parkinsonian syndromes

1. If an individual has severe postural instability but good stride length, consider progressive supranuclear palsy rather than Parkinson's.
2. Frequent backward falls are a red flag for atypical Parkinsonian syndromes.
3. Atypical Parkinsonian syndromes are progressive conditions; therefore one must anticipate change and plan for the future.
4. The person, not the condition, is to be treated.
5. Owing to the speed of deterioration and difficulty with communication that can occur, early discussions regarding advanced care planning, feeding tubes and end of life should be considered.
6. Record a voice bank, capturing the individual's voice for posterity or for future use in electronic communication.
7. Refer for equipment such as a wheelchair in a timely manner.
8. Access resources and guidance from the Progressive Supranuclear Palsy Association and Multiple System Atrophy Trust, or CurePSP in the US.

References

Armstrong, M. J., Litvan, I., Lang, A. E., Bak, T. H., Bhatia, K. P., Borroni, B., et al. (2013). Criteria for the diagnosis of corticobasal degeneration. *Neurology*, *80*(5), 496–503.

Bjornsdottir, A., Gudmundsson, G., Blondal, H., & Olafsson, E. (2013). Incidence and prevalence of multiple system atrophy: a nationwide study in Iceland. *J Neurol Neurosurg Psychiatry*, *84*(2), 136–140.

Calvert, M., Pall, H., Hoppitt, T., Eaton, B., Savill, E., & Sackley, C. (2013). Health-related quality of life and supportive care in patients with rare long-term neurological conditions. *Qual Life Res*, *22*(6), 1231–1238.

Cortelli, P., Calandra-Buonaura, G., Benarroch, E. E., Giannini, G., Iranzo, A., Low, P. A., et al. (2019). Stridor in multiple system atrophy: Consensus statement on diagnosis, prognosis, and treatment. *Neurology*, *93*(14), 630–639.

Gaig, C., & Iranzo, A. (2012). Sleep-disordered breathing in neurodegenerative diseases. *Curr Neurol Neurosci Rep*, *12*(2), 205–217.

Ghosh, B. C., Carpenter, R. H., & Rowe, J. B. (2013). A longitudinal study of motor, oculomotor and cognitive function in progressive supranuclear palsy. *PLoS ONE*, *8*(9), e74486.

Gilman, S., Wenning, G. K., Low, P. A., Brooks, D. J., Mathias, C. J., Trojanowski, J. Q., et al. (2008). Second consensus statement on the diagnosis of multiple system atrophy. *Neurology*, *71*(9), 670–676.

Graham, N. L., Bak, T. H., & Hodges, J. R. (2003). Corticobasal degeneration as a cognitive disorder. *Mov Disord*, *18*(11), 1224–1232.

Higginson, I. J., Gao, W., Saleem, T. Z., Chaudhuri, K. R., Burman, R., McCrone, P., et al. (2012). Symptoms and quality of life in late stage Parkinson syndromes: a longitudinal community study of predictive factors. *PLoS ONE, 7*(11), e46327.

Hoglinger, G. U., Respondek, G., Stamelou, M., Kurz, C., Josephs, K. A., Lang, A. E., et al. (2017). Clinical diagnosis of progressive supranuclear palsy: The movement disorder society criteria. *Mov Disord, 32*(6), 853–864.

Kim, H. J., Jeon, B., & Fung, V. S. C. (2017). Role of Magnetic Resonance Imaging in the Diagnosis of Multiple System Atrophy. *Mov Disord Clin Pract, 4*(1), 12–20.

Litvan, I., Mangone, C. A., McKee, A., Verny, M., Parsa, A., Jellinger, K., et al. (1996). Natural history of progressive supranuclear palsy (Steele-Richardson-Olszewski syndrome) and clinical predictors of survival: a clinicopathological study. *J Neurol Neurosurg Psychiatry, 60*(6), 615–620.

Mahapatra, R. K., Edwards, M. J., Schott, J. M., & Bhatia, K. P. (2004). Corticobasal degeneration. *Lancet Neurol, 3*(12), 736–743.

Massey, L. A., Jager, H. R., Paviour, D. C., O'Sullivan, S. S., Ling, H., Williams, D. R., et al. (2013). The midbrain to pons ratio: a simple and specific MRI sign of progressive supranuclear palsy. *Neurology, 80*(20), 1856–1861.

McCrone, P., Payan, C. A., Knapp, M., Ludolph, A., Agid, Y., Leigh, P. N., et al. (2011). The economic costs of progressive supranuclear palsy and multiple system atrophy in France, Germany and the United Kingdom. *PLoS ONE, 6*(9), e24369.

MSA Trust. *Factsheets [online]*. Available at: https://www.msatrust.org.uk/support-for-you/fact-sheets/.

MSA Trust (2015). Multiple System Atrophy Care Pathway.

NHS Rightcare (2019). Progressive Neurological Conditions Toolkit. https://www.england.nhs.uk/rightcare/wp-content/uploads/sites/40/2019/08/progressive-neuro-toolkit.pdf.

Pillas, M., Selai, C., Quinn, N. P., Lees, A., Litvan, I., Lang, A., et al. (2016). Development and validation of a carers quality-of-life questionnaire for parkinsonism (PQoL Carers). *Qual Life Res, 25*(1), 81–88.

PSP Association. (2011). Pathway of Care for PSP: A Guide for Health and Social Care Professionals [online]. Available at: https://pspassociation.org.uk/app/uploads/2018/06/PT009-13-6-Pathway-Guide-web-2013.pdf.

PSP Association. (2018). *A Professional's Guide to Corticobasal Degeneration* [online]. Available at: https://pspassociation.org.uk/app/uploads/2018/11/PSPA-CBD-Guide-A5-LR.pdf.

PSP Association. (2019a). *Red Flags for Corticobasal Degeneration (CBD)* [online]. Available at: https://pspassociation.org.uk/app/uploads/2019/01/CBD-Red-Flags-1-Final-LR.pdf.

PSP Association. (2019b). Red Flags for Progressive Supranuclear Palsy (PSP). Retrieved October 28, 2020, from https://pspassociation.org.uk/app/uploads/2019/02/PSP-Red-Flag-Final-LR.pdf.

PSP Association. (2020). A Guide to PSP & CBD for Occupational Therapists. Available at: https://pspassociation.org.uk/app/uploads/2020/10/OT-guide-2020-LR-Final.pdf.

Schmotz, C., Richinger, C., & Lorenzl, S. (2017). High Burden and Depression Among Late-Stage Idiopathic Parkinson Disease and Progressive Supranuclear Palsy Caregivers. *J Geriatr Psychiatry Neurol, 30*(5), 267–272.

Schrag, A., Ben-Shlomo, Y., & Quinn, N. P. (1999). Prevalence of progressive supranuclear palsy and multiple system atrophy: a cross-sectional study. *Lancet, 354*(9192), 1771–1775.

Schrag, A., Selai, C., Mathias, C., Low, P., Hobart, J., Brady, N., et al. (2007). Measuring health-related quality of life in MSA: the MSA-QoL. *Mov Disord, 22*(16), 2332–2338.

Schrag, A., Selai, C., Quinn, N., Lees, A., Litvan, I., Lang, A., et al. (2006). Measuring quality of life in PSP: the PSP-QoL. *Neurology, 67*(1), 39–44.

Chapter 14

Remote Assessments for Parkinson's

Richard Genever

Chapter Outline

Introduction

The onset of the COVID-19 outbreak had a sudden impact on every aspect of healthcare. At the end of March 2020, seeing people face-to-face in clinic instantly became impossible or, at the very least, risky. The severity of this problem necessitated rapid and widespread change, leading to different ways of diagnosing and supporting people with many conditions. When clinicians were faced with the possibility of not being able to make an assessment, the telephone or a computer became a much more appealing option.

Assessing people remotely presents two types of challenge. The first of these is practical; the second is the need to develop new skills. This chapter looks at the various options for the remote assessment of people with Parkinson's and the merits and potential issues involved. It also considers the ways in which we communicate face-to-face and how that approach might have to be modified for remote assessments.

Remote assessment: the options

Telephone assessment

The simplest way to conduct a remote assessment is by telephone, which has the great advantage of being almost universally available. It is familiar and does not require any training for the service user. Telephone clinics are extremely easy to implement from an organisational point of view. All that is needed is a list of the individuals' telephone numbers. As the only requirement for the person with Parkinson's is to be near a phone, there is more flexibility about exactly when a telephone assessment might take place. This can allow services to be maintained even during a time of unpredictable inpatient demands and can be delivered from anywhere. Some thought must be given to the pre-clinic information that is sent out. Service users would have to know in advance if there could be some uncertainty about when they might be called. Some would need a more fixed time especially if they were going to be supported during the call by another person.

The flexibility about where and when a telephone clinic could be delivered opens up possibilities that might not previously have been considered. For example, an evening clinic might be popular with working people and might also suit a clinician who wanted to work over a smaller number of days. Another factor that might be of relevance during a pandemic is that a remote clinic can be delivered by someone who is self-isolating but well.

There are some obvious disadvantages with a telephone clinic. The inability to see the person that you are assessing means that examination is not possible. This limits telephone consultations to follow-up appointments (at least in the realm of movement disorders). Being restricted to what you can hear means that you are relying on interpreting those messages correctly. Also, there is no opportunity to pick up on other useful pieces of non-verbal "intelligence," such as noticing a person's partner shaking their head when you hear the service user saying that all is well.

Video assessment

Video assessment is not new. However, until recently, it was mainly the preserve of teams that supported remote communities. During the time of COVID-19, many more people have used video conferencing as a way of maintaining contact with family and friends. According to the Online Nation survey (Ofcom, 2020), the number of online adult consumers using video calling weekly doubled to 71% between February and May of 2020. This means that video calling has been socialised to a much greater extent.

The most common way for people to access healthcare remotely is from their own homes. Any internet-enabled device with a camera can be used. This means that anyone with a smartphone, tablet computer, laptop or personal computer with a webcam can receive a review using such a device.

There are a number of National Health Service (NHS)–approved systems that can be used for remote assessment. These include AccuRx, EMIS, TPP, Near

Me (Scotland only) and NHS Attend Anywhere. The advantage of using one of these products is the assurance that it has reached all the required standards for use in this area. NHS England and Improvement procured 12 months' access to Attend Anywhere as a means of accelerating the process (British Medical Association, 2020). Using a platform that is designed for healthcare, rather than videoconferencing, can have additional benefits such as built-in waiting areas or the ability to message service users to update them about delays.

In 2020, NHSX issued guidance that video conferencing applications— such as WhatsApp, Skype, or FaceTime—could be used to communicate with patients. You are permitted to use your own device, but you should make sure that you use strong passwords and should have the same regard for the protection of confidential information as with any other clinical situation (NHSX, 2020). One additional consideration if you are not using an approved healthcare application with your own device is that you may be sharing direct contact information, such as your phone number.

In the early days of telehealth, during which video-enabled devices were not as commonplace, another option was to attend a telemedicine room. Such venues were often located in a local healthcare facility, such as a primary health centre, and some still exist. Users book a time in the telemedicine room, where camera operation and the link to the assessment centre are all taken care of. This approach means that the technical aspects are facilitated by an expert. Issues such as having the right camera angle for any situation will be managed for you. It does mean that there will be an additional person in the room at the time of assessment and does not necessarily reduce the risks of viral transmission. This approach is mainly seen in large countries, such as Canada, where distance can be an obstacle to effective healthcare delivery Ontario Telemedicine Network, 2020).

How safe is video assessment?

Overall, video assessment has been shown to be safe and acceptable to service users (Wherton, 2020). Some situations lend themselves more naturally to video than others. Monitoring people with a long-term condition, such as Parkinson's, is particularly conducive to remote assessment. Clinical scenarios that would require palpation to make an effective assessment would not be appropriate. This means that making a new diagnosis of Parkinson's might be possible by video but not telephone. However, there might be times when a face-to-face review might still be necessary to make a clear diagnosis.

General tips on providing remote assessments

The basic principles of a remote assessment are the same as those for face-to-face reviews. There is a clinical conversation, problems are recognised, and a plan is agreed on. However, there are also some differences. A successful traditional review involves a combination of verbal and non-verbal communication.

When one is assessing a person remotely, some of this will have to be replaced by verbal communication. It is worth giving some thought to the different types of communication that you might have to get across.

Preparation

Before the assessment, it is important to familiarise yourself with information about the other person's health. This is particularly necessary for remote assessments, as breaking away from the discussion can lead to a disjointed experience. Make sure that you have reviewed recent correspondence and test results. If the person has previously consented to access, it will be helpful to look at his or her medication through the Summary Care Record (or an alternative).

For video consultations you should think about what the other person can see. Your background should be simple, to avoid distractions. You should check that no confidential information is visible. The room should be well lit. Usually, you will be able to see yourself during the consultation, and that can be a source of distraction. Having the camera at eye level gives the least distorted view of your face.

Before starting a video call, make sure that you have written down a telephone number that will enable you to call the service user in the event of a problem with the video connection.

Welcoming

With a remote assessment, there may be more uncertainty on the part of the service user about who you are; therefore you must provide a clear introduction at the very start of the call. Start any call with, "Hello! My name is …."

This will reassure the service user before any questions or conversations arise around his or her identity.

A few words of explanation about how the assessment works will be helpful. This will help the other person to feel more at ease and will give some structure to the consultation. It is worth taking a moment to make sure that you can see the individual you are assessing. Ideally you should be able to see his or her upper body, including the arms and face. For certain assessments (such as looking at walking), you may have to ask the caller to more or to move the camera. Having a second person in the room with the caller will make this much easier.

During a consultation

It is important to remember that the person you are speaking with may not be able to see what you are doing at all times, even during a video consultation. Try to get into the habit of explaining why you have stopped talking for any reason, including when you are making notes or looking at other information, such as test results. This will help the other person not to feel ignored or to wonder whether there is a technical problem.

Making the consultation count

The objectives of a remote consultation are the same as those of a face-to-face review. There are the overt goals, such as identifying issues and exploring potential solutions. There are also less obvious objectives, such as building trust—also helping service users to have more control over their medical conditions and to set goals. As remote assessments are likely to be less familiar to service users, they may be reluctant to ask more difficult questions or to persevere with a line of inquiry if they did not feel that they have been given satisfactory answers to their questions. For the clinician, this could easily lead to the sensation that the consultation has been completed quickly and to everyone's satisfaction even if that is not the case. There is a shift in the power dynamic toward the clinician, which potentially allows him or her to "shut down" the discussion.

Being aware of this potential can help the clinician to think about the way in which questions are asked. It may be necessary to ask more closed questions than usual, particularly if the service user offers the view that everything is fine.

Sara Riggare, a person with Parkinson's, blogs about living with the condition. She describes seeing her specialist about twice a year. This means that she spends 8765 hours a year in self-care (see Fig. 14.1) (Riggare, 2021). This

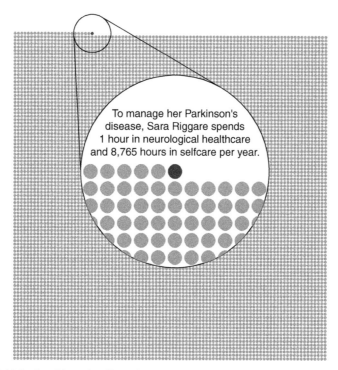

FIGURE 14.1   Sara Riggare's self-care hours.

observation offers us a way of helping to make remote consultations more rewarding. We can use the time before the appointment to ask service users to complete a simple questionnaire designed to explore the motor and non-motor symptoms that they may be experiencing. This could be then be considered once the person's own priorities have been explored. It could also act as a safety net to ensure that important questions, such as checking for medication side effects or asking about driving, are not forgotten.

The time after the appointment can also be used to increase the reach and effectiveness of the consultation. The clinic letter is an opportunity to include a summary of the information that has been discussed. It can point to sources of help and provide important reminders about things to look out for. A well-written letter can be of use to service users and clinicians alike throughout the time to next review.

Coaching

Another way to help people to get the most from remote appointments is to make sure that you are all speaking the same language; for example, it is possible that someone could use the same words to describe both tremor and dyskinesia. *Freezing* and *wearing off* are two other problems that could be described using similar terms but have very different meanings. Spending a little time to describe the common symptoms of Parkinson's and some of the medical terminology used will help people to benefit more from future appointments. It is especially important to ask enough questions to understand what a service user is describing during a remote assessment.

Remote therapy

Delivering therapy interventions remotely can be a challenge for both the therapist and the service user, but many aspects of therapy can be successfully delivered without a face-to-face encounter. The subjective elements of an initial assessment can be carried out by telephone or video, thus shortening the time required for a subsequent face-to-face encounter. During the remote consultation, it is essential that the therapist listen carefully to the individual, as the intervention plan will be reliant on what the individual reports (Russell & Trutter, 2010). Following a remote assessment, the therapist should summarise the findings of the assessment and make sure that the individual is asked whether he or she has any questions. Shared goals and the intervention plan, as well as next steps, can then be agreed.

Baseline measures can be difficult to carry out remotely, but therapists may be able to use outcome tools that can be adapted in such circumstances. It may be necessary for the therapist to time the individual while the task is observed on video, or the individual may be able to time it and report back to the therapist. For example, the Five Times Sit to Stand Test could be used in a physiotherapy video session if the service user's computer camera is correctly positioned for the therapist to observe and time the task.

Physiotherapy

Although it may be preferable to see an individual face to face when freezing of gait (FOG) and falls are at issue, a telephone or video consultation may still be of use. That is, it is often possible for the clinician to ascertain enough detail, such as where and when FOG occurs, to formulate advice, cues and strategies. This can be followed up with written information posted or emailed to the individual after the session. If FOG is the reason for the falls, the remote session may resolve the situation; but if there are other reasons for falls, it is likely that the person will have to be seen face to face.

The benefits of delivering therapy by video sessions include the therapist's ability to:

- Observe gait and posture
- See how the individual is carrying out his or her home exercise programme
- Demonstrate any new exercises or interventions

Challenges include

- Difficulty assessing muscle strength and tone
- Difficulty assessing balance and posture
- Limited range of suitable outcome measures

The Chartered Society of Physiotherapy (www.csp.org) has developed guidance for physiotherapists on decision making regarding offering remote or face-to-face consultations.

Occupational therapy

One advantage of conducting a video consultation is that the occupational therapist (OT) can carry out a virtual home assessment rather than having to make a home visit. Advice regarding moving hazards can be given and observations made to enable referral for equipment such as rails. Advice regarding the placement of visual cues around the home can be offered and the caregiver can be encouraged to follow through on it.

Assessment of upper limb function—for instance, when eating or writing—can be carried out remotely in a video session, with advice and intervention tailored to the individual's home environment.

Assessment and intervention for non-motor symptoms—including advice regarding sleep, fatigue and anxiety—can be delivered remotely; but the assessment of cognition may be more challenging. The Montreal Cognitive

Assessment (MoCA) can be carried out in a video session with some adjustments. The version of the MoCA that has been adapted for use with people who are blind can be used with someone with Parkinson's in a video session. This version omits the visuospatial element of the assessment. Alternatively, the visuospatial section can be posted to the individual in advance of the video session, but he or she should then be advised not to look at it until asked to do so during the session. Any adaptation of the assessment changes the validity of the tool. Nevertheless, these adaptations offer the opportunity to assess cognition when the individual cannot be seen in a face-to-face consultation.

The Royal College of Occupational Therapists offers advice and resources for OTs delivering remote interventions. These include guidance on developing digital skills, offering occupational therapy remotely, and ensuring clinical safety (www.rcot.co.uk).

Speech and language therapy

Voice and swallowing assessments can be offered via video consultation with some adjustments. Any changes in speech, voice quality, and communication skills can be assessed, as can swallowing skills, signs of aspiration and cough strength.

However, a remote session does not lend itself to observing abdominal breathing, recording and playing back the voice to aid self-monitoring or accurately measuring vocal loudness.

The Royal College of Speech and Language Therapists advises SLTs to consider, in advance of a remote session, what they will not be able to assess, such as neck tension or laryngeal elevation. It also recommends that the SLT use his or her clinical judgment after the session when scores are being interpreted, considering the margin for error as well as individual and contextual factors (www.rcslt.org).

Challenges for the health professional's activity levels

Challenges for health care professionals in delivering remote interventions include a reduction in their own physical activity levels. Telephone or video clinics with back-to-back appointments for sessions that can last up to 3 hours can greatly reduce the professional's daily activity and step count. They can also affect posture and have implications for eye health, concentration levels and fatigue for clinicians who spend long periods of time looking at a screen.

Currently no guidelines regarding this issue exist, but we would recommend the use of a standing desk, taking short breaks away from the computer in between appointments, engaging in exercise "bullets" such as 5 minutes of a Pilates-type exercise, and incorporating a stretch routine. These can be fitted in between appointments.

TABLE 14.1 Technology and internet access

	Household access		Personal access	
	Non-disabled	Disabled	Non-disabled	Disabled
Smartphone	81%	53%	75%	45%
Any computer	85%	64%	77%	54%
Internet	NA	NA	92%	67%

NA, Not applicable.
Source: Ofcom (2019).

Access to devices and the internet

It is important to remember that not everyone has access to devices such as smartphones, tablets or computers. Even today, internet access is not universal. This must be considered when services are being planned. Everyone should be able to have access to specialist healthcare even if they do not have technological resources such as these.

The Ofcom Access and Inclusion Report (2018) found that, although mobile phone use is increasing among persons 75 years of age and over, they remain least likely to have access to this technology. Around 1 in 5 people in this age group own a smartphone, but they are less likely than others to use it as a main way of accessing the internet. Larger devices, such as tablets, are preferred by these older individuals. In 2018, only about half of persons 75 years of age or older had broadband installed at home.

People with disabilities also have less access to technology. The survey found that those with a disability were less likely to have a smartphone, computer or access to the internet (Table 14.1). These disparities were most exaggerated in the least affluent groups.

Sources of guidance and additional information on remote assessment

Shortly after COVID restrictions were put in place, numerous bodies recognised that remote assessment would expand rapidly. It was clear that clinicians would be stepping outside of their comfort zones and would benefit from guidance on how to set up remote assessment services and carry out such reviews.

The Royal College of General Practitioners has published "The Top 10 Tips for Successful GP Video Consultations." This covers a range of subjects, from setting up for video to techniques to employ during an assessment (Royal College of General Practitioners, 2020).

Remote assessment did not begin with COVID-19. In 2012, The Royal College of Nursing produced a guide called "Using Telephone Advice for Patients with Long-Term Conditions." It includes useful questions to ask yourself before setting up a remote assessment service. There are also recommendations on the documentation of telephone consultations (Royal College of Nursing, 2012).

The University of Oxford has produced "Video Consultations—a Guide for Practice." It is aimed at primary care, but many of the principles apply equally well to remote specialist reviews. It deals with setting up the service and also offers advice for clinicians and service users on how to carry out video assessments. The guidance is published in BJGP Life (BJGP Life, 2020).

Top tips for using remote consultations

1. Long-term conditions like Parkinson's are suited to a degree of remote management.
2. Prepare before the consultation.
3. Be aware of how you may have to use words to explain things that might not require explanation in a face-to-face assessment.
4. Think about what the other person can see behind you during a video consultation.
5. Consider ways in which to help the other person get the most from the consultation, such as preclinic questions and additional information in letters.
6. For video assessments, it is often better to have a second person assisting at the other end to help with things such as camera position.
7. Take opportunities to coach individuals on how to describe changes in their condition.
8. Be mindful of the ease with which a remote consultation can be ended by the health professional and make sure that this does not lead to a failure to address issues.
9. Make time to be active during a day of remote consultations.
10. Sometimes there will be no alternative to a face-to-face review.

References

BJGP Life. (2020). Video consultations: a guide for practice. Retrieved January 5, 2021, from https://bjgplife.com/2020/03/18/video-consultations-guide-for-practice/

British Medical Association, (2020). COVID-19: video consultations and homeworking. Retrieved January 5, 2021, from https://www.bma.org.uk/advice-and-support/covid-19/adapting-to-covid/covid-19-video-consultations-and-homeworking.

Chartered Society of Physiotherapy. (2020) Face-to-face or remote consultations: supporting you to make safe decisions about patient contact. Retrieved January 25, 2021, from https://www.csp.org.uk/news/coronavirus/clinical-guidance/reopening-your-services/guidance-advice-implementation.

NHSX (2020). COVID-19 IG Advice. Retrieved January 5, 2021, from https://www.nhsx.nhs.uk/information-governance/guidance/covid-19-ig-advice/

Ofcom. (2019). Access and Inclusion Report, 2018. Retrieved January 6, 2021, from https://www.ofcom.org.uk/research-and-data/multi-sector-research/accessibility-research/access-and-inclusion.

Ofcom. (2020). Online Nation 2020 Report. Retrieved January 5, 2021, from https://www.ofcom.org.uk/__data/assets/pdf_file/0027/196407/online-nation-2020-report.pdf.

Ontario Telemedicine Network. (nd). Ontario Telemedicine Network. Retrieved January 25, 2021, from https://otn.ca/

Riggare, S. (2021). 1 vs 8765. Retrieved January 5, 2021, from https://www.riggare.se/1-vs-8765/

Royal College of General Practitioners. (2020) Top 10 tips for successful GP video consultations. Retrieved January 5, 2021, from https://www.rcgp.org.uk/about-us/rcgp-blog/top-10-tips-for-successful-gp-video-consultations.aspx.

Royal College of Nursing. (2012). *Using telephone advice for patients with long-term conditions.* 1st ed. London: RCN.

Royal College of Occupational Therapists. (2021). Retrieved January 25, 2021, from https://www.rcot.co.uk/coronavirus-covid-19-0.

Royal College of Speech and Language Therapists. (2021) Telehealth Guidance. RCSLT. Retrieved January 25, 2021, from https://rcslt.org/members/delivering-quality-services/telehealth/tele-health-guidance#section-8.

Russell, T., & Trutter, P. (2010). The diagnostic accuracy of tele-rehabilitation for non-articular lower-limb musculoskeletal disorders. *Telemedicine & e-health*doi: 10.1089/tmj.2009.0163.

Wherton, J., Shaw, S., & Papoutsi, C. (2020). Guidance on the introduction and use of video consultations during COVID-19: important lessons from qualitative research. *BMJ Leader, 4*, 120–123.